HEALTH
PROMOTION

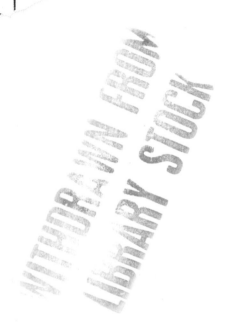

For Baillière Tindall:

Senior Commissioning Editor: Jacqueline Curthoys
Project Development Manager: Karen Gilmour
Project Manager: Jane Shanks
Design Direction: George Ajayi

HEALTH
PROMOTION
Foundations for Practice

Jennie Naidoo
Principal Lecturer, Health Promotion,
University of the West of England, Bristol, UK

Jane Wills
Senior Lecturer, Health Promotion,
South Bank University, London, UK

SECOND EDITION

431880
N613

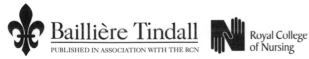
Baillière Tindall
PUBLISHED IN ASSOCIATION WITH THE RCN

Royal College
of Nursing

Edinburgh London New York Oxford Philadelphia St Louis Sydney Toronto 2000

BAILLIÈRE TINDALL
An imprint of Elsevier Limited

First edition 1994
Second edition 2000
    Reprinted 2000, 2001, 2002, 2003 (twice), 2004, 2005, 2006, 2007

ISBN 978 0 7020 2448 1

British Library Cataloguing in Publication Data
A catalogue record for this book is available from the British Library

Library of Congress Cataloguing in Publication Data
A catalogue record for this book is available from the Library of Congress

Note
Medical knowledge is constantly changing. As new information becomes
available, changes in treatment, procedures, equipment and the use of drugs
become necessary. The authors and the publishers have taken care to ensure that
the information given in this text is accurate and up to date. However, readers
are strongly advised to confirm that the information, especially with regard to
drug usage, complies with the latest legislation and standards of practice.

The Publisher

ELSEVIER
your source for books,
journals and multimedia
in the health sciences
www.elsevierhealth.com

Working together to grow
libraries in developing countries
www.elsevier.com | www.bookaid.org | www.sabre.org
ELSEVIER   BOOK AID International   Sabre Foundation

Printed in China
C/09

Contents

*P*reface to the second edition

This second edition has been comprehensively updated and expanded to reflect recent research findings and organizational and policy changes, many of which have been introduced by the new UK government elected in 1997. This government has announced its commitment towards a new public health and to tackling inequalites in health. Health promotion is now a central strategy within a raft of interlinked policies designed to foster a fairer, healthier society. An increasing number of practitioners from fields as diverse as public health nursing, health care service provision, environmental health and voluntary agencies now have health promotion as a core aspect of their work.

Additions to this edition include a new chapter on public health work (Ch. 9) and a new Section 3 which examines the settings approach in health promotion to reflect the focus of the World Health Organization. Four key settings (workplaces, schools, neighbourhoods and health services) are discussed and the dilemmas of promoting health in particular settings are explored. Other chapters have been substantially revised to acknowledge recent developments in the theory and practice of health promotion. For example, the role of epidemiology is considered in Chapter 3 on measuring health and Chapter 4 now reflects recent advances in health promotion. Chapter 18 on planning discusses the strategic planning role of many health promoters as well as considering in detail the planning of small-scale interventions.

This second edition retains the strengths which proved so popular in the first edition, combining an academic critique with a readable and accessible style which both informs the reader of recent debates and engages their attention through linked activites. The intention, as always, is to encourage readers to develop their practice and thus contribute to the challenge of promoting people's health.

2000

Jennie Naidoo
Jane Wills

Authors' acknowledgements

We wish to acknowledge the contribution colleagues and students at the University of the West of England and South Bank University have made to this book. Their experience, ideas and commitment to furthering the practice of health promotion prompted us to write this book, and have contributed to this new edition.

Finally, we would like to thank our families and partners for their support and patience.

Publisher's acknowledgements

Figure 1.3 a-f, from McKeown & Lowe (1974), *An Introduction to Social Medicine*, reproduced with permission from Blackwell Scientific Publications, Oxford, UK.

Figure 1.5, from Seedhouse (1986), *Health: Foundations for Achievement*, reproduced with permission from Wiley, Chichester, UK.

Figure 2.4, from Drever & Whitehead (1997), *Health Inequalities, Decennial Supplement*, reproduced with permission from the Office for National Statistics © Crown Copyright 1999.

Figure 2.5, from OPCS (1995), *Mortality Statistics: Perinatal and Infant*, reproduced with permission from the Office for National Statistics © Crown Copyright 1999.

Figure 3.1, from Gray & Payne (1993), *World Health and Disease*, reproduced with permission from Open University Press, Buckingham, UK.

Figure 3.2, from Andrews & Withey (1976), *Social Indications of Well-being: American Perceptions of Life Quality*, with kind permission from Plenum Publishing Corporation, NY, USA.

Figure 4.1, The Development of Health Promotion, from Bunton & McDonald (1992), *Health Promotion, Discipline and Diversity*, reproduced with permission from Routledge, London, UK.

Figure 5.4, adapted from Tones & Tilford (1994), *Health Education: Effectiveness, Efficiency and Equity*, Stanley Thorne, Cheltenham, UK, with permission from Keith Tones.

Figure 6.1, The Ethical Grid, from Seedhouse (1988), *Ethics, the Heart of Health Care*, p. 141, reproduced with permission from John Wiley & Sons Ltd, Chichester, UK.

Figure 11.2, from Ajzen & Fishbein (1990), *Understanding Attitudes and Predicting Social Behaviour*, reproduced with permission from Prentice Hall, New Jersey, USA.

Figure 11.3, from Ajzen (1991), The theory of planned behaviour. Organizational Behaviour and Human Decision Processes 50: 179-211, reproduced with permission from Academic Press, Orlando, USA.

Figure 12.2, from the National Smoking Educational Campaign (1999), reproduced with permission from the Health Education Authority, London, UK.

Figure 12.3, created by BUGA UP (Billboard Utilising Graffitists Against Unhealthy Promotions) and reproduced courtesy of Cecilia Farren.

Figure 12.4, created by AGHAST (Action Group to Halt Advertising & Sponsorship by Tobacco) and reproduced courtesy of Cecilia Farren.

Figure 15.1, from Appleyard & Lintel (1972), 'The Environmental Quality of City Streets' the Residents' Viewpoint. *Journal of the American Institute of Planners* 38: 84-101, with permission from the Regents of the University of California, USA. Reprinted by permission of the *Journal of the American Planning Association*.

Figure 16.1, from Taylor et al (1998), *A Public Health Model of Primary Care*, reproduced with permission from the Public Health Alliance, Birmingham, UK.

Figure 16.3, adapted from HEA (1998), *Promoting Health Through Primary Care Nursing*, with permission from the Health Education Authority, London, UK.

Figure 16.5, from MacHardy, Kerr & Thomas (1998), 'The Health Promoting Health Service'. International Conference Paper. Health Promotion Wales, Cardiff, UK, reproduced with permission from the Health Education Board for Scotland, UK.

Figure 17.2, from Annett & Rifkin (1990), *Improving Urban Health*, reproduced with permission from WHO, Geneva, Switzerland.

Figure 18.1, Rational Health Planning, McCarthy (1982), from *Epidemiology and Policies for Health Planning*, reproduced with kind permission of the King's Fund Centre.

Figure 18.4, from Ewles & Simnett (1999), *Promoting Health*, reproduced with permission from Baillière Tindall, Edinburgh, UK.

Figure 18.5, from Green et al (1980), *Health Education Planning: a Diagnostic Approach*, by kind permission of Mayfield Publishing Co., Mountain View, CA, USA.

Figure 18.6, adapted from Ewles & Simnett (1999), *Promoting Health*, with permission from Baillière Tindall, Edinburgh, UK.

Introduction

Health promotion is an important part of the work of a wide range of health care workers and those engaged in education and social welfare. It is an emerging area of practice and study, still defining its boundaries. This book aims to provide a theoretical framework which is vital if health promoters are to be clear about their intentions and desired outcomes when they embark on interventions designed to promote health. It offers a foundation for practice which encourages practitioners to see the potential for health promotion in their work.

The book is divided into four main sections. The first section provides a theoretical background, exploring the concepts of health, health education and health promotion. The section concludes that health promotion is the working towards positive health and well-being of individuals, groups and communities. Health promotion includes health education but also acknowledges that it is social and economic factors which determine health status. Ethical and political values influence practice. Those who promote health thus need to be clear about their intentions and how they perceive the purpose of health promotion. Is it, for example, to encourage healthy lifestyles? Or is it to redress health inequalities and empower people to take more control over their lives? We shall be asking readers to reflect on these and other questions in the context of their own work.

The second section discusses strategies to promote health and some of the dilemmas that they pose. What are the benefits and problems of working in partnership to promote health? How can practitioners broaden their work towards promoting the public health? How can health promoters work with communities and what are the strengths and limitations of a community development approach? What influences individual health behaviour and how can we help people to change? Is it effective to use the mass media to promote health?

Section 3 looks at the settings in which health promotion interventions take place and how these can be oriented towards health. This reflects the recent focus on settings for health promotion in both international and national policy documents. The chapters in this section discuss the rationale for workplaces, schools, neighbourhoods and the health services being targeted by government policies as key settings for health promotion. Reference is made in these chapters to specific target groups such as young people, adults and older people.

Section 4 is concerned with the implementation of health promotion. How do we assess clients' needs? Should health promotion interventions be targeted to particular groups? What strategies have been successful and what needs to be taken into account when planning an intervention or health promotion programme? Above all, how will we know if health promotion works?

This book is suitable for a wide range of professional groups and the examples have been chosen to reflect the diversity of people who practise health promotion. It includes many interactive exercises to encourage reflection and debate and to enable readers to apply their knowledge and increased understanding to practice situations. Where appropriate, feedback has been given but on many occasions this is not possible because the issues are open ended and contested. The aim is to allow and encourage readers to consider these issues for themselves, and not have their views prescribed or limited.

The book is clearly structured and signposted for ease of reading and study. Each chapter starts with an overview outlining the contents of that chapter and its links with other chapters and a few key points. A chapter summary acts as an *aide-mémoire* of the main points covered. Interspersed throughout the text are a number of helpful **Example**, **Activity** and **Discussion** boxes:

 = content input as an **Example**

 = **Activity**, in general more linked to text and some responses discussed

 = **Discussion** point, broader and more open ended.

Each chapter includes recommendations for further reading, and questions to encourage further discussion and debate either by the individual reader or student groups.

An aid for the reflective practitioner, this book will help the student in basic or post-basic training and qualified professionals who want to include health promotion in their work.

SECTION 1

The Theory of Health Promotion

This section explores the concepts of health, health education and health promotion. Those who promote health need to be clear about their intentions and how they perceive the purpose of health promotion. Is it to encourage healthy lifestyles? Or is it to redress health inequalities and empower people to take control over their lives?

1. *Concepts of health*
2. *Influences on health*
3. *Measuring health*
4. *Defining health promotion*
5. *Models and approaches to health promotion*
6. *Ethical issues in health promotion*
7. *The politics of health promotion*

1 *Concepts of health*

OVERVIEW

Everyone engaged in the task of promoting health starts with a view of what health is. However, there is a wide variety of these views, or concepts, of health. It is important at the outset to be clear about the concepts of health which are personally adhered to, and to recognize where these differ from those of your colleagues and clients. Otherwise, you may find yourself drawn into conflicts about appropriate strategies and advice that are actually due to different ideas concerning the end goal of health. This chapter introduces different concepts of health, and traces the origin of these views. Working your way through this chapter will enable you to clarify your own views on the definition of health and to locate these views in a conceptual framework.

Defining health, disease, illness and ill health

Health

Health is a broad concept which can embody a huge range of meanings, from the narrowly technical to the all-embracing moral or philosophical. The word 'health' is derived from the Old English

 What are your answers to the following?

- I feel healthy when . . .
- I am healthy because . . .
- To stay healthy I need . . .
- I become unhealthy when . . .
- My health improves when . . .
- (A person) affected my health by . . .
- (An event) affected my health by . . .
- (A situation) affected my health by . . .
- . . . is responsible for my health

word for heal (*hael*) which means 'whole', signalling that health concerns the whole person and his or her integrity, soundness, or well-being. There are 'common-sense' views of health which are passed through generations as part of a common cultural heritage. These are termed 'lay' concepts of health, and everyone acquires a knowledge of them through their socialization into society. Different societies or different groups within one society have different views on what constitutes 'common sense'.

Health has two common meanings in everyday use, one negative and one positive. The negative definition of health is the absence of disease or illness. This is the meaning of health within the western scientific medical model, which is explored in greater detail later on in this chapter. The positive definition of health is a state of well-being, interpreted by the World Health Organization in its constitution as 'a state of complete physical, mental and social well-being, not merely the absence of disease or infirmity' (WHO 1946).

Some authors argue that health is holistic and includes different dimensions, each of which needs to be considered (Aggleton & Homans 1987, Ewles & Simnett 1999). Holistic health means taking account of the separate influences and interaction of these dimensions. Figure 1.1 shows a diagrammatic representation of the dimensions of health.

The inner circle represents individual dimensions of health.

- Physical health concerns the body, e.g. fitness, not being ill.
- Mental health refers to a positive sense of purpose and an underlying belief in one's own worth, e.g. feeling good, feeling able to cope.
- Emotional health concerns the ability to express feelings and to develop and sustain relationships, e.g. feeling loved.
- Social health concerns the sense of having support available from family and friends, e.g. having friends to talk to, being involved in activities with other people.

Figure 1.1
Dimensions of health. Adapted from Aggleton & Homans (1987) and Ewles & Simnett (1999).

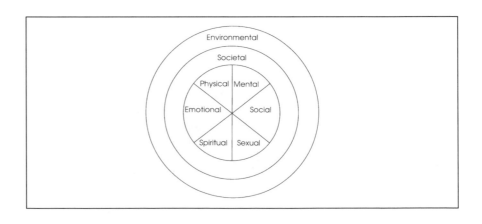

■ Spiritual health is the recognition and ability to put into practice moral or religious principles or beliefs.

■ Sexual health is the acceptance and ability to achieve a satisfactory expression of one's sexuality.

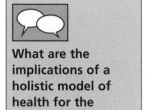

What are the implications of a holistic model of health for the professional practice of health workers?

The two outer circles are broader dimensions of health which affect the individual. Societal health refers to the link between health and the way a society is structured. This includes the basic infrastructure necessary for health (for example, shelter, peace, food, income), and the degree of integration or division within society. We shall see in Chapter 2 how the existence of patterned inequalities between groups of people harms health. Environmental health refers to the physical environment in which people live, and includes things such as housing, transport, sanitation and pure water facilities and pollution.

Disease, illness and ill health

Disease, illness and ill health are often used interchangeably although they have very different meanings. Disease derives from *'desaise'* meaning uneasiness or discomfort. Illness indicates a condition causing harm or pain. Nowadays, disease implies an objective state of ill health, which may be verified by accepted canons of proof. In our society, these accepted canons of proof are couched in the language of scientific medicine. For example, microscopic analysis may yield evidence of changes in cell structure, which may in turn lead to a diagnosis of cancer or disease. Disease is the existence of some pathology or abnormality of the body which is capable of detection.

Illness is the subjective experience of loss of health. This is couched in terms of symptoms, for example the reporting of aches or pains, or loss of function. Illness and disease are not the same, although there is a large degree of coexistence. For example, someone may be diagnosed as having cancer through screening, even when there have been no reported symptoms. That is, a disease may be diagnosed in someone who has not reported any illness. When someone reports symptoms, and further investigations such as blood tests prove a disease process, the two concepts, disease and illness, coincide. In these instances, the term ill health is used. Ill health is therefore an umbrella term used to refer to the experience of disease plus illness.

Social scientists view health and disease as socially constructed entities. Health and disease are not states of objective reality waiting to be uncovered and investigated by scientific medicine. Rather, they are actively produced and negotiated by ordinary people. This process becomes most apparent when doctors and their patients disagree about the significance or meaning of symptoms. For example, someone can feel ill but after investigations nothing medically wrong can be found. The subjective experience of feeling ill is not always matched by an objective diagnosis of disease. When this happens, doctors and health workers may label such sufferers 'malingerers', denying the validity of subjective illness. This can have important consequences, for example a sick certificate may be withheld if a doctor is not convinced that someone's reported illness is genuine.

In November 1993 Judge John Prosser QC decided that RSI (repetitive strain injury, a work-related condition) does not exist and dismissed a claim for compensation. Judge Prosser said that RSI is 'meaningless' and 'has no place in the medical books'. He described RSI sufferers as 'eggshell personalities who need to get a grip on themselves'.

Can you think of other examples of a disease or condition which has been experienced by people but not been readily diagnosed? Do you know anybody who has experienced symptoms without being given a diagnosis?

It is also possible to experience no symptoms or signs of disease, but to be labelled sick as a result of examination or screening. Hypertension and precancerous changes to cell structures are two examples where screening may identify a disease even though the person concerned may feel perfectly healthy. Figure 1.2 gives a visual representation of these discrepancies. The central point is that subjective perceptions cannot be overruled, or invalidated, by scientific medicine.

Instead of questioning whether a certain blood sugar level accurately differentiates between diabetics and non-diabetics, consider these questions:

■ Why is it important to make this distinction?
■ Who stands to gain from such a process?
■ Whose livelihood depends on the business of investigation, diagnosis and treatment?
■ How does the person receiving a diagnosis of diabetes experience the process?
■ Why do not all diabetics comply with a prescribed treatment regime?

The western scientific medical model of health

In modern western societies, and in many other societies as well, the dominant professional view of health adopted by most health care

Figure 1.2 *The relationship between disease and illness.*

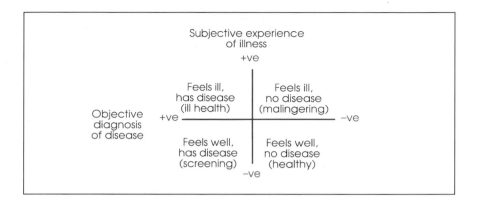

workers during their training and practice is labelled western scientific medicine. Western scientific medicine operates with a narrow view of health, which is often used to refer to no disease or no illness. In this sense, health is a negative term, defined more by what it is not than by what it is.

This view of health is extremely influential, as it underpins much of the training and ethos of a wide variety of health workers. These definitions become powerful because they are used in a variety of contexts, not just in professional circles. For example, the media often present this view of health, disease and illness in dramas set in hospitals or in documentaries about health issues. By these means, professional definitions become known and accepted in society at large.

The scientific medical model arose in western Europe at the time of the Enlightenment, with the rise of rationality and science as forms of knowledge. In earlier times, religion provided a way of knowing and understanding the world. The Enlightenment changed the old order, and substituted science for religion as the dominant means of knowledge and understanding. This was accompanied by a proliferation of equipment and techniques for studying the world. The invention of the microscope and telescope revealed whole worlds which before had been invisible. Observation, calculation and classification became the means of increasing knowledge. Such knowledge was put to practical purposes, and applied science was one of the forces which accompanied the Industrial Revolution. In an atmosphere when everything was deemed knowable through the proper application of scientific method, the human body became a key object for the pursuit of scientific knowledge. What could be seen, and measured, and catalogued, was 'true' in an objective and universal sense.

This view of health is characterized as:

■ **Biomedical** – health is assumed to be a property of biological beings.

Key milestones in the development of scientific medicine

1543 Vesalius publishes *On the Structure of the Human Body* based on his own dissections
1628 Harvey publishes his discoveries concerning the blood circulatory system
1674 Leeuwenhoek produces lenses powerful enough to enable him to observe bacteria
1796 Jenner first uses vaccine derived from cowpox to successfully immunize a person against smallpox
1847 James Simpson uses chloroform as an anaesthetic
1854 Florence Nightingale, founder of modern nursing, and her team nurse victims of the Crimean War
1858 Virchow publishes a book on cellular pathology which introduces the concept of the cell as the centre of all pathological changes
1864 Pasteur isolates organisms under the microscope
1865 Lister begins the practice of antisepsis during surgery, which is followed by a dramatic reduction in mortality rates
1882 Koch isolates the tubercle bacillus
1883 Koch isolates the cholera bacillus
1895 Roentgen discovers X-rays
1900 Landsteiner discovers the four human blood types A, B, AB and O
1902 Alexis Carrel demonstrates a method of joining blood vessels that makes organ transplantation feasible
1928 Alexander Fleming discovers penicillin
1954 First kidney transplant operation performed
1956 The first flexible endoscope for seeing inside the body is built
1967 First heart transplant operation performed
1978 First IVF baby in Britain

- **Reductionist** – states of being such as health and disease may be reduced to smaller and smaller constitutive components of the biological body.
- **Mechanistic** – it conceptualizes and treats the body as if it were a machine.
- **Allopathic** – it works by a system of opposites. If something is wrong with a body, treatment consists of applying an opposite force to correct the sickness, e.g. pharmacological drugs which combat the sickness.
- **Pathogenic** – it focuses on why people become ill.

Doyal & Doyal (1984) develop the machine analogy further, and refer to five basic assumptions underpinning western scientific medicine. These are:

1. The body is like a machine, in which all the parts are interconnected but capable of being separated and treated separately.
2. Health equals all the parts of the body functioning properly.
3. Illness equals some malfunction of the parts of the body, which is measurable.
4. Disease is caused by internal processes such as degeneration through ageing or the failure of self-regulation, or by external processes such as the invasion of pathogens into the body.
5. Medical treatment aims to restore normal functioning or health to the body system.

This view sees health and disease as linked, as if on a continuum, so that the more disease a person has the further away he or she is from health and 'normality'. It also conveys a notion of morality, so that normal equals good. Sontag (1988) describes how metaphors were used to describe AIDS in the 1980s. Terms such as 'invasion', 'sin' and 'plague' signalled AIDS as a punishment for unhealthy (immoral) sexual behaviour.

The pathogenic focus on finding the causes for ill health has led to an emphasis on risk factors. Antonovsky (1993) has called for a *salutogenic* approach which looks instead at why some people remain healthy. He identifies coping mechanisms which enable some people to remain healthy despite adverse circumstances, change and stress. An important factor for health, which Antonovsky labels a 'sense of coherence', involves the three aspects of understanding, managing and making sense of change. These are human abilities which are in turn nurtured or obstructed by the wider environment.

 One of the principles of the Ottawa Charter (see p. 78) is to 'create supportive environments'.

What might this mean in professional practice?

New developments in medicine and nursing recognize the importance of social factors in the causation of health and disease, and the necessity of treating the whole person. However, the legacy of western scientific medicine is pervasive, and elements of this approach still underpin the professional training of many health workers.

There is a dichotomy between therapeutic medicine and preventive medicine which exists both at community level and clinical level. One of the main reasons for the dichotomy must be the traditional undergraduate and postgraduate training which produces doctors who are largely unaware of the potential for prevention of chronic disease but who have an exaggerated view of the benefits of treatment.

(National Forum for CHD Prevention 1990, p. 46)

A critique of the medical model

The role of medicine in determining health

What effect do medical advances in knowledge have on death rates?

What other reasons could account for declining death rates?

The view that health is the absence of disease and illness, and that medical treatment can restore the body to good health has been criticized. The distribution of health and ill health has been analyzed from a historical and social science perspective. It has been argued that medicine is not as effective as is often claimed. The 20th century has seen a steady reduction in mortality and increased longevity amongst people living in the industrialized West, and it is often assumed that medical advances have been responsible for this. McKeown & Lowe (1974) set out to test this assumption by undertaking a historical analysis (see Fig. 1.3, p. 13).

McKeown & Lowe (1974) concluded that social advances in general living conditions, such as improved sanitation and nutrition, have been responsible for most of the reduction in mortality achieved during the last century. The contribution of medicine to reduced mortality has been minor, when compared with the major impact of improved environmental conditions.

Cochrane (1972) argues that most medical interventions have not been proved effective prior to their widespread adoption. The randomized controlled trial is the scientific method of validating a medical treatment as effective. This method relies on randomly dividing people with the same disease or illness into two groups. One group receives the medical treatment, whilst the other group does not. The two groups are then compared, and only when the group receiving medical treatment fares significantly better is the treatment deemed effective. Cochrane (1972) argues that it is relatively rare for experimental treatments to be properly evaluated using randomized controlled trials. Often the demand for treatment or a cure makes such trials impossible. A recent example of this was the demand by people with AIDS to receive the new drug AZT whilst it was still at the experimental stage. Medical treatments may be adopted even when they have not been shown to be effective. For example, coronary care units have grown in number, although there is no evidence that hospital care produces better outcomes than home care (Skrabanek & McCormick 1992).

The role of social factors in determining health

The modern UK is characterized by profound inequalities in income and wealth (Rowntree 1995). These in turn are associated with persistent inequalities in health (Wilkinson 1996). The impact of

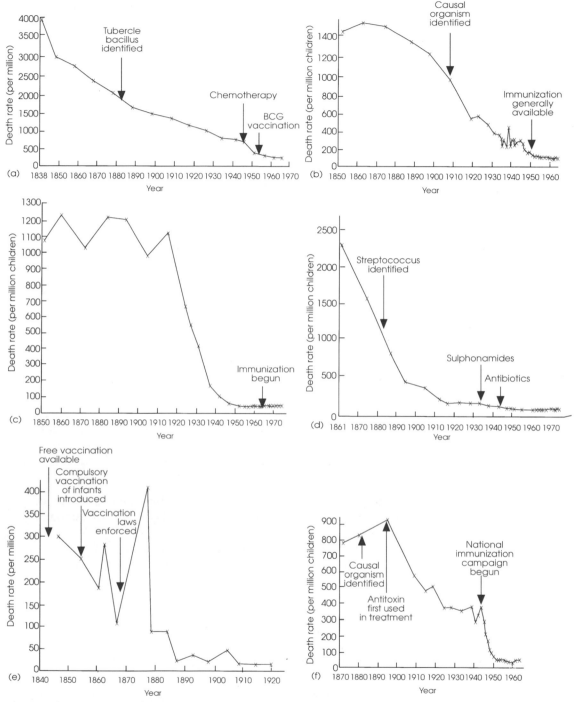

Figure 1.3   *The role of medicine in reducing mortality.*
(a) Respiratory tuberculosis: death rates, England and Wales.
(b) Whooping cough: death rates of children under 15, England and Wales.
(c) Measles: death rates of children under 15, England and Wales.
(d) Scarlet fever: death rates of children under 15, England and Wales.
(e) Smallpox: death rates, England and Wales.
(f) Diphtheria: death rates of children under 15, England and Wales.
*   From McKeown & Lowe (1974).*

scientific medicine on health is marginal when compared to major structural features such as the distribution of wealth, income, housing and employment. Tarlov (1996) has claimed that medical services have contributed only 17% to the gain in life expectancy in the 20th century. As Chapter 2 will show, the distribution of health mirrors the distribution of material resources within society. In general, the more equal a society is in its distribution of resources, the more equal, and better, is the health status of its citizens (Wilkinson 1996).

Medicine as a means of social control

Social scientists argue that medicine is a social enterprise closely linked with the exercise of professional power (Stacey 1988). This derives from its role in legitimizing health and illness in society and the socially exclusive and autonomous nature of the profession. Although it faces challenges from a number of recent developments, such as managerialism in the NHS and the rise of self-help and complementary therapies, medicine remains a powerful institution (Gabe et al 1994). Medicine is a powerful means of social control, whereby the categories of disease, illness, madness and deviancy are used to maintain a status quo in society.

Doctors who make the diagnosis are in a powerful position. Access to such power is controlled by professional associations with

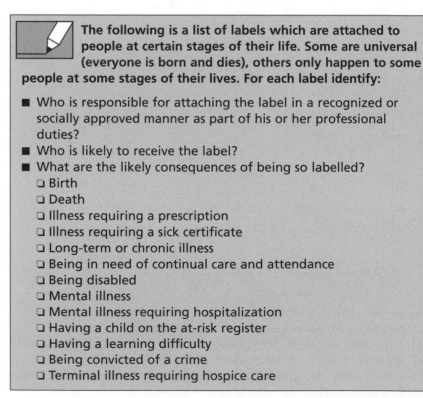

The following is a list of labels which are attached to people at certain stages of their life. Some are universal (everyone is born and dies), others only happen to some people at some stages of their lives. For each label identify:

- Who is responsible for attaching the label in a recognized or socially approved manner as part of his or her professional duties?
- Who is likely to receive the label?
- What are the likely consequences of being so labelled?
  - ❏ Birth
  - ❏ Death
  - ❏ Illness requiring a prescription
  - ❏ Illness requiring a sick certificate
  - ❏ Long-term or chronic illness
  - ❏ Being in need of continual care and attendance
  - ❏ Being disabled
  - ❏ Mental illness
  - ❏ Mental illness requiring hospitalization
  - ❏ Having a child on the at-risk register
  - ❏ Having a learning difficulty
  - ❏ Being convicted of a crime
  - ❏ Terminal illness requiring hospice care

their own vested interests to protect (Freidson 1986). The 1858 Medical Act established the General Medical Council which was authorized to regulate doctors, oversee medical education, and keep a register of qualified practitioners. Medical colleges resisted the entry of women to the profession for many years (Stacey 1988). In 1901 there were 36 000 medical practitioners, of which 212 were women. There is evidence that Black and Asian doctors face discrimination in their medical careers (Esmail & Everington 1993, Skellington & Morris 1992). This implies that ability is not the sole criterion for gaining a place to train in medicine or in subsequent career progression. Medicine may be seen as a social activity which concentrates professional power amongst an elite.

A stronger form of this argument says that medicine upholds a specific form of economy (capitalism), and/or patriarchy (the institutionalized power of men over women). For a capitalist state to thrive, social order and healthy workers are needed, and the National Health Service (NHS) provides the means to achieve both (Doyal with Pennell 1979). Some feminists argue that the NHS primarily serves the needs of men, and that women's health needs tend to be subordinated to their role as mother, wife and carer. These issues are discussed in greater detail in Chapter 2.

Health as autonomy

It has been claimed that health means autonomy and that autonomy or health is subverted by the medicalization of life (Illich 1975). This critique argues that medicine has acquired an authority beyond its legitimate area of operation. The medicalization of life is the encroachment of medical decisions and techniques into ordinary stages of the life cycle, such as birth and death. Doctors are called upon to make life and death decisions; yet they have no particular training which qualifies them to make these moral choices. Illich argues that this kind of power does not naturally belong to technical experts but is a fundamental human right which should be exercised by everyone in relation to their own lives, if they are to be healthy.

For Illich, health is a personal task which people must be free to pursue autonomously. Doctors and health workers contribute to ill health by taking over people's responsibility for their health. In addition, the practice of medicine leads to iatrogenic ill health caused by doctors and health workers. Illich identifies three types of iatrogenesis. Clinical iatrogenesis is ill health caused by medical intervention, for example side-effects caused by prescribed medicine, dependency on prescribed drugs and cross-infection in medical settings such as hospitals. Social iatrogenesis is the loss of coping and the right to self-care which has resulted from the medicalization of everyday life. Cultural iatrogenesis is the loss of the means whereby people cope with pain and suffering, which results from the unrealistic expectations generated by medicine.

 Two recent campaigns organized by a health promotion department were:

■ 'A pill for every ill?' – a campaign to persuade people not to ask their GP for a prescription.
■ 'Is it an emergency?' – a campaign to persuade people not to call out GPs at night.

To what extent do you think society has become dependent on medicine? Is this true of developing countries?

Health workers come to be seen as disabling elements in the lives of ordinary people. Whilst it is possible to agree with Illich that doctors and health workers wield enormous power in people's lives, which is not always exercised in accordance with their patients' wishes or beliefs, it does not follow that we would all be better off without any health care system at all. Medicine has made some remarkable contributions to people's health (for example the widespread use of antibiotics discovered in the 1950s). The caring function of health workers is also important for many people when they are ill, especially for those without close ties of family and friends. To argue, as Illich does, for the abolition of professional health workers seems to be a case of throwing the baby out with the bath water.

The view that people should make their own decisions about their own health and that of their dependants is widespread amongst both the general public and government circles. The rise of self-help groups dating from the 1970s is an example of the popularity of this view (Kelleher 1994). The huge increase in the number of people involved in self-help health activities indicates a general belief that people know what is best for them, and that other people in similar circumstances are often more helpful and supportive than medical experts.

The emergence of alternative or complementary therapies reflects the growing number of people who are dissatisfied with invasive, impersonal and mechanical medicine or who have conditions that have not been successfully treated by medicine.

Practitioners and users of complementary therapies argue that they:

■ have a more holistic approach
■ operate outside the orthodox profession of medicine and therefore are able to develop more equal patient/therapist relationships

How might alternative therapies address these critiques of the medical model?

■ recognize the relationship between mind and body, challenging the dualism of medicine.

Lay concepts of health

For people concerned with the promotion of health, there is another problem with the dominance of scientific medicine. This is the focus within medicine on illness and disease, and the neglect of health as a positive concept in its own right. Many researchers have studied the general public's beliefs about health or lay concepts of health. The findings present an interesting picture, where there are continuities in definitions but also differences attributable to age, sex and class.

Herzlich (1973) studied a group of middle-class Parisians and Normans, and found that they described health in three different ways:

■ as a state of being and the absence of illness
■ as something to have, an inner strength or resistance to ill health
■ as a state of doing and being able to fulfil the maximum potential for life.

Older people are more likely to define health as wholeness or integrity, inner strength and ability to cope (Williams 1983). Young people are more likely to define health in terms of fitness, energy or strength (Blaxter 1990).

Other researchers have identified a social class difference in concepts of health (Blaxter 1990, Calnan 1987, d'Houtaud & Field 1986). Middle-class respondents typically have a more positive view of health, as something which is linked to enjoying life, and being fit and active. Working-class respondents tend to see health as more functional, to do with getting through the day and not being ill.

Functional health means being able to do those normal social tasks which are expected of someone and is: 'the state of optimum capacity of an individual for the effective performance of the roles and tasks for which (s)he has been socialised' (Parsons 1972, p. 117). Blaxter (1990) identifies a gender difference, with men having a more positive notion of health as being fit, and women having a more negative notion of health as not being ill and being able to carry out everyday tasks.

One way of thinking about these differences is in terms of internal and external locus of control. These terms are used in psychology to refer to people's beliefs about how much choice and self-determination they have, and are explored in more detail in Chapter 11. People with a strong internal locus of control believe they have the power to make decisions which will affect their life. They will therefore be strongly motivated to make recommended changes to improve their health. By contrast, people with a strong external locus of control believe they are relatively powerless to make changes which will affect their life. They are more likely to be fatalistic about the future and will not be strongly motivated to make recommended changes to improve their health.

Researchers have found that these differing views are linked to social class. Typically, middle-class people are more likely to have a strong internal locus of control. Working-class people are more likely to have a strong external locus of control.

What explanations can you think of to account for this finding?

Part of the explanation might be that, compared to working-class people, middle-class people have more control over their lives because of higher income, better housing and more job security. This in turn can lead to different social classes holding different beliefs about autonomy or fatalism, which are then passed on to their children.

There is then a difference between lay and professional concepts of health. The gap between the two has been identified by health workers as a problem, giving rise to concern. The concern centres around two issues: the perceived lack of communication or poor communication between health worker and client; and clients' lack of compliance with prescribed treatment regimes. However, there is a crossover between lay and professional beliefs about health. Health workers acquire their professional view of health during training. These beliefs overlie their original views of health adopted at an early age from family and society, so professionals are familiar with both. The general public is also aware of, and operates with, both sets of beliefs. So the two sets of beliefs, scientific medicine and lay public, are not discrete entities but overlap each other and exist in tandem.

Cornwell (1984) describes how people operate with both official and lay beliefs about health. Cornwell's study of London's Eastenders found that accounts of health were either public or private. Public accounts are couched in terms of scientific medicine and reflect these dominant beliefs. Health and illness are related to

People's explanations for their health and illness are complex. Why is it important for health promoters to understand the health beliefs of those with whom they work?

How might they do this?

Consider the well-known phrase 'feed a cold, starve a fever'.

■ What do you think are the origins of this saying?
■ What do the public believe to be the causes of a cold or chill?
■ What is popularly believed to be the cause of a fever?
■ What is regarded as appropriate treatment for each?

This is discussed further in Helman (1986).

medical diagnosis and treatment, and medical terms and events are used to explain health status. These public accounts were offered first in Cornwell's interviews. What Cornwell terms private accounts reflect lay views of health, which typically use more holistic and social concepts to explain health and illness. For example, private accounts related health to general life experiences, such as employment, housing and perceived stress. Private accounts were offered in subsequent interviews, when a relationship had been established between Cornwell and the women she was interviewing. Cornwell suggests that people are therefore aware of both systems of beliefs and can use either when asked to talk about health. In encounters with strangers who are perceived as professionals, people use public accounts. However, in more informal settings, people use private accounts.

Thorogood (1993) similarly describes how Caribbean women's use of bush and other home remedies is a dynamic, active resource which is used to manage their families' lives and health. Whilst the use of bush and other home remedies is rooted in Caribbean culture and history, it is also part of current social relationships. Both Cornwell and Thorogood describe lay health beliefs which are used to make sense of the experience of health and illness and to suggest positive strategies for coping with and managing ill health.

 How would your account of your health over the last month differ if you were talking to:

■ Your doctor?
■ Your friend?
■ A member of your family?
■ A researcher?

Cultural views of health

We are able to think about health using the language of scientific medicine because that is part of our cultural heritage. We do so as a matter of course, and think it is self-evident or common sense.

However, other societies and cultures have their own common-sense ways of talking about health which are very different. The Ashanti view disease as the outcome of malign human or supernatural agencies, and diagnosis is a matter of determining who has been offended. Treatment includes ceremonies to propitiate these spirits as an integral part of the process. Ways of thinking about health and disease reflect the basic preoccupations of society, and dominant views of society and the world. Anthropologists refer to this phenomenon as the cultural specificity of notions of health and disease.

> The Gnau of New Guinea refer to illness and other general misfortunes by the same word, *wala*. They also use the pidgin English *sik* to refer to bodily misfortunes. Sickness is a particular type of misfortune which is caused by evil beings or by magic and sorcery. People who are sick act in certain ways (shunning certain foods, eating alone) which oblige others to find out and treat the illness.
>
> Source: Lewis (1986)

In any multicultural society such as the UK, a variety of cultural views coexist at any one time. For example, traditional Chinese medicine is based on the dichotomy of Yin and Yang, female and male, hot and cold, which is applied to symptoms, diet and treatments, such as acupuncture and Chinese herbal medicine. Alternative practitioners offer therapies based on these cultural views of health and disease alongside (or increasingly within) the National Health Service, which is based on scientific medicine.

The influence of culture on views of health is most apparent when other societies are being studied. However, Crawford (1984) applies the same analysis to western society, with provocative results. Crawford argues that capitalism is the bedrock of western society. Capitalism is an economic system centred on maximum production and consumption of goods through the free market. These economic goals have their parallel in views about health. Health is concerned with both release (consumption) and discipline (production) (Fig. 1.4). Hence the coexistence of apparently opposite beliefs in relation to health.

A unified view of health

Is there any unifying concept of health which can reconcile these different views and beliefs? Attempts at such a synthesis have come from philosophers such as Seedhouse (1986) and from organizations concerned with health such as the World Health Organization.

Figure 1.4 *Cultural views about health in capitalist society. Adapted from Crawford (1984).*

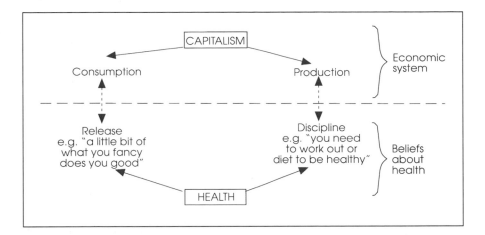

Figure 1.5 shows four theories of health:

■ Health as an ideal state
■ Health as mental and physical fitness
■ Health as a commodity
■ Health as a personal strength.

What problems can you identify with each of these four views of health?

1. *Health as an ideal state* provides a holistic and positive definition of health. It is important in showing the interrelationship of different dimensions of health. A medical diagnosis of ill health does not necessarily coincide with a sense of personal illness or feeling unwell. Equally, a person free from disease may be isolated and lonely. However, it has been argued that this definition is too idealistic and vague to provide practical guidance for health promoters. Health in this sense is probably unattainable.

2. *Health as mental and physical fitness* is a perspective developed by Talcott Parsons (1951), a functional sociologist. It suggests that health is when people can fulfil the everyday tasks and roles expected of them. The functional view of health imposes social norms without regard to individual variation. It excludes people who, owing to a chronic illness or disability, are unable to fulfil normal social roles such as that of being an employee. Using a functional definition of health, a contented and coping person who has a disability is not counted as healthy.

3. *Health as a commodity* leads to unrealistic expectations of health as something which can be purchased. Health cannot be

The theory that health is an ideal state:

■ A "Socratic" goal of perfect well-being in every respect.

■ An end in itself.

■ Disease, illness, handicap, and social problems must be absent.

A group of theories which hold that health is a personal strength or ability – either physical, metaphysical or intellectual:

■ These strengths and abilities are not commodities which can be given or purchased. Nor are they ideal states. They are developed as personal tasks. They can be lost. They can be encouraged.

The theory that health is the foundations for achievement of potentials

"A person's optimum state of health is equivalent to the state of the set of conditions which fulfil or enable a person to work to fulfil his or her realistic chosen and biological potentials. Some of these conditions are of highest importance for all people. Others are variable dependent upon individual abilities and circumstances." (p. 61)

– Created by removing obstacles

The theory that health is a commodity which can be bought or given:

■ The rationale which lies behind medical theory and practice.

■ Usually an end for the provider, a means for the receiver.

■ Health is lost in the presence of disease, illness, pain, malady. It might be restored piecemeal.

The theory that health is the physical and mental fitness to do socialized daily tasks (i.e., to function normally in a person's own society):

■ A means towards the end of normal social functioning.

■ All disabling disease, illness and handicap must be absent.

Figure 1.5 *A summary of theories of health. Adapted from Seedhouse (1986).*

guaranteed by paying a higher price for health care. This view also tends to compartmentalize the total experience of health or ill health into different activities which can be costed. This is at odds with how people experience health and illness.

4. *Health as a personal strength* is a view which derives from humanistic psychology and suggests that an individual can become healthy through self-actualization and discovery (Maslow 1970). This approach encourages individuals to define their own health but it does not address the social environment which creates health and ill health.

Seedhouse suggests that these four views can be combined in a unified theory of health as the foundation for human achievement. Health is thus a means to an end rather than a fixed state that a person should aspire to. Provided certain central conditions are met, people can be enabled to achieve their potential. Working for health is to create these conditions:

■ basic needs of food, drink, shelter, warmth
■ access to information about the factors influencing health
■ skills and confidence to use that information.

This definition acknowledges that people have different starting points which set limits for their potential for health. It encompasses a positive notion of health which is applicable to everyone, whatever their circumstances. However, it could be argued that this definition does not acknowledge the social construction of health sufficiently. People as individuals have little scope to determine optimum conditions for realizing their potential.

> By health I mean the power to live a full, adult, living, breathing life in close contact with what I love … I want to be all that I am capable of becoming.
>
> (Mansfield 1977, p. 278)

The view of health as personal potential is attractive because it is so flexible, but this very flexibility causes problems. It leads to relativism (health may mean a thousand different things to a thousand different people), which makes it impracticable as a working definition for health promoters.

The World Health Organization (WHO) has been responsible for progressing the debate about definitions of health.

> [Health is] the extent to which an individual or group is able, on the one hand, to realise aspirations and satisfy needs; and, on the other hand, to change or cope with the environment. Health is, therefore, seen as a resource for everyday life, not an object of living; it is a positive concept emphasising social and personal resources, as well as physical capacities.
>
> (WHO 1984)

This definition is important for several reasons. It establishes health as a social as well as an individual product, and it emphasizes the dynamic and positive nature of health. Health is viewed as both a fundamental human right and a sound social investment. This view has been publicly affirmed by the Jakarta Declaration which linked health to social and economic development (WHO 1997). This definition provides a variety of reasons for supporting health, which are likely to meet the concerns of a range of groups. It establishes a broad consensus for prioritizing health, and legitimizes a range of activities designed to promote health. For example, in addition to the more acceptable strategies of primary health care and personal skills development, the WHO also identified in the Ottawa Charter the more radical strategies of community participation and healthy public policy as essential to the promotion of health (WHO 1986). However, it could still be argued that such a broad definition makes it difficult to identify practical priorities for health promotion activities.

There is no agreement on what is meant by health. Health is used in many different contexts to refer to many different aspects of life. Given this complexity of meanings, it is unlikely that a unified concept of health which includes all its meanings will be formulated.

Conclusion

There are no rights and wrongs regarding concepts of health. Different people are likely to hold different views of health and may operate with several conflicting views simultaneously. Where people are located socially, in terms of social class, gender, ethnic origin and occupation, will affect their concept of health. The medical model has, however, dominated western thinking about health. Yet its value for health promotion is limited:

- it relies on a concept of normality that is not widely accepted
- it ignores broader societal and environmental dimensions of health
- it ignores people's subjective perceptions of their own health
- the focus on pathology and malfunction leads to practitioners responding to ill health rather than being proactive in promoting health.

There is such a range of meaning attached to the notion of health, that in any particular situation, it is important to find out what views are in operation. Clarifying what you understand about health, and what other people mean when they talk about health, is an essential first step for the health promoter.

Questions for further discussion

- How would you describe your own concept of health?
- What have been the most important influences on your views?

Summary

Definitions of health arise from many different perspectives. Whilst scientific medicine is the most powerful ideology in the West, it is not all-embracing. Social sciences' perspectives on health produce a powerful critique of scientific medicine, and point to the importance of social factors in the construction and meaning of health. Lay concepts of health derived from different cultures coexist alongside scientific medicine. Attempts to produce a unified concept of health appear to founder through overgeneralization and vagueness.

Further reading

Aggleton P 1990 Health. Routledge, London. *A readable introduction to a social science perspective on health.*

Seedhouse D 1986 Health: the foundations for achievement. John Wiley, Chichester. *A clear account of different views of health which attempts to provide a unified concept of health.*

Beattie A, Gott M, Jones L, Sidell M (eds) 1993 Health and wellbeing: a reader. Macmillan/Open University, Basingstoke. *An edited selection of accounts from different perspectives and disciplines.*

Nettleton S 1995 The sociology of health and illness. Polity Press, Oxford. *An accessible introduction to the sociology of health and illness which explores the social construction of medical knowledge, lay health knowledge, concepts of lifestyle and risk and the newly emerging sociology of the body.*

References

Aggleton P, Homans H 1987 Educating about AIDS. NHS Training Authority, Bristol

Antonovsky A 1993 The sense of coherence as a determinant of health. In: Beattie A, Gott M, Jones L, Sidell M (eds) Health and wellbeing: a reader. Macmillan/Open University, Basingstoke, pp 202–214

Blaxter M 1990 Health and lifestyles. Tavistock/Routledge, London

Calnan M 1987 Health and illness. Tavistock, London

Cochrane A L 1972 Effectiveness and efficiency. Nuffield Provincial Hospitals Trust, London

Cornwell J 1984 Hard-earned lives. Tavistock, London

Crawford R 1984 A cultural account of 'health': control, release and the social body. In: McKinley J (ed) Issues in the political economy of health care. Tavistock, London, pp 60–103

d'Houtaud A, Field M 1986 New research on the image of health. In: Currer C, Stacey M (eds) Concepts of health, illness and disease: a comparative perspective. Berg, Leamington Spa, pp 235–255

Doyal L, Doyal L 1984 In: Birke L, Silvertown J (eds) More than the parts: biology and politics. Pluto Press, London

Doyal L, with Pennell I 1979 The political economy of health. Pluto Press, London

Esmail A, Everington S 1993 Racial discrimination against doctors from ethnic minorities. British Medical Journal 306: 691

Ewles L, Simnett I 1999 Promoting health: a practical guide to health education, 4th edn. Harcourt, Edinburgh

Freidson F 1986 Professional powers: a study of the institutionalization of formal knowledge. University of Chicago Press, Chicago

Gabe J, Kelleher D, Williams G (eds) 1994 Challenging medicine. Routledge, London

Helman C 1986 Feed a cold, starve a fever. In: Currer C, Stacey M (eds) Concepts of health, illness and disease: a comparative perspective. Berg, Leamington Spa, pp 213–231

Herzlich C 1973 Health and illness. Academic Press, London

Illich I 1975 Medical nemesis, part I. Calder and Boyers, London

Kelleher D 1994 Self-help groups and medicine. In: Gabe J, Kelleher D, Williams G (eds) Challenging medicine. Routledge, London

Lewis G 1986 Concepts of health and illness in a Sepik society. In: Currer C, Stacey M (eds) Concepts of health, illness and disease: a comparative perspective. Berg, Leamington Spa, pp 119–135

McKeown T, Lowe C R 1974 An introduction to social medicine. Blackwell Scientific Publications, Oxford

Mansfield K 1977 In: Stead C K (ed) The letters and journals of Katherine Mansfield: a selection. Penguin, Harmondsworth

Maslow A H 1970 Motivation and personality, 2nd edn. Harper and Row, New York

National Forum for Coronary Heart Disease Prevention 1990 CHD prevention in undergraduate medical education. National Forum for Coronary Heart Disease Prevention, London

Parsons T 1951 The social system. Free Press, Glencoe, Illinois, USA

Parsons T 1972 Definitions of health and illness in the light of American values and social structure. In: Jaco E, Gartley E (eds) Patients, physicians and illness: a sourcebook in behavioural science and health. Collier-Macmillan, London, pp 97–117

Rowntree Foundation 1995 Inquiry into income and wealth. Joseph Rowntree Foundation, York

Seedhouse D 1986 Health: foundations for achievement. John Wiley, Chichester

Skellington R, Morris P 1992. Race in Britain today. Sage, London

Skrabanek P, McCormick J 1992 Follies and fallacies in medicine. Tarragon Press, Glasgow

Sontag S 1988 AIDS and its metaphors (published with illness as metaphor). Penguin, London

Stacey M 1988 The sociology of health and healing. Unwin Hyman, London

Tarlov A R 1996 Social determinants of health: the sociobiological translation. In: Blane D, Brunner E, Wilkinson R (eds) Health and social organisation: towards a health policy for the 21st century. Routledge, London

Thorogood N 1993 Caribbean home remedies and their importance for black women's health care in Britain. In: Beattie A, Gott M, Jones L, Sidell M (eds) Health and wellbeing: a reader. Macmillan/Open University, Basingstoke, pp 23–33

Townsend P, Davidson N, Whitehead M 1988 Inequalities in health: the Black Report and The Health Divide. Penguin, Harmondsworth

Wilkinson R G 1996 Unhealthy societies: the afflictions of inequality. Routledge, London

Williams R G A 1983 Concepts of health: an analysis of lay logic. Sociology 17: 183–205

World Health Organization 1946 Constitution. WHO, Geneva

World Health Organization 1984 Health promotion: a discussion document on the concept and principles. WHO Regional Office for Europe, Copenhagen

World Health Organization 1986 Ottawa charter for health promotion. Journal of Health Promotion 1: 1–4

World Health Organization 1997 4th International conference on health promotion. New players for a new era – leading health promotion into the 21st century. WHO, Jakarta

2 *Influences on health*

OVERVIEW

The previous chapter showed that there is a wide range of meanings attached to the concept of health, and different perspectives offered by the scientific medical model and social science. It emphasized the importance of social factors in the construction and meaning of health. This chapter shows how the major influences on mortality and morbidity are social and environmental factors. It summarizes recent research which suggests that there are inequalities in health status between groups of people which reflect structural inequalities in society such as social class, gender and ethnicity.

Determinants of health

Since the decline in infectious diseases in the 19th and early 20th centuries, the major causes of sickness and death are now cardiovascular (now accounting for nearly 48% of deaths) and cancers (now accounting for 25% of deaths) (OPCS 1993). Increased longevity and the current life span of women to 80 years and men to 75 years accounts for the increase in degenerative diseases in the population as a whole. Despite the increase in life expectancy, epidemiologists who study the pattern of diseases in society have found that not all groups have the same opportunities to achieve good health and there are population patterns which make it possible to predict the likelihood that people from different groups will die prematurely.

In trying to determine what affects health, social scientists and epidemiologists will seek to compare at least two variables: firstly, a measure of health, or rather ill health, such as mortality or morbidity; and, secondly, a factor such as gender or occupation that could account for the differences in health. Of course, effects on health can be due to several variables interacting together. For example, research into coronary heart disease (CHD) has linked a large number of factors with the incidence of the disease: high levels of blood cholesterol, high blood pressure, obesity, cigarette smoking and low levels of physical activity. Other research indicates there may be links between CHD and psychosocial factors, such as stress and lack of social support, environmental factors such as hard tap water, and family history (WHO 1982). Many studies have also tried to establish whether there is a coronary-prone personality (known as Type A) (Marmot 1980). We also know that mortality from CHD is higher among lower social classes, among men rather than women, and among people from the Indian sub-continent (DoH 1992). Figure 2.1 illustrates in a simple form how health status can be accounted for not by one variable, but by many factors which interact together. It shows that some factors have an independent effect on health or they may be mediated by other intervening variables.

What is clear is that ill health does not happen by chance or through bad luck. The Lalonde Report published in Canada in 1974 was influential in identifying four 'fields' in which health could be promoted:

- genetic and biological factors which determine an individual's predisposition to disease
- lifestyle factors in which health behaviours such as smoking contribute to disease
- environmental factors such as housing or pollution
- the extent and nature of health services.

Genetic factors are largely unalterable and what limited scope there is for intervention lies in the medical field. The previous chapter outlined McKeown and Lowe's work (1974) which showed that medical interventions in the form of vaccination had remarkably little impact on mortality rates. This suggests that factors other than the purely biological determine health and well-being.

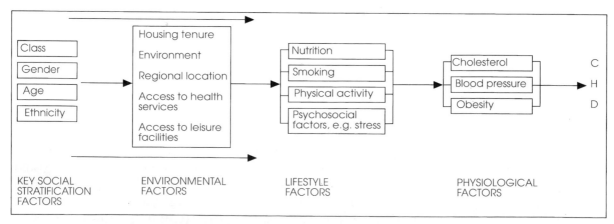

Figure 2.1 *Factors influencing the development of coronary heart disease (CHD).*

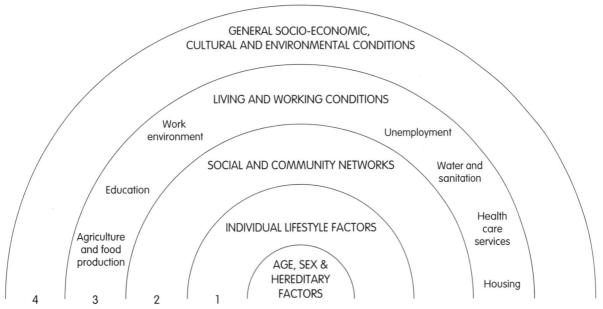

Figure 2.2 *The main determinants of health. From Dahlgren & Whitehead 1991.*

Lifestyles are frequently the focus of health promotion interventions. Figure 2.3 shows a whole range of factors that may influence smoking behaviour. Take another of the factors implicated in coronary heart disease such as nutrition and identify the influences on that health behaviour.

Dahlgren & Whitehead (1991) thus talk of 'layers of influence on health' that can be modified (see Fig. 2.2):

■ personal behaviour and lifestyles
■ support and influence within communities which can sustain or damage health
■ living and working conditions and access to facilities and services
■ economic, cultural and environmental conditions such as standards of living or the labour market.

Social class and health

Most research which has sought to identify the major determinants of health and ill health has focused on the links between social class and health. In 1980 a report was published of a Department of Health and Social Security working group on inequalities in health (Townsend & Davidson 1982). The report which is known as the Black Report after the group's chairman, Sir Douglas Black, provided a detailed study of the relationship between mortality and morbidity, and social class.

The terms social class, social disadvantage, socio-economic status and occupation are often used interchangeably. The classification of social class derives from the Registrar General's scale of five occupational classes ranging from professionals in class I to unskilled manual workers in class V. This has been largely unchanged since 1921 (class III was divided into manual and non-manual work in 1971). Because people are allocated to social

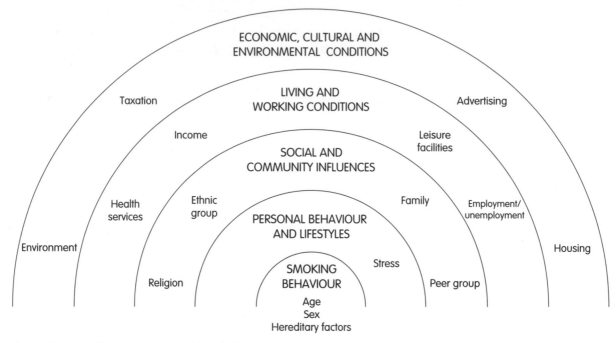

Figure 2.3   *Influences on smoking behaviour.*

classes on the basis of the occupation of the head of the household, the classification is more suited to men of working age than the elderly, the unemployed or women. The Office of National Statistics will introduce eight new categories for the census in 2001 to take account of changes in the labour market with a social class for the self-employed and one for people who have never worked or who are long-term unemployed (Table 2.1).

Table 2.1   *Social class classification*

1	Higher managerial and professional
1.1	e.g. company directors, bank managers, senior civil servants
1.2	e.g. doctors, barristers and solicitors, teachers, social workers
2	Lower managerial and professional
	e.g. nurses, actors and musicians, police, soldiers
3	Intermediate
	e.g. secretaries, clerks
4	Small employers and own account workers
	e.g. publicans, play group leaders, farmers, taxi drivers
5	Lower supervisory, craft and related occupations
	e.g. printers, plumbers, butchers, train drivers
6	Semi-routine occupations
	e.g. shop assistants, traffic wardens, hairdressers
7	Routine occupations
	e.g. waiters, road sweepers, cleaners, couriers
8	Never worked and long-term unemployed

Although social class classification is not a perfect tool, it does serve as an indicator of the way of life and living standards experienced by different groups. It correlates with other aspects of social position such as income, housing, education and working and living environments.

The Black Report and a later report commissioned by the Health Education Authority, *The Health Divide* (Whitehead 1988) found significant differences in death rates between socio-economic classes. More recent reports (Acheson 1998, Benzeval et al 1995) draw together data which show that far from ill health being a matter of bad luck, health and disease are socially patterned with the more affluent members of society living longer and enjoying better health than disadvantaged social groups. This gap in health may even be getting worse. Economic growth has been accompanied by widening income differentials which is reflected in widening differences in mortality rates between the social classes (Phillimore et al 1994).

 The extent and nature of health inequalities

LIFE EXPECTANCY

■ A man in social class I is likely to live around 7 years longer than a man in social class V.

Infant mortality

■ A child born into social class V is twice as likely to die before the age of 15 as a child born into social class I.

Causes of death

■ Of the 66 major causes of death in men, 62 were more common among social classes IV and V combined than in other social classes.
■ Of the 70 major causes of death in women, 64 were more common in women married to men in social classes IV and V.

Long-standing illness

■ There are twice as many reports of long-standing illness among men and women from social class V compared to social class I.

Source: DoH (1996)

Figure 2.4 shows that there are substantial differences in male mortality with a step-wise increase with decreasing social class. Social class differences are at their most marked in the first year of life. Although infant mortality rates are declining, children in social class V are still nearly twice as likely to die before their first birthday compared to children in social class I or II (see Fig. 2.5). Low birth

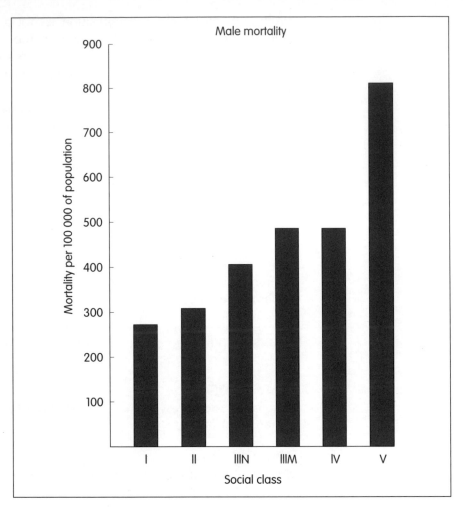

Figure 2.4   *Male mortality by social class. From Drever & Whitehead (1997).*

weight is probably the most important predictor of death in the first month of life and this is clearly class-related with two-thirds of babies under 2500 g born to mothers in social class V (OPCS 1995). Although it is common to talk of 'diseases of affluence' such as coronary heart disease being the major killers in contemporary Britain, most disease categories are more common among social classes IV and V. Particularly large differentials have developed for respiratory disease, lung cancer, accidents and suicide. People from lower social classes also experience more sickness and ill health. The General Household Survey each year reports that men and women from social classes IV and V experience more limiting long-standing illness than people in social classes I and II.

Although there is a clear pattern linking social class and health, there is no consensus about what it is about social class that is the most important factor. Those factors most commonly cited are income, housing, and employment.

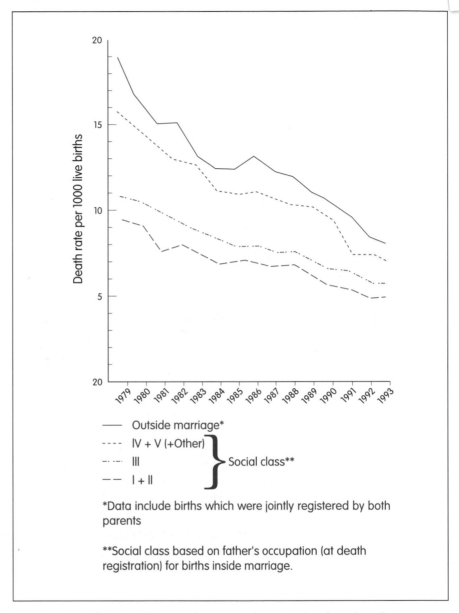

Figure 2.5 *Infant death rates by social class: England and Wales 1979–1993. From OPCS (1995).*

Income and health

Income is a major determinant of standard of living and variations in ill health and premature mortality reflect differences in levels of income and material deprivation. According to the Rowntree Report, in 1990 24% of the population had incomes below half the national average after allowing for housing costs (Rowntree Foundation 1995). Those most likely to be in this category are the unemployed, pensioners, lone parents, families with three or more children and the low paid. The British Household Panel Survey found that 5% of people had sustained financial hardship and poverty in the period 1991–1995.

Blackburn (1991) suggests that there are three ways in which low income can affect health:

- *Physiological* – inadequate or unfit housing, lack of food, lack of fuel
- *Psychological* – stress and lack of social support
- *Behavioural* – health-damaging behaviours such as smoking or drinking or giving children sweets are ways of helping people to cope with the demands of disadvantage.

Poverty also reduces people's choices of a healthier lifestyle. Healthy food, for example, not only costs more but when money is short, families buy food which is high in calories and filling rather than necessarily nutritious.

Housing and health

Health can be damaged by housing quality and its lack of availability. In 1991/2 local authorities accepted 169 966 housing applications from homeless families with children or pregnant women. A further 2827 people were rough sleepers and 19 417 were hostel dwellers. An unknown number of families share unsuitable or inadequate accommodation (Connelly & Crown 1994). The particular problems of homelessness, which include respiratory illness, depression, high rates of infection among children, accidents, and difficulties in gaining access to health services, have been well-documented (Arblaster & Hawtin 1993, Standing Conference on Public Health 1994).

Cold and damp housing have been shown to contribute to illness. Children living in damp houses are likely to have higher rates of respiratory illness, symptoms of infection and stress (Martin et al 1987). These will be exacerbated by overcrowding. The high accident rates to children in social class 5 are associated with high-

Linda visits her GP with Alex aged 4 who has a chronic wheeze. Linda has two other children under 7 whom she is bringing up alone on a high-rise estate which is due for demolition in the next 5 years. The flats are damp with condensation running down the walls. There has been a recent infestation of cockroaches. Linda last visited her GP 6 weeks ago for her own bronchitis. The GP told her to stop smoking.

What would you expect the GP to advise regarding Alex's health? How effective do you think this advice would be?

density housing where there is a lack of play space and opportunities for parental supervision. Psychological and practical difficulties accompany living in high-rise flats and isolated housing estates which may adversely affect the health of women at home or older people.

Employment and health

Work is important to consider as a social determinant of health:

- it determines income levels
- it affects self-esteem
- the type of employment may itself directly affect health.

The traditional focus of occupational health has been to consider how particular types of employment carry high occupational health risks. This may be because of the risk of accidents (for example in mining), exposure to hazardous substances or because of stress. Some occupations encourage lifestyles which may be damaging to health. Publicans, for example, are at high risk of developing cirrhosis.

 Consider how the following differences between manual and non-manual occupations can influence health:

- Pay
- Hours of work
- Occupational pension and sickness scheme
- Holiday entitlements
- Accidents at work
- Exposure to toxic substances and environmental hazards
- Job security
- Occupational mobility
- Prestige and status
- Autonomy.

There has been considerable interest in how the psychosocial environment of work can affect health (Marmot & Feeney 1996). Most research has identified high demands and low control over work decisions as contributing to job stress and cardiovascular risk. These factors together with the amount of social support people get at work have been confirmed in workplace studies in many developed countries (see Ch. 13 for further discussion). There is also a considerable body of evidence that unemployment can damage health (Bethune 1997, Moser et al 1990), although it is far from clear whether unemployment itself can lead to a deterioration in health or whether it is the poverty associated with unemployment which contributes to the poor health of the unemployed.

Consider the following evidence concerning the effects of unemployment on health. What could account for this relationship?

1. The unemployed report higher rates of mental ill health including depression, anxiety, sleep disturbance.
2. Suicide and parasuicide rates are twice as high among the unemployed as the employed.
3. The death rates among the unemployed are at least 20% higher than expected after adjustment for social class and age.
4. The unemployed have higher rates of bronchitis and ischaemic heart disease than the employed.
5. Over 60% of unemployed people smoke compared to 30% of employed people.

It seems that unemployment has a profound effect on mental health, damaging a person's self-esteem and social structure. Part of its effect on health must also arise from the material disadvantage of living on a low income.

Source: Bartley (1994), Moser et al (1990), Smith (1987)

Gender and health

Gender refers to the social categorization of people as men or women, and the social meaning and beliefs about sexual difference.

What could account for the following evidence of gender differences in health?

■ Women live on average 6 years longer than men and yet women record higher levels of morbidity in both chronic and acute illness.
■ Women account for 51% of the population in the United Kingdom but account for between 60% and 65% of NHS expenditure.
■ Over 60% of general practice consultations involve women.
■ Over 60% of hospital beds are occupied by women.
■ Admissions to psychiatric hospitals are three times higher for women than for men for some disorders.

Source: DoH (1996), Miles (1991)

Some of the sex differences in morbidity have been attributed as an artefact of measurement of the use of health services. Women are more likely to report illness as they are less likely to be in full-time employment or because they are more inclined to take care of their health, resulting in increased consultation rates. However, this does not explain the sex difference in mortality. Nor is there a consistent tendency for women's greater willingness to consult.

The natural selection or genetic explanation suggests that women are more resistant to infection and benefit from a protective effect of oestrogen accounting for their lower mortality rates. Paradoxically, female hormones and the female reproductive system are claimed to render women more liable to physical and mental ill health. Biological explanations are unable to account for the social class difference in women's health whereby women in social classes I and II experience better health than women in social classes IV and V (Bridgewood & Savage 1993). It is also important to note that greater female longevity has only arisen in the 20th century and is mostly attributable to the dramatic decline in infectious disease mortality and a decline in the number of births.

Lifestyle explanations argue that women are socialized to be passive, dependent and sick. Women readily adopt the sick role because it fits with preconceived notions of feminine behaviour. Men, by contrast, are encouraged to be aggressive and risk-taking both at work and in their leisure time. The higher rates for accidents and alcoholism amongst men are cited as evidence for this. Although it is often said that women rate their health less positively and report more physical and psychosocial symptoms, there is no blanket difference between men and women. More women report headaches, tiredness, depression, varicose veins, haemorrhoids, arthritis and rheumatism. But younger males report digestive troubles, asthma and back trouble. At older ages, more men report heart disease. Until the age of 74 similar numbers of men and women report a chronic illness.

 Many explanations have been offered to account for women's ill health. With which of the following do you most agree?

1. Women consult their GPs more frequently than men and so will appear to have greater morbidity.
2. Women acknowledge their feelings of illness.
3. In the same situation, a man would be told to get on with things. A woman is labelled as ill.
4. Many women are workers inside and outside the home and have care responsibilities.
5. Much of women's ill health is due to depression from their social isolation at home.
6. Much of women's ill health relates to their reproductive organs.
7. The patriarchal control of medicine has deprived women of control over natural processes such as childbearing and child rearing, producing more problems.
8. Women have less access to material resources than men.

Finally, it has been argued that women's social position as both carers and workers inside, and increasingly outside the home, is a dual burden which leads to increased stress and ill health. 42% of the employed workforce is female and yet women receive on average two-thirds of the male wage for equal work. Most women work part time with less security and benefits than full-time workers, and working conditions at home and in the workplace may be hazardous, especially for poorer women in social classes IV and V (Doyal 1995). Employment outside the home does have a protective benefit for some women but this seems to be dependent on material circumstances (Arber 1990).

Health of ethnic minorities

Race is another way in which social and health inequalities are structured. Race should be understood as a political not biological category. We therefore use the term 'ethnic minority' to identify those who share a cultural heritage and who also share experience of discrimination.

Research comparing the mortality rates of immigrants from the Indian sub-continent, Africa and the Caribbean with people born in England and Wales found higher rates for tuberculosis, accidents and cancer of the liver but lower than average rates for bronchitis and most other cancers in the migrants. There was strikingly high mortality from hypertension and strokes among those from the Caribbean and African Commonwealth and those born in South Asia were much more likely than average to die from ischaemic heart disease. Mortality statistics show disturbingly high infant mortality rates as well as high maternal mortality among women from Pakistan.

Black and ethnic minority groups also experience more ill health, particularly chronic and mental ill health. Schizophrenia is diagnosed more commonly among African Caribbeans, and there are higher rates of suicide and parasuicide and chronic conditions such as asthma and rheumatism among a range of black and minority ethnic groups (Nazroo 1998, Smaje 1995).

Professional and public attention has tended to focus not on this association between ethnicity and ill health, but on the tiny minority of ill health which can be attributed to diseases specific to certain ethnic minority groups such as sickle cell anaemia, thalassaemia and Tay–Sachs disease.

There is still very little information on the health of ethnic minorities. Until 1991 ethnic origin was not recorded in census information or official statistics. The country of birth recorded on birth and death certificates has therefore formed the basis for the association between health and ethnic origin. This clearly does not account for British-born ethnic minorities (approximately 50% of black and ethnic minority groups were born in the UK). It is important then not to put all members of ethnic minorities into one disadvantaged category. More data would enable us to find out how many people from ethnic minority groups are disadvantaged, and how. It would also then be possible to determine whether the poor health of black and ethnic minority groups is associated with the low income, poor working conditions or unemployment, and poor housing shared by those in lower social classes, or whether there is, in addition, ill health resulting from the experience of racism and institutionalized discrimination in health care and other services (Ahmad 1993, Smaje 1995). Research shows that whilst black and ethnic minority groups make above average use of GP services and average use of childhood immunization services, there is a lower than average use of community, screening and hospital services (Rudat 1994, Smaje 1995).

 Consider the following possible explanations for the high rates of hypertension in older generation black and minority ethnic communities. Which do you consider to be the most likely explanation(s)?

■ Greater consumption of saturated fats in the United Kingdom.
■ High cost of imported African, Caribbean and Asian foods.
■ Stress associated with chronic situations, such as poverty and racism.
■ Lack of exercise, which is not incorporated into daily life as it is in Africa and the Caribbean.
■ Retention of excess salt because of a different climate and lifestyle.

Place of residence and health

The Health Divide (Whitehead 1988) showed how mortality rates increase steadily moving from the Southeast to the Northwest and that a North–South divide is present for most diseases. Dorling (1997) has reported that in the early 1990s a resident of Glasgow was 31% more likely to die than someone of the same age and sex living in Bristol and 66% more likely to die than someone living in rural Dorset. Even within cities and regions there are significant variations. The greatest health disparities are in regions with the poorest mortality rates – the North, Wales, Scotland and the Northwest (Townsend et al 1988). One obvious explanation for the geographic differences in death rates might be differences in social class distribution, those areas with high mortality rates being those areas with a greater proportion of people in social classes IV and V. Yet the regional mortality differences remain even after adjustment for social class, and people in each social class do better in the healthier regions. Although a North–South divide does exist, it is not clear cut. The healthiest areas of the North compare favourably with those in the South.

Social cohesion and exclusion

There is a growing body of evidence demonstrating that it is *relative* inequalities in income and material resources, coupled with the resulting social exclusion and marginalization which is linked to poor health (Blane et al 1996, Wilkinson 1996). The key evidence on this comes from the international data on income distribution and national mortality rates. In the developed world it is not the richest countries which have the best health but the most egalitarian. Whilst the exact mechanisms linking social inequality to ill health are uncertain, it is likely that both physiological pathways (e.g. the effect of chronic stress on the immunological process) and social pathways (e.g. support networks) are relevant. Healthy, egalitarian societies are more socially cohesive and have a stronger community life. The need to invest in 'social capital' is now being acknowledged by policy makers and the Department of Health. (See Ch. 15 for more discussion of the ways in which communities can build social capital.)

'The quality of the social life of a society is one of the most powerful determinants of health (and this, in turn, is very closely related to the degree of income equality)' (Wilkinson 1996, p. 5).

Which of the following, in your view, reflects the quality of life of a society?
■ High level of civic activities
■ High gross national product
■ Low crime rates
■ High percentage of adults receiving a university education
■ Availability and accessibility of information exchange mechanisms
■ High levels of employment

The degree to which an individual is integrated into society and has a social support network has been shown to have a significant impact on health. Research has shown that those with few friends or family are more likely to die early, less likely to survive a heart attack

Which groups in society do you regard as 'socially excluded'?

'Health is an important dimension of social exclusion which involves not only social but also economic and psychological isolation. Although people may know what affects their health, they can find it difficult to act on what they know, setting up a downward spiral of deprivation and poor health' (DoH 1999, p. 44).

or stroke and more likely to develop a cold when exposed to a cold virus in experimental conditions (Bloom 1990, Kawachi et al 1996). Being well supported enables someone to draw on a network for resources and encouragement. It is also likely that those who are more isolated have greater stress, which has been shown to affect the immune system.

Explaining health inequalities

What explanation would you offer for the inequalities in health between social classes?

We have seen that there are inequalities in health relating to social class, geographic location, gender and ethnic origin.

You may believe that people in the lower social classes choose more unhealthy ways of living, or you may believe that people in social classes IV and V have low incomes which prevent them adopting a healthy lifestyle and cause them to live in unhealthy conditions. There is a continuing debate over this question and no simple answer. Explanations have tended to be of four broad types: artefact, social selection, cultural/behavioural and materialist/structural.

Health inequalities as an artefact

The artefact explanation argues that the widening gap in mortality figures between the social classes is not real, but an effect of the way in which class and health are measured. Because there have been changes in the classification of occupations and in the structure of social classes, it makes it impossible to make comparisons over time. For example, the assignment of occupations to social classes has changed over several decades as has the relative size of the classes. There is now a much smaller proportion of the population in class V and comparisons between class I and class V over 30–50 years are not comparing similar-sized segments of the population. There may have been changes in the relative status of the classes also. The smaller class I before 1945 may be very different from the expanded class I in the 1980s when the Black Report was published. It is also argued that the mortality rates of class V are skewed because, as social mobility continues, this class contains a greater proportion of older people at risk from dying.

Establishing a relationship between social class and health, particularly over time, is difficult. However, a considerable amount of research supports the view that the relationship is a real phenomenon and not merely an artefact of the data. When other indicators of disadvantage are used, such as housing, access to a car, education, household possessions and income, they all show a similar pattern of health inequalities between the top and bottom of the social scale (Goldblatt 1990).

Health inequalities as a selection process

Social selection theory argues that the relationship between class and health is a causal one, but that it is health which determines people's class and not vice versa. The healthy experience upward social mobility and mortality rates are kept low in the upper classes. People with higher levels of illness drift down the social scale and thus inflate the rates of death and disability among social classes IV and V. There is some evidence that health can affect social status. A study of women in Aberdeen found that those who were taller tended to marry into a higher social class. As height may be taken as an indicator of health, this evidence suggests some sort of health selection taking place at marriage (Illsley 1986). Chronic illness can also account for downward social mobility. Manual workers with failing health are often moved into other jobs because of sickness and are more likely to have difficulty finding new work.

The argument suggests that health is a static property rather than a shifting state of being which is influenced by social and economic circumstance. Thus some people, because of their genetic health potential, are able to overcome disadvantage and 'climb out of poverty'. Whilst this may be true for some people, the extent of social mobility is not sufficient to account for the overall scale of social-class differences in health (Wilkinson 1986).

Health inequalities as a result of lifestyles

This argument suggests that the social distribution of ill health is linked with differences in risk behaviours. These behaviours – smoking, high alcohol consumption, lack of exercise, high-fat and high-sugar diets – are more common among lower social classes.

For example, while smoking has decreased in all social classes over the last 2 decades, there are still major differences in the proportion of smokers in classes I to V. In 1992, only 14% of professional men and 13% of professional women smoked, against 35% of women and 42% of men in unskilled manual occupations (Thomas et al 1994). In 1990, 6 out of 10 lone parents smoked, the same proportion as in 1976 (Marsh & McKay 1994).

According to Wilkinson (1986) the current distribution of coronary heart disease, stroke and lung cancer and the so-called 'diseases of affluence' among the lower social classes can be attributed in part to the downward social shift in the consumption of tobacco and refined foods.

Behaviour cannot, however, be separated from the social context in which it takes place. Hilary Graham (1992) has shown how the decision to smoke by many working-class women is a coping strategy to deal with the stress associated with poverty and isolation. The decision to smoke *is* a choice but it is not taken through recklessness or ignorance; it is rather a choice between 'health evils' – stress versus smoking.

Do you agree with those people who say that people who die from lung cancer caused by smoking have only themselves to blame?

Now consider these extracts from interviews with lone parents who have made a positive choice to smoke because it allows them to cope with parenting in adverse circumstances.

'Sometimes I put him outside the door and put the radio on at full blast, then I've sat down and had a cigarette, calmed down and fetched him in again.'

'If I was economizing I'd cut down on cigarettes but I wouldn't give them up. I'd stop eating. That sounds terrible doesn't it? Food just isn't that important to me, but having a cigarette is the one thing I do for myself.'

Source: Graham (1992)

Health inequalities and cultural explanations

Some writers claim that there are cultural differences between social groups in their attitudes towards health and protecting their health for the future. Thus giving up cigarettes, as a form of deferred gratification, is more likely to appeal to middle-class people who, as we saw in Chapter 1, may have a stronger locus of control and may believe that they determine the course of their life. Working-class people who may have to struggle to get by each day do not make long-term plans and have a fatalistic view of health, believing it to be a matter of luck. Thus attitudes are passed on from generation to generation. This phenomenon is referred to as the 'culture of poverty' or 'cycle of deprivation'. According to such views, ill health can be explained in terms of the characteristics of poor people themselves and their inadequacy and incompetence. In 1986, Edwina Currie, a newly appointed health minister, caused a storm of controversy by suggesting that the high levels of premature death, permanent sickness and low birth weights in the northern regions were due to ignorance and people failing to realize that they had some control over their lives.

A behavioural explanation which sees lifestyles and cultural influences determining health has considerable appeal to any government that is concerned to reduce public expenditure. If individuals are seen as responsible for their own health, government inactivity is legitimized. Such viewpoints, which are particularly associated with the Thatcherite years of the 1980s and early 1990s, have been widely criticized as victim blaming, in that people are seen as being responsible for factors which disadvantage them but over which they have no control.

Cultural explanations of behaviour may be seen as an extension of individual victim blaming to cultural victim blaming – attitudes and behaviour which are different and may be perfectly rational are seen as in some way socially deficient. Thus poor people are viewed as ignorant, feckless or too apathetic to do anything about changing their lives. Women may be seen as negligent in their care for others as reflected in this speech from the turn of the century.

'The problem of infant mortality is not one of sanitation alone, or housing or, indeed, of poverty as such, but is mainly a question of motherhood . . . death in infancy is probably more due to such ignorance and negligence than any other cause' (George Newman, Chief Medical Officer, 1906).

Health inequalities as a result of material disadvantage

This explanation argues that the distribution of health and ill health in the population reflects a profoundly unequal distribution of resources in society. Thus those who experience ill health are those who are lower in the social hierarchy, who are least educated, who have least money and have fewest resources. Low income may be the result of unemployment or ill-paid hazardous occupations; it can lead to poor housing in polluted and unsafe environments with few opportunities to build social support networks; and in turn such conditions lead to poor health. Lack of money can make it difficult for households to implement what they may know to be healthy choices. Blaxter (1990), analysing data from the largest health and lifestyle survey completed in the UK, found that the health of low-income groups improves substantially as income increases.

Access to health services

The inequalities in health that we have considered in this chapter are all the more remarkable because the National Health Service has

Consider the following evidence on the nature and extent of childhood accidents.

■ Accidents are the leading cause of death among children aged 1–4.
■ A child from social class IV or V is twice as likely to suffer a fatal accident as a child from social class I or II.

To what do you attribute this?

■ Children from lower social classes are more accident prone or more reckless.
■ Parents from lower social classes do not exercise due care in safeguarding their home and supervising their children.
■ The physical environment in which poor children play has less space and is less likely to have safety features such as stairgates and fireguards. Poor children are more likely to have to play outside in environments lacking safety features.

been in existence for more than 40 years. Its intention to provide a universal service freely available to all might have been expected to reduce inequalities in health status. Yet in the early 1970s a GP writing in *The Lancet* put forward a radical view that good health care tends to vary inversely with the need of the population (Tudor Hart 1971).

'In areas with most sickness and death, GPs have more work, larger lists, less hospital support and inherit more clinically ineffective traditions of consultation than in the healthiest areas; and the hospital doctors shoulder heavier caseloads with less staff and equipment, more obsolete buildings and suffer recurrent crises in the availability of beds and replacement of staff. These trends can be summed up as the Inverse Care Law: that the availability of good medical care tends to vary inversely with the needs of the population served.' (Tudor Hart 1971).

Nearly 3 decades later, differential access to and quality of health services still exist. Rural and inner city areas have more single-handed general practices and fewer services. In addition, poorer groups and ethnic minority groups make less use of immunization, screening and antenatal care (Benzeval et al 1995).

What reasons can you offer for the low take-up of preventive services by working-class people?

Some of the reasons may relate to ease of access. Working-class and older people who do not have cars may find public transport difficult, especially those with young children. Clinics may lack play space. For hourly paid workers, attendance at primary health care clinics may mean loss of earnings. The use of appointment systems by clinics and GP surgeries causes difficulties for households without a telephone. There is also evidence that health care workers respond differently to different social groups. Thus working-class people may have low expectations of primary health care. Or is the most likely explanation to do with cultural attitudes? As discussed earlier in this chapter, some writers suggest that working-class people do not value their health and have a fatalistic attitude towards prevention.

There is evidence of variation in the quality and quantity of care available to people in different social groups, between regions and between different ethnic groups. However, since medical care has had little impact on the overall death rate from heart disease or cancers, and probably only about 5% of deaths are preventable through medical treatment, it must be concluded that differences in health status are not wholly attributable to variations in the amount and type of care received.

Tackling inequalities in health

Although the extent of health inequalities has been highlighted for nearly 20 years, the centrality of social deprivation as a cause of ill health has been down-played. The emphasis of government strategy has been to change individual lifestyles through high-profile media campaigns and health screening. Benzeval et al (1995) proposed a range of broad policy initiatives based on key action areas identified in the Ottawa Charter (WHO 1986):

■ *Strengthening individuals*. This means ensuring that people have information and skills so that they are supported and enabled to make informed choices. It means taking account of different material circumstances and constraints on choice, e.g. parenting programmes, assertiveness skills for problem drinkers.
■ *Strengthening communities*. This means supporting people in their communities to make decisions about health issues affecting them, e.g. training and education programmes, cookery clubs and community cafes.
■ *Improving access to facilities and services*. This involves mediating between people and service providers in order to ensure that needs are met, e.g. providing outreach services in local or community settings, supporting advocacy and linkworker agencies which advocate on behalf of client groups, such as people with learning difficulties or those for whom English is not their mother tongue, who find accessing services difficult.
■ *Encouraging a healthy public policy*. A healthy public policy underpins other areas. Wider social and economic change reduces poverty and ensures that the environment and living conditions are conducive to health, e.g. tobacco taxation, integrated transport systems.

 Our Healthier Nation

To achieve its aims (of improving the health of the population as a whole and improving the health of the worst off in society and narrowing the health gap) the Government is setting out its third way between the old extremes of individual victim blaming on the one hand and nanny state social engineering on the other . . .

Connected problems require joined-up solutions. This means tackling inequality which stems from poverty, poor housing, pollution, low educational standards, joblessness and low pay. Tackling inequalities generally is the best means of tackling health inequalities in particular.

(DoH 1998, pp. 5, 12)

Although many health promoters may feel powerless to effect change at a macro level, it is possible to address health inequalities in planning health promotion interventions as the above examples illustrate. One of the central tasks for health promoters is to acknowledge socio-economic factors as crucial in determining individual and population health (Naidoo & Wills 1998).

Conclusion

Health promotion is not a purely technical activity. As we have seen, even identifying the causes of ill health will lead to political judgements being made.

Consider the following points of view about the causes of health and illness. Which comes closest to your own?

■ Ill health is the result of people's unhealthy lifestyles. No one makes people live this way and so it is up to individuals to take responsibility for their own health. The role of the health promoter is to provide information to encourage people to be concerned about their health and make healthier decisions.

■ Ill health is the result of the social and economic conditions in which people live. It is not people's fault if they become ill. People may have unhealthy lifestyles but this is because it is difficult to make healthy choices on a low income. The role of the health promoter is to try to empower people to take charge of their lives by raising awareness of the factors that influence their health. Health promoters need to draw the attention of policy makers to the influence of social and economic conditions on their clients' health.

In any area of work or discipline, there will always be debate about what constitutes good practice. It is important to clarify your thinking and where you stand because it will affect your views on the purpose of health promotion and what would be appropriate health promotion activities. It is also important that you share these thoughts with colleagues and clients to reach a common understanding of the ideals upon which health promotion activities are based.

In practice, behavioural and structural explanations are often aligned to the right or left of the political spectrum, and have become linked with very different policies and approaches to health promotion. The behavioural approach which focuses on individual lifestyles has informed much of health education because it suggests that information, advice or mass media messages can change behaviours such as smoking or sexual activity. A structural approach which sees health as determined by social and economic conditions, and reflecting the unequal distribution of power and resources in society, requires the health promoter to become involved in political activity.

Questions for further discussion

■ Is it fair or effective to encourage individuals to change their health behaviour?
■ Good health depends on adequate income. Do you agree?
■ What long-term social policy initiatives would most bring about an improvement in the health of your clients?
■ What are the implications for professional practice of the links between health and wealth?

Summary

This chapter has reviewed the evidence concerning health differences in the population and the physical, social and environmental variables that are implicated in ill health: poverty, unemployment, inadequate housing, stressful and dangerous working conditions, lack of social support, air and water pollution. It goes on to consider the ways in which risk factors associated with personal behaviour – smoking, nutrition, exercise – are influenced by the social environment.

Several explanations for inequalities in health have been discussed. None offers a complete explanation, but the chapter concludes that there is sufficient evidence to point to social and economic factors determining health. It argues that disadvantage can give rise to or exacerbate health-damaging behaviours such as smoking or poor nutrition, and so health behaviours should not be separated from their social context.

Further reading

Acheson D 1998 Independent inquiry into inequalities in health: a report. Stationery Office, London. *Brings together recent research on continued inequalities in health and identifies a number of key areas for action to tackle inequalities in health.*

Benzeval M, Judge K, Whitehead M (eds) 1995 Tackling inequalities in health: an agenda for action. King's Fund, London. *A comprehensive summary of data on health inequalities, which considers ways in which policy initiatives can address housing, family poverty and service provision.*

Drever F, Whitehead M (eds) 1997 Health inequalities. Stationery Office, London. *A summary of trends and patterns in ill health and death among adults and children and for ethnic minority groups. Includes historical and international findings.*

Townsend P, Davidson N, Whitehead M 1992 Inequalities in health, 2nd edn. Penguin, Harmondsworth. *The Black Report and The Health Divide published in one volume. The most significant reports on health status and still essential reading.*

References

Acheson D 1998 Independent inquiry into inequalities in health: a report. Stationery Office, London

Ahmad W I U (ed) 1993 'Race' and health in contemporary Britain. Open University, Buckingham

Arber S 1990 Opening the black box: inequalities in women's health. In Abbott P, Gilbert N (eds) New directions in the sociology of health. Falmer, Basingstoke

Arblaster L, Hawtin M 1993 Health, housing and social policy. Socialist Health Association, London

Bartley M 1994 Unemployment and ill health: understanding the relationship. Journal of Epidemiology and Community Health 48: 333–337

Benzeval M, Judge K, Whitehead M (eds) 1995 Tackling inequalities in health: an agenda for action. King's Fund, London

Bethune A 1997 Unemployment and mortality. In: Drever F, Whitehead M (eds) Health inequalities. Decennial supplement. Stationery Office, London

Blackburn C 1991 Poverty and health: working with families. Open University, Buckingham

Blane D, Brunner E, Wilkinson R (eds) 1996 Health and social organisation: towards a health policy for the 21st century. Routledge, London

Blaxter M 1990 Health and lifestyles. Tavistock/Routledge, London

Bloom J R 1990 The relationship of social support and health. Social Science and Medicine 30(5): 635–637

Bridgewood A, Savage D 1993 General household survey 1991. HMSO, London

Connelly J, Crown J (eds) 1994 Homelessness and health. Royal College of Physicians, London

Dahlgren, Whitehead M 1991 Policies and strategies to promote social equity in health. Institute for Future Studies, Stockholm

Department of Health (DoH) 1992 On the state of the public health 1991. HMSO, London

Department of Health (DoH) 1996 Variations in health. What can the Department of Health and the NHS do? HMSO, London

Department of Health (DoH) 1998 Our healthier nation: a contract for health. Stationery Office, London

Dorling D 1997 Death in Britain. Rowntree Foundation, York

Doyal L 1995 What makes women sick? Gender and the political economy of health. Macmillan, Basingstoke

Drever F, Whitehead M (eds) 1997 Health inequalities Decennial supplement. Office for National Statistics, London © Crown Copyright 1999

Goldblatt P 1990 Longitudinal study: mortality and social organisation 1971–81 England and Wales. OPCS Series LS No. 6. HMSO, London

Graham H 1992 Smoking among working class mothers with children. Department of Applied Social Studies, University of Warwick

Illsley R 1986 Occupational class, selection, and the production of inequalities. Quarterly Journal of Social Affairs 2(2): 151–165

Kawachi et al 1996 A prospective study of social networks in relation to total mortality and CVD in men in the USA. Journal of epidemiology and Community Health 50: 245–251

Lalonde M 1975 A new perspective on the health of Canadians. Ministry of Supply and Services, Ottawa, Canada

McKeown T, Lowe CR 1974 An introduction to social medicine. Blackwell Science, Oxford

Marmot M G 1980 Type A personality and ischaemic heart disease. Psychological Medicine 10: 603–606

Marmot M, Feeney A 1996 Work and health: implications for individuals and society. In: Blane D, Brunner E, Wilkinson R (eds) Health and social organisation: towards a health policy for the 21st century. Routledge, London

Marsh A, McKay S 1994 Poor smokers. Policy Studies Institute, London

Martin C J, Platt S D, Hunt S M 1987 Housing and ill health. British Medical Journal 294: 1125–1127

Miles A 1991 Women, health and medicine. Open University, Milton Keynes

Moser K, Goldblatt P, Fox J, Jones D 1990 Unemployment and mortality. In: Goldblatt P (ed) Longitudinal study: mortality and social organisation. OPCS Series LS No. 6. HMSO, London

Naidoo J, Wills J 1998 Practising health promotion: dilemmas and challenges. Baillière Tindall, London

Nazroo J 1998 The health of Britain's ethnic minorities. Policy Studies Institute, London

Office of Population Censuses and Surveys (OPCS) 1993 Mortality statistics: cause 1991. HMSO, London

Office of Population Censuses and Surveys (OPCS) 1995 Mortality statistics: perinatal and infant. Office for National Statistics, London © Crown Copyright 1999

Phillimore P, Beattie A, Townsend P 1994 Widening inequality of health in northern England. British Medical Journal 308: 1125–1128

Rowntree Foundation 1995 Inquiry into income and wealth. Rowntree Foundation, York

Rudat K 1994 Black and minority ethnic groups in England: health and lifestyles. HEA, London

Smaje C 1995 Health, 'race' and making sense of the evidence. King's Fund, London

Smith R 1987 Unemployment and health. Oxford University Press, Oxford

Standing Conference on Public Health 1994 Housing, homelessness and health. Nuffield Provincial Hospitals Trust, London

Thomas M, Goddard E, Hickman M, Hunter P 1994 General household survey 1992. HMSO, London

Townsend P, Davidson N 1982 Inequalities in health: the Black Report. Penguin, Harmondsworth

Townsend P, Phillimore P, Beattie A 1988 Health and deprivation: inequalities and the North. Croom Helm, London

Tudor Hart J 1971 The inverse care law. Lancet 1: 405

Whitehead M 1988 The health divide. HEC, London

Wilkinson R 1986 Class and health: research and longitudinal data. Tavistock, London

Wilkinson R 1996 Unhealthy societies: the afflictions of inequality. Routledge, London

World Health Organization 1982 Prevention of coronary heart disease, report of a WHO expert committee. Technical Report Series. WHO Geneva

World Health Organization 1986 Ottawa charter for health promotion. Journal of Health Promotion 1: 1–4

3 *Measuring health*

OVERVIEW

We have seen in Chapter 1 how people define health in different ways and in Chapter 2 how there are different determinants of health. This would suggest that measuring health is not a simple task. This appears to be borne out by the existence of a number of ways of measuring health and a lack of clear agreement about which are the best ways to measure health. This chapter looks first at why we might want to measure health. It goes on to investigate the different means of measuring health currently in use and unpacks some of the assumptions underlying their use. Finally, the uses of the different kinds of measures are explored. The practical uses of measuring health are discussed further in Chapters 17 and 18 on needs assessment and programme planning, and in Chapter 19 on evaluation.

Why measure health?

Finding a means to measure health is an important practical task for health promoters. There are several reasons why this is so.

1. *To establish priorities.* The collection and evaluation of information about the health status and health problems of a community is an important way of identifying needs.
2. *To assist planning.* Health promoters need information to assist the planning and evaluation of health promotion programmes. It is important to establish baseline data in order to plan priorities and to have a standard against which health promotion interventions can be evaluated.
3. *To justify resources.* Health promotion is often in competition with other activities for scarce resources. To make a claim for resources and to prove that their activities are effective, health promoters need information on the health status of populations.
4. *To assist the development of the profession.* Measurements of health gain are important to the professional development of

health promoters. Unless there is a means of measuring the effect of our actions, health promotion work will remain invisible, underfunded and low priority. By demonstrating the efficacy of health promotion interventions, it is possible to argue for resources, credibility and funding.

Ways of measuring health

Depending on the purpose, different measures of health may be used or developed. The means of measuring health depend primarily on the view of health which is held. If health is basically about physical functioning, then measures of physical fitness will be an adequate measure of health. If health is defined as having no disease, then measures of the extent of disease may be used (in reverse) as measures of health. However, if health is defined as including social and mental aspects and as meaning something other than being not ill, specific measurements of health will need to be developed.

 If you wanted to describe the health of the people where you live or work, what information would you need?

It is likely that you included:

■ Information about the health status of the community (e.g. the number of deaths and the main causes of death; the number of episodes of illness and the main types of illness)
■ Information on the determinants of health (e.g. people's lifestyles; the quality of housing; levels of employment; the adequacy and accessibility of health services)
■ Information about the community itself (e.g. the age, gender, ethnic and socio-economic breakdown of the population).

Community health workers who profile their communities have many different ways of building a picture of their area. Some of these are described in Chapter 17 on needs assessment. In this chapter we look at sources of information available to describe a community's health.

We shall look next at the contribution of epidemiology through the measurement of health as a negative variable, and move on to consider the measurement of health as a positive variable. Measuring health as a negative variable means measuring the opposite to health (e.g. disease or death) and using these results to infer the degree of health. Health is therefore being defined as a negative (health is not being ill or dead), not as a positive (health in its own right).

Epidemiology and health promotion – measuring health as a negative variable (e.g. health is not being diseased or ill)

Epidemiology is the study of the occurrence and spread of diseases in the population. It is concerned with the health status (or more usually the ill-health status) of populations. Health promoters use epidemiological evidence to identify health problems, at-risk groups and the effectiveness of preventive measures. The most common means of assessing a population's health are through mortality and morbidity rates. This reflects the reductionist model of health which sees health as a simple matter of illness or its absence. Thus data on deaths and illnesses are often used as surrogate measures of health. There are obviously shortcomings to this approach. Measuring conditions which limit health, such as illness, is not the same as measuring health itself. Measuring mortality rates does not reflect the extent of illness in the population nor does it say anything about the quality of health experienced by people when they were alive. Conditions such as arthritis or schizophrenia cause considerable suffering and pain but do not lead to premature death and so are not reflected in mortality rates.

If you wished to develop a health promotion intervention to improve food hygiene, why would mortality rates be a poor indicator of its priority?

■ How else could you find out about the extent of poor food hygiene in your area?
■ Why might mortality statistics be a good indicator in a developing country of the necessity of health promotion around food hygiene?

On the plus side, statistics concerning mortality are readily obtainable in developed countries. A death certificate is sent to the Director of Public Health in every health authority and the total number of deaths, the geographic and population variations and the causes of death are all collated in each district's annual public health report. The statistics can also be used in international comparisons because most countries hold some form of database on deaths and disease rates.

Although these statistics are often presented as if they were objective facts, it is important to remember that statistics are devised by people in a social context, subject to assumptions, bias and error. At every stage of the data-collecting process, decisions are taken which help shape the ultimate form of information presented.

It is often suggested that suicide is under-reported as a cause of death. Can you think of any reasons why this might be the case?

Suicide and mental illness tend to be stigmatized, that is, they have negative meanings which become attached to the person affected, their relatives and friends. Suicide may be contrary to cultural or religious beliefs, and a diagnosis of suicide as a cause of death may also have repercussions in terms of insurance. For all these reasons, suicide is likely to be under-reported.

The International Classification of Diseases, injuries and causes of death (ICD) classifies death according to diagnosed diseases which cause death, e.g. cancer of the lung. Death certificates which use the ICD thus give no information about contributory risk factors such as smoking or diet.

■ What impact do you think this has on our perception of risk factors and causes of disease, and on suitable strategies for prevention and treatment?
■ Is it likely to foster understanding of social, environmental or biological causes of disease?

Mortality statistics

There are several different ways of expressing death rates. The crude death rate is the number of deaths per 1000 people per year. However, this figure is obviously affected by the age structure of the population which may vary over time and region. An area with a high proportion of elderly, such as a south coast retirement town, would have consistently higher death rates than a more deprived area with a higher percentage of premature deaths, such as an inner city area. The standardized mortality ratio (SMR) measures the death rate taking into account differences in age structure. It is the number of deaths experienced within a population group (which may be defined by geographic or socio-economic factors) compared to what would be expected for this group if national averages applied, taking age differences into account. The overall average for England and Wales is 100, so SMRs of below 100 indicate a lower than average mortality rate, whilst SMRs of more than 100 indicate higher than average mortality rates.

The infant mortality rate (IMR) is another commonly used statistic. The IMR is the number of deaths in the first year of life per 1000 live births. The IMR is strongly associated with adult mortality rates. It reflects maternal health, particularly nutrition, and the provision of social care and child welfare. The IMR is therefore capable of being used as an indicator of the general health of the population, particularly when comparisons between countries are being drawn. The perinatal mortality rate (PMR) is the number of stillbirths and deaths in the first 7 days after birth per 1000 births. The neonatal death rate is the number of deaths occurring in the first 28 days after birth per 1000 live births. Both the SMR and the IMR are readily available statistics, and therefore easy to use as surrogate measures of health. Table 3.1 compares key health indicators for different countries in Europe.

Table 3.1 *Key health indicators for countries in Europe (1990)*

Country	Life expectancy	Infant mortality rate	Crude death rate	Birth rate
Belgium	M72.0 W78.9	8.4	10.6	12.0
Denmark	M72.6 W78.2	7.5	11.9	12.4
France	M73.4 W81.8	7.2	9.2	13.3
Germany	M72.0 W78.1	7.5	11.5	11.2
Greece	M74.6 W79.8	9.7	9.2	10.1
Ireland	M72.0 W77.7	8.2	8.9	14.9
Italy	M73.6 W80.4	8.6	10.1	10.0
Luxembourg	M71.8 W79.2	7.3	9.9	13.0
Netherlands	M73.9 W80.3	6.5	8.6	13.2
Portugal	M69.8 W77.3	9.8	9.7	11.0
Spain	M73.4 W80.5	7.7	8.5	10.2
United Kingdom	M73.3 W78.8	7.4	11.3	13.8

Source: World Health Statistics Annual (1990)

- **Which country has the lowest life expectancy for men and women?**
- **Which country has the highest IMR?**
- **Which country has the highest crude death rate?**
- **What reasons can you give to explain these findings?**

Death rates are also available broken down by gender, social class and cause. In Britain, it is well established that death rates are related to social class and gender (Townsend et al 1988). People in the lower social classes have higher than average death rates at all ages and for virtually all causes. Women on average live longer than men, so their premature death rate is lower than that of men. This is discussed in greater detail in Chapter 2.

Reductions in mortality for selected causes among targeted groups in the population constituted the majority of the targets in 'The Health of the Nation' (DoH 1992) strategy and in the new proposed 'Our Healthier Nation' (DoH 1999) strategy for England.

 'Our Healthier Nation' targets

By 2010, reductions in mortality in the following areas:

1. Heart disease and stroke
   Reduce the death rate in people under 65 years by at least two fifths.
2. Accidents
   Reduce the death rate by at least a fifth and serious injury by at least a tenth.
3. Cancers
   Reduce the death rate amongst people under 75 years by at least a fifth.
4. Mental illness
   Reduce the death rate from suicide and undetermined injury by at least a fifth.

Baseline: 1996; Source: DoH (1999)

 No targets have been set to reduce mortality rates from sexual ill health. What explanations might there be for this?

Possible reasons include: low numbers of deaths, long time lag between preventive action and outcome of reduced mortality, and concern with morbidity rather than mortality.

■ Are any of these factors relevant?
■ Are there any other relevant factors?

Morbidity statistics

Statistics measuring illness and disease are more difficult to obtain. This is due in part to the difficulty in establishing a hard and fast line between health and disease. There is no one source of data for the whole population concerning disease and illness. Instead, there are a number of different sources of relevant information. These are summarized below.

Sources of health information

These sources of data may be accessed from public health departments, health authority purchasing plans, annual public health reports, local authority community care plans, local authority planning departments and environmental health departments and the Office for National Statistics.

Mortality
■ Death by cause, age, sex and area of residence
■ Infant deaths (in children under 1 year)
■ Perinatal deaths (after 28th week of pregnancy and in the first 7 days after birth)
■ Neonatal deaths (within first 28 days of birth)

Morbidity
■ General Household Survey (annual survey of health behaviour and experience of illness)
■ Health service records on consultation and treatment episodes
■ Registers for specific conditions such as cancers, disability, blindness and partial sight, people at risk of harm, drug addiction
■ Notification systems for infectious (communicable) diseases, congenital malformations, abortion
■ National General Practice Morbidity Survey
■ Sickness absence from work records

Information on health status and behaviour
■ GP records on height, weight, body mass index, smoking and drinking behaviour of individuals and profiles of practice populations
■ Dental health records
■ Child health surveillance records
■ National surveys for the Office for National Statistics, e.g. the annual National Food Survey, Children and Smoking survey and occasional surveys, e.g. Allied Dunbar National Fitness Survey

Demographic data
■ Census information on the whole population is collected every 10 years (information includes numbers in household by age, sex, marital status, place of birth, occupation, ethnicity (since 1991) educational level, house type and tenure, accommodation and facilities)
■ Register of births including birth weight and mother's occupation
■ Claimants of unemployment benefit, free school meals, housing benefit, income support

Environmental indicators
■ Services available
■ Levels of pollution: air, water and noise
■ Crime statistics
■ Type of housing
■ Leisure facilities
■ Road traffic accidents

The health services collect routine data on the use of their services and activity rate. These data can be used to express the disease experience of different populations but there are several problems with adopting this approach. The main problem with using many of the health authority measurements is that they were developed primarily for administrative, planning or management tasks, and reflect available services and use of these services, rather than health itself. Health authority data are primarily collected as a management tool. To some extent, this determines what data are collected. Routinely available morbidity data represent only the tip of the illness iceberg. Many people who are ill do not seek help from primary care services or hospitals. However, the advantage of using data of this kind is that they are routinely collected, are consistent across regions and are easily accessed.

 Hospital activity analysis (HAA) data record episodes of treatment, not patients treated.

■ What will these data tell you about the health status of the local population?
■ What do they not tell you?
■ Why do you think they are collected in this way?

The General Household Survey (GHS) is a continuous government survey of a sample of the population. The GHS includes questions on people's experience of illness, both long term (chronic) and within the last fortnight (acute). GHS data are difficult to use comparatively over time as the wording of the questions changes occasionally. The following are examples of questions used in the GHS (Foster et al 1995).

■ Over the last 12 months would you say your health has on the whole been good, fairly good or not good?
■ Do you have any long-standing illness, disability or infirmity? By long-standing I mean anything that has troubled you over a period of time or that is likely to affect you over a period of time.
■ Now I'd like you to think about the 2 weeks ending yesterday. During those 2 weeks, did you have to cut down on any of the things you usually do (about the house/at work or in your free time) because of (any chronic condition cited earlier in the interview) illness or injury?

The GHS is useful in providing information on people's subjective experience of illness, because it relies on people's self-reported illness rather than use of services. It also collects information on people's health-related behaviour such as smoking, drinking and exercise.

A number of proxy measures of health are used such as the number of days at work lost due to sickness. However, such data are available only for people in paid employment. The large section of the population who are not in paid employment, and their experience of illness, is therefore invisible. It is known that unemployment is associated with a marked increase in mortality and psychological and physical ill health (Bethune 1997, Moser et al 1990, White 1991).

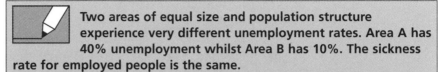 **Two areas of equal size and population structure experience very different unemployment rates. Area A has 40% unemployment whilst Area B has 10%. The sickness rate for employed people is the same.**

■ Numerically, which area will have the greatest ill health if days lost at work due to sickness is the measure used?
■ Will this reflect the likely extent of ill health in the two areas?

Area B will have the highest sickness rate, but it is likely that the actual extent of ill health will be greater in Area A.

Various government research studies have developed measures to assess disability and to produce estimates of the number of people with disabilities in the population. These disability indices are based on the results of questionnaires asking people what, if any, difficulty they experience in daily life. The onus is therefore placed on the individual being unable to perform certain tasks such as taking a bath or walking unaided up flights of stairs. The reason for these difficulties could be located in housing design and might be capable of being remedied by modifying the home environment. However, by treating disability as an inherent individual attribute, the effect of the social environment in generating and maintaining disability is rendered invisible. Abberley (1992) criticizes disability indices for reinforcing the social production of disability, by treating social factors which produce disability as given and unalterable. In this way, he argues, they fail to address the real concerns of people with disabilities.

 A typical question from disability surveys is: 'Does your health problem/disability affect your work in any way at present?

■ How many different reasons can you think of for someone answering 'yes' to this question?
■ How many of these reasons refer to physical diseases?
■ How many of these reasons refer to mental illnesses?
■ How many of these reasons refer to social factors?

The uses of epidemiology

Epidemiological studies examine the distribution and patterns of health and disease in populations. Epidemiological data help to build up a picture by:

1. showing the scale of the problem
2. showing the natural history and aetiology of the condition
3. showing causation and association
4. identifying risk
5. showing effectiveness.

Scale of the problem:

- *Incidence*. The number of people developing a disease over a specified period, e.g. in 1999 there were 22 000 newly diagnosed cases of breast cancer.
- *Prevalence*. The number of people with a condition or characteristic at a specified time, e.g. in 1999, 27% of the population were regular smokers.
- How the condition is distributed by gender, age, socio-economic class, ethnicity, etc., e.g. obesity is most common in women aged 55–64.

Natural history and aetiology of the condition:

- Indicates if primary prevention is possible.
- Shows severity of the problem and ways in which individuals, families or communities may be affected.

Causation and association:

- Is there evidence that exposure to a particular environmental, lifestyle or socio-economic factor contributes to ill health.

 Asthma and air pollution

The prevalence of asthma in young children in Greenwich, London, in 1996 was well above the national average. Hospital admissions were particularly clustered from the area around Trafalgar Road, a major trunk road through London to the South. This suggests an association between air pollution from traffic and asthma. However, it is not possible to suggest traffic pollution is the *cause* of asthma as the existence of pollution is neither necessary for children to get asthma (asthma can be associated with other factors such as stress or pet allergies) nor sufficient to cause asthma (many children are exposed to high levels of pollution but do not get asthma). Causation is hard to prove as it must be established that exposure to a risk factor is both necessary and sufficient to cause disease.

Identifying risk:

- Assessing the chance or probability of a disease or condition occurring.
- Assessing how much illness is due to a particular factor (*the attributable risk*).

Effectiveness:

- Showing trends in mortality and morbidity over time.
- Evaluation studies can show whether any changes can be attributed to particular interventions.

Epidemiological studies of mortality, illness, disease and disability are often used to talk about health. Such usage reinforces, albeit in an indirect way, the definition of health as 'not disease'. But the advantage of such statistics is that they are already collected, are relatively consistent and are readily available. Recognizing the limitations of such measures has prompted health promoters to develop new means of measuring health as an independent phenomenon distinct from illness or disease. These measures may be conveniently divided into those describing health as an objective quality which is an attribute of people or environments, and those describing health as a subjective reality which is socially produced.

Measures of health as an objective attribute

There are a number of ways of measuring health as an objective factor including:

- health measures
- health behaviour indicators
- environmental indicators
- socio-economic indicators.

Health measures

There are measures of the health status of people, including vital statistics such as height and weight, and dental health status (the decayed, missing and filled teeth, or DMF, index). Floud (1989) argues that the average height of a population may be taken as a measure of health, as it represents a proxy for nutritional status and therefore welfare. In the same way, Townsend et al (1987) use the percentage of low birth weight babies as an indicator of health.

Health behaviour indicators

Increasingly common are measurements of people's behaviour which are then used as a measure of health. For example, the number of people smoking, drinking alcohol, using drugs, taking regular exercise, eating a healthy diet, practising safer sex or planned fertility, may all be used to describe different populations, and to make comparisons between them regarding relative health status. This information may be routinely collected, such as smoking prevalence in young people, or it may be obtained from commissioned surveys (e.g. Rudat 1994). These lifestyle measures are sometimes narrowed down to more specific behaviour in relation to the health services. For example, the percentage of children immunized against childhood illnesses, or the percentage of women screened for cervical and breast cancer, may be used to describe the health status of a population.

Environmental indicators

The same method may be applied to physical and social environments. Measurements of the physical environment include air and water quality, and housing type and density. These measures are routinely collected by the environmental health departments of local authorities.

Socio-economic indicators

The social environment may also be measured in terms of its 'healthiness'. One of the measures most commonly used to assess the social environment is wealth. Figure 3.1 compares Human Development Index scores (which include three components – life expectancy, educational attainment and income) and the gross national product (GNP; a measure of a country's wealth) of different countries. If GNP rank and human development rank are the same, the country will be on the diagonal line. Below the line, countries are doing worse in human development terms than their GNP rank would suggest. Above the line, countries are doing better in human development terms than their GNP rank would suggest.

The evidence suggests that countries with a more equitable distribution of wealth enjoy better health and that countries with a very unequal distribution of wealth suffer poorer health (Wilkinson 1996).

Objective measurements of people's health status, health-related behaviour and the environment may be combined to provide an overall picture of health. The health of different populations, from neighbourhoods to nations, may be assessed and compared using this method. Targets for improvements in health may also be set using these measurements.

Improvements in the social and physical environment, such as an increase in the number of smoke-free places, an increase in the number, accessibility and safety of play areas and sports centres, or improvements in housing amenities and density, may also be added

Figure 3.1
Scattergram showing relationship between GNP rank and Human Development Index rank, 1992. Rank ordering: best = 1; worst = 160. (Data derived from United Nations Development Programme 1992 Human development report 1992. Oxford University Press, Oxford and New York, Table 1.) From Gray & Payne (1993).

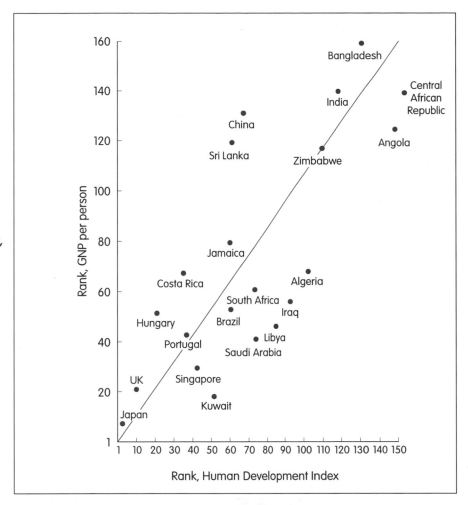

■ **What might account for those countries whose human development rank is better than their GNP rank?**
■ **What might account for those countries whose human development is worse than their GNP rank?**

into the equation (Catford 1983, WHO 1985). People's health-related beliefs and attitudes, and the extent to which they conform to professional beliefs, have also been considered to be a measure of health (Catford 1983). For example, the percentage of the population seeking to make recommended lifestyle changes, or having an understanding of basic health issues, has been suggested as a positive health measure. Combining a number of discrete elements to measure health is attractive because it gives a more rounded picture of health, and provides a clear basis and direction for health promoters.

Measuring deprivation

Much of the evidence which finds that people who are most disadvantaged experience more illness and premature death has derived from the link between occupational class and health status. Occupational class is still the main measure of socio-economic status. Its limitations were discussed in Chapter 2. The classification of classes is derived from census information on type of employment. Two new categories will be included in the 2001 census (unemployed and self-employed), and the Office for National Statistics is working to harmonize social class categories with market research social grades.

Researchers working in Britain have developed measures of health which aggregate socio-environmental data. The Jarman index is a formula which is said to express the health needs of communities served by health authorities. The impetus for the development of these indicators was administrative; to attempt to find a fairer means of remuneration for general practitioners (GPs) serving deprived communities. The Jarman index (Jarman 1983) combines census data with factors identified by GPs as increasing workload and pressure of work. Some factors, such as the percentage of people over 65 years in the population, were excluded because this is already included in determining levels of remuneration for GPs.

 The Jarman factors are:

- Percentage of pensioners living alone
- Percentage of children under 5 years old
- Percentage of lone-parent families
- Percentage of unskilled workers
- Percentage of unemployed
- Percentage of people with recent changes of address
- Percentage of people of minority ethnic origin
- Percentage of housing which is overcrowded.

Consider each of these factors, and provide a reason why it has been included. Are there any other factors which might be added?

Indices of deprivation differ in the indicators they include and will therefore show different areas as deprived. The Townsend index, for example, uses proxy measures of deprivation including not owning a car and electricity disconnection (Townsend et al 1987).

Subjective health measures

The previous section has outlined means of measuring health as if it were an objective property of beings, societies, or environments, capable of scientific scrutiny. However, it is apparent that health is not such a simple or uncontested attribute. Chapter 1 highlighted the importance of subjective interpretations of health and the multiple meanings health may have in different contexts. This has led some researchers to attempt to devise measurements of health which incorporate subjective reporting of health. Measurements of subjective health may be broadly divided into four different types (Bowling 1992):

- measures of physical well-being (indicated by physical function) and health status
- measures of psychological well-being
- measures of social well-being
- measures of quality of life.

Jeff is 78 years old. His wife died last year after several years of Alzheimer's disease during which he cared for her. He has one son who visits rarely. Jeff has been in good physical health and used to walk to the local shops every day. He lives in the same terraced house in which he was born. The area is now full of young working couples. Jeff has been to see his GP for the first time in 8 years because he is suffering from acute headaches.

What indicators could be used to assess Jeff's:
- physical well-being?
- psychological well-being?
- social well-being?
- quality of life?

Physical well-being, functional ability and health status

Measures of functional ability use people's self-reports of physical activity, such as the ability to perform everyday activities, e.g. personal care, degree of mobility, domestic activities (Hunt 1988, Stewart et al 1981). A health assessment questionnaire is regularly used for people with arthritis (Chambers et al 1982). Such scales are widely used to assess eligibility for benefits among elderly or disabled people. They clearly fit a functionalist model of health but ignore quality of life issues.

The Nottingham Health Profile (Hunt et al 1986) is an example of a broader measure of health status. This health profile arose from research examining the most important aspects of health cited by the general public. It has been used extensively, and is claimed to be both reliable and valid. The profile consists of six separate dimensions which are scored independently. These are:

- physical mobility
- pain
- sleep
- social isolation
- emotional reactions
- energy level.

All of these items are scored by respondents on a standard questionnaire. The profile is therefore a subjective assessment of people's health status, and one which places equal emphasis on mental and physical health. However, the scale only measures negative aspects of health, and only measures traits which an original sample deemed important to their quality of life. It does not tap into each individual's unique view of his or her health. Hunt et al (1986) claim that the profile is more useful as a predictor of subsequent health outcomes than more objective measurements of health status. The Nottingham Health Profile is a means of rigorously assessing health and it is increasingly being used in conjunction with other socio-environmental measures to create health profiles of areas (e.g. University of Bristol Medical School 1989).

Other measures of subjective health include the Sickness Impact Profile (Bergner et al 1981) and the General Health Questionnaire (Goldberg & Hillier 1979).

Psychological well-being

Psychological well-being scales have measured the presence or absence of symptoms such as anxiety or depression (Dupuy 1984). The Edinburgh Postnatal Depression questionnaire is, for example, widely used. Measuring positive health has proved problematic (Kemm 1993). McDowell & Newell (1987) refer to life satisfaction and happiness as possible measures. Other measures include self-esteem, a sense of coherence and perceived control over one's life. Together, these attributes have been said to constitute a psychological immune system which protects against psychological morbidity (Antonovsky 1987).

Social health

Health includes the dimension of social health, which has been defined as the degree to which people function adequately as members of the community (Greenblatt 1975, Renne 1974). A key characteristic of social health is social support, incorporating both the extent of a person's social networks and their perceived adequacy (Antonovsky 1987). More recently, the concept of 'social capital' has been used to describe these networks and the trust

What examples can you think of where social support may have an effect on health?

which links people together in a community (Wilkinson 1996). In a 20-year study in Italy, social capital has been associated with some measures of health status such as infant mortality and life expectancy (Putnam et al 1993).

Quality of life

Quality of life has been used by some researchers to encompass the broader notion of health and is also increasingly being used by researchers evaluating the effect of health care services. Quality of life includes an objective evaluation of life circumstances and a subjective evaluation of these circumstances. Fallowfield (1990) proposes four core domains in the quality of life:

- psychological (e.g. depression)
- social (e.g. engagement in social and leisure activities)
- occupational (e.g. ability to carry out paid and/or domestic work)
- physical (e.g. pain, sleep, mobility).

Andrews & Withey (1976) have devised a nonverbal quality of life scale, the delighted–terrible faces (Fig. 3.2).

QALYs

The desire to include a measurement of health in evaluating health care outcomes has led to the development of quality-adjusted life years (QALYs). QALYs are an explicit attempt to include not just years of life saved but also the quality of life, when making resource allocation decisions regarding different medical procedures. The quality of life includes things such as freedom from pain and discomfort, and the ability to live independently. The assessment of quality of life is made by both health professionals and lay people. The QALY is the arithmetic product of life expectancy and an adjustment for the quality of the remaining life years gained (Baldwin et al 1990). These two components are quite separate.

Figure 3.2
Delighted–terrible faces: a nonverbal scale to assess self-ratings of quality of life and life satisfaction. Here are some faces expressing various feelings . . . Which face comes closest to expressing how you feel about your health? From Andrews & Withey (1976).

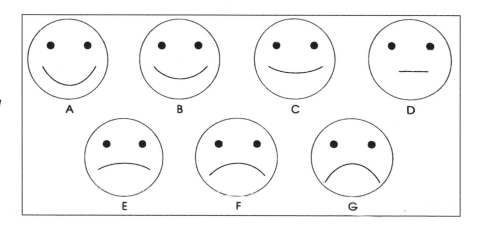

QALYs are an important tool in making decisions about how to ration health care resources.

There is much theoretical and methodological confusion in attempts to measure different aspects of positive health and a lack of consensus in how this may best be achieved. It is an area which is currently being refined and researched, and is undoubtedly important to any adequate conceptualization and measurement of health.

Conclusion

Measuring health is an important activity for health promoters, and is · integral to the planning and evaluation of health promotion programmes. Yet there is no consensus on the best means to measure health, and a wide variety of methods have been used. Some are opportunistic, relying on data already collected and available such as the Jarman index and QALYs. The drawback of using these methods is that they use data which have been collected for specific reasons, often managerial or administrative. Other methods such as the Nottingham Profile have arisen from research which has addressed the issue of how to measure health. The fact that the concept 'health' can have so many different meanings, as outlined in Chapter 1, also contributes to the variety of different methods used. Some methods focus on one dimension of health, whereas others try to span different dimensions. It is also the case that different measures may suit different purposes. It is unlikely that any one method will ever prove to be a comprehensive measure of health, even if it combines different measurements within a weighted index. What is important then is to be specific about *why* you wish to measure health, and to then go on to select the most appropriate means of doing so, bearing in mind constraints on the time and money you have at your disposal.

 You are putting together a proposal to justify a health promotion intervention around the following conditions. In each case, what sorts of information would you need? Where would you obtain this information?

■ Young people with mental health problems
■ Parenting for lone mothers
■ Older people and drinking

Questions for further discussion

What are the advantages and disadvantages of measuring health as:

■ a negative variable (health is not being ill)
■ a positive variable (health is positive well-being)?

Thinking of your own work, how can you must usefully measure health?

Summary

This chapter has examined the reasons for attempting to measure health, and demonstrated that the most commonly used measures of health are in fact measures of ill health, disease and premature death. Recently there has been more activity directed towards trying to find ways of measuring health as an independent positive variable in its own right. Different approaches have been taken, ranging from measuring health as an objective property of people or environments, to measuring health as it is subjectively experienced and interpreted by people. These different approaches have been identified and described.

Further reading

Bowling A 1992 Measuring health. Open University Press, Milton Keynes. *A useful summary of the different ways of measuring health.*

Katz J, Peberdy A 1997 Promoting health: knowledge and practice. Macmillan/Open University Press, Basingstoke, ch 13. *A good summary of the application of epidemiology to health promotion.*

Unwin N, Carr S, Leeson J, Pless-Mulloli T 1997 An introductory study guide to public health and epidemiology. Open University Press, Buckingham. *A basic introduction to epidemiology which explains core concepts in a simple and readable form.*

References

Abberley P 1992 A critique of the OPCS disability surveys. Radical Statistics 51: 7–21

Andrews F M, Withey S B 1976 Social indicators of well-being: Americans' perception of life quality. Plenum Press, New York

Antonovsky A 1987 Unravelling the mystery of health: how people manage stress and stay well. Jossey-Bass, San Francisco

Baldwin S, Godfrey C, Propper C 1990 Quality of life: perspectives and policies. Routledge, London

Bergner M, Bobbitt R A, Carter W B, Gibson B S 1981 The sickness impact profile: development and final revision of a health status measure. Medical Care 19: 787–805

Bethune A 1997 Unemployment and Mortality. In: Drever F, Whitehead M (eds) Health inequalities. Decennial supplement. Stationery office, London

Bowling A 1992 Measuring health: a review of quality of life measurement scales. Open University Press, Milton Keynes

Catford J 1983 Positive health indicators – towards a new information base for health promotion. Community Medicine 5: 125–132

Chambers L W et al 1982 The McMaster health index questionnaire as a measure of quality of life for patients with rheumatoid disease. Journal of Rheumatology 9: 780–784

Department of Health (DoH) 1992 The health of the nation. HMSO, London

Department of Health (DoH) 1999 Saving lives: Our healthier nation (white paper). Stationery office, London

Dupuy H J 1984 The psychological general well-being (PGWB) index. In: Wenger N K et al (eds) Assessment of quality of life in clinical trials of cardiovascular therapies. Le Jacq, New York, pp 170–183

Fallowfield L 1990 The quality of life: the missing measurement in health care. Souvenir Press, London

Floud 1989 Measuring European inequality: the use of height data. In: Fox J (ed) Health inequalities in European countries. Gower, Aldershot, pp 231–249

Foster K, Jackson B, Thomas M, Hunter P, Bennett N 1995 General household survey 1993. HMSO, London

Goldberg D P, Hillier J F 1979 A scaled version of the general health questionnaire. Psychological Medicine 9: 139–145

Gray A, Payne P, with U20S Course Team 1993 World health and disease. Open University, Buckingham

Greenblatt H N 1975 Measurement of social well-being in a general population survey. Human Population Laboratory California State Department of Health, Berkeley

Hunt S M 1988 Subjective health indicators and health promotion. Health Promotion 3: 3–34

Hunt S M, McKenna S P, McEwan J et al 1986 Measuring health status. Croom Helm, London

Jarman B 1983 Identification of underprivileged areas. British Medical Journal 286: 1705–1709

Kemm J R 1993 Towards an epidemiology of positive health. Health Promotion International: 8(2): 129–134

McDowell I, Newell C 1987 Measuring health: a guide to rating scales and questionnaires. Oxford University Press, New York

Moser K A, Goldblatt P, Fox J, Jones D 1990 Unemployment and mortality. In: Goldblatt P (ed) Longitudinal study: mortality and social organisation. OPCS Series LS No. 6. HMSO, London

Putnam R D, Leonardi R, Nanetti R Y 1993 Making democracy work: civic traditions in modern Italy. Princeton University Press, Princeton, NJ

Renne K S 1974 Measurement of social health in a general population survey. Social Sciences Research 3: 25–44

Rudat K 1994 Black and minority ethnic groups in England: health and lifestyles. HEA, London

Stewart A L et al 1981 Advances in the measurement of functional status: construction of aggregate indexes. Medical Care 19: 473–488

Townsend P, Phillimore P, Beattie A 1987 Health and deprivation: inequality and the North. Croom Helm, London

Townsend P, Davidson N, Whitehead M 1988 Inequalities in health: the Black Report and The Health Divide. Penguin, Harmondsworth

University of Bristol Medical School 1989 Avon County health survey 1989: county report. Department of Epidemiology and Public Health Medicine, University of Bristol, Bristol

White M 1991 Against unemployment. Policy Studies Institute, London

Wilkinson R G 1996 Unhealthy societies: the afflictions of inequality. Routledge, London

World Health Organization 1985 Targets for health for all. WHO Regional Office for Europe, Copenhagen

World Health Organization 1990 World Health Statistics Annual. WHO, Geneva

4 *Defining health promotion*

Key points

- The development of health promotion
- Definitions of health education and health promotion and the relationship between them
- The role of the World Health Organization in health promotion

OVERVIEW

The process of attempting to promote health may include a whole range of interventions including:

- those which foster healthy lifestyles
- those which encourage access to services and involvement in health decisions
- those which seek to promote an environment in which the healthy choice becomes the easier choice
- those which educate about the body and keeping healthy.

Until the 1980s most of these interventions were referred to as 'health education' and the practice was almost exclusively located within preventive medicine or, to a lesser extent, education. In recent years, the term 'health promotion' has become widely used. There is no agreed consensus on what health promotion is or what health promoters do when they try to promote health, nor what a successful outcome might be. Many professions including nursing have found health promotion to be part of an expanding job description. This development reflects the arguments presented in this book, that it is health and not illness or disease which should underpin health care work. Yet what practitioners do in the name of health promotion varies enormously. This chapter outlines the historical development of health promotion and considers different views on the purpose, the nature and the scope of health promotion practice.

The development of health promotion (Table 4.1)

The term health promotion is used in a number of different ways, often without any clarification of meaning. In 1985 when the term was becoming widely adopted, Tannahill described it as a meaningless concept because it was used so differently. Over a decade later, Seedhouse (1997) describes the field of health promotion as muddled, poorly articulated and devoid of a clear philosophy. These different understandings reflect the origins of health promotion and range from:

■ 'Slick salesmanship of health' (Williams 1984)
■ 'Attempts to persuade, cajole or otherwise influence individuals to alter their lifestyle' (Gott & O'Brien 1990)
■ 'Any combination of education and related legal, fiscal, economic, environmental and organisational interventions designed to facilitate the achievement of health and the prevention of disease' (Tones 1990)
■ 'An approach and philosophy of care which reflects awareness of the multiplicity of factors which affect health and which encourages everyone to value independence and individual choice' (Wilson Barnett 1993).

■ **What do you consider to be the main features of health education?**
■ **And what do you consider the main features of health promotion?**
■ **Is your work mostly health education or health promotion?**

The origins of health promotion lie in the 19th century when epidemic disease eventually led to pressure for sanitary reform for the overcrowded industrial towns. Alongside the public health movement emerged the idea of educating the public for the good of its health. The Medical Officers of Health appointed to each town under the Public Health legislation of 1848 frequently disseminated everyday health advice on safeguards against 'contagion'. Voluntary associations were also formed including the London Statistical Society (1839), the Health of Towns Association (1842) and the Sanitary Institute (1876). The temperance movement held Band of Hope mass meetings, and through schools and churches lectured to young people on the virtue of abstinence. By the 1920s health education had become associated with diarrhoea, dirt, spitting and venereal disease! The evidence that between 10% and 20% of soldiers in the First World War had contracted venereal disease led to propaganda, one-off lectures and the first of 'shock-horror' techniques in which soldiers were shown lurid pictures of diseased genitals to dissuade them from having sex (Blythe 1986, Welshman 1997).

Changing patterns of morbidity and mortality shifted attention away from disease to personal behaviour. The Central Council for Health Education was established in 1927, paid for by local authority public health departments, and public health doctors formed the

Health education slogans were produced in the 1920s by insurance companies keen to reduce health insurance claims:

■ 'Have a hot bath at least once a week'
■ 'Moderation in all things – every hour you steal from digestion will be reclaimed by indigestion'
■ 'Cultivate cheerfulness, hopefulness of mind and evenness of temper which are the most wonderful of remedial agencies'
■ 'Do not spit – it dries in the dust and other people breathe it in'.

majority of its membership. An extract from some of the tasks listed as important reflects an emphasis on information, and education to bring about change in personal habits and behaviour:

■ The provision of better and cheaper posters and leaflets
■ The provision of exhibits for exhibition
■ The production of a readable monthly bulletin
■ The provision of a panel of lecturers who really could lecture and hold an audience.

The Central Council was principally concerned with propaganda and instruction. During the Second World War it delivered 3799 lectures on sex education and venereal disease which were attended by 340 000 people (Amos 1993).

The Health Education Council (HEC) which was set up in 1968 as a quango – a quasi-autonomous nongovernmental organization – reflected the Department of Health and Social Security's, as it then was, medical model of health. The members were drawn from public health, and the medical and dental professions with the inclusion of advertising and consumer affairs representatives. Its brief was to create a 'climate of opinion generally favourable to health education, develop blanket programmes of education and selected priority subjects' (Cohen Committee 1964). Similar health education agencies were set up in Wales, Scotland and Northern Ireland.

The HEC came to be associated with mass publicity campaigns such as 'Look After Yourself' (LAY) which was launched in 1978. LAY reflected the view that people could be encouraged to adopt lifestyles which would lead to better health. The lead agency for health education in England consistently emphasized such mass campaigns and short-term initiatives. Sutherland, the first director of education and training at the Health Education Council, has vividly described the pressures and lobbying which led the HEC away from confrontation with vested interests, such as agriculture or tobacco, and kept it confined to mass-media campaigns despite evidence of their limited effect (Sutherland 1987).

Table 4.1 *The development of health promotion in the 20th century*		
	1900	Concern for infant and child health: health visitors, mother and baby clinics, school medical service (1908)
	1906–1914	Liberal Government reforms including national insurance and old age pensions
	1919	Ministry of Health. Numerous voluntary organizations producing leaflets and posters including National Association for the Prevention of Tuberculosis, Health and Cleanliness Council, British Red Cross
	1927	Central Council for Health Education of medical officers of health, local authority associations and health insurance committees
	1940–1945	Major campaigns, e.g. to promote diphtheria immunization. Rates rose from 8% to 62%. Emphasis on venereal disease education during the Second World War
	1946	Responsibility for health education transferred to Ministry of Health from local authorities
	1948	Establishment of National Health Service
	1957	First course of training for health education specialists at London University Institute of Education. First health education officers employed by local authorities
	1964	Cohen Committee to consider the future of health education recommended a strong central body
	1968	Health Education Council set up, funded and appointed by the newly established Department of Health and Social Security (DHSS)
	1970s	High-profile mass-media campaigns on smoking, immunization, family planning. Employment of Saatchi and Saatchi advertising agency. Support for curriculum development work in schools. Support for training and research
	1974	NHS reorganization: regional, area and district health authorities, consensus management by multidisciplinary district management team. Creation of community health councils
	1976	'Prevention and Health: Everybody's Business' published by DHSS followed by numerous reports on prevention
	1977	World Health Organization Declaration at Alma Ata committing members to the principles of 'Health for All 2000'
	1980	Publication of the Black Report on inequalities in health
	1982	Reorganization of the NHS to offer more local community structure: district health authorities

Table 4.1 *Cont'd*	1984	Griffiths Report recommended general managers for the NHS, reducing health professionals' role in management
	1986	World Health Organization 1st International Conference on Health Promotion. Publication of Ottawa Charter
	1987	White Paper 'Promoting Better Health'. Culmination of reports on primary health care and neighbourhood nursing (Cumberledge Report). Family doctors to be encouraged to carry our health promotion linked to financial incentives for health checks and reaching targeted vaccination levels
		Health Education Council disbanded. Health Education Authority established as a special health authority within the NHS in England. The Health Promotion Authority for Wales and the Health Education Board (1991, renamed) in Scotland are set up
		Ministerial groups focus on the issues of HIV/AIDS and drug misuse. These issues receive relatively large sums of money. Major advertising campaigns, including the first AIDS awareness campaign 'Don't die of ignorance'
		'Look after your heart' campaign to raise awareness of coronary heart disease
	1988	2nd International Conference on Health Promotion in Adelaide focusing on healthy public policy
		Acheson Report on public health in England
	1990	NHS and Community Care Act divided the NHS into purchaser and provider units. The purchasing authority has responsibility for determining health needs and commissioning services from provider units
	1991	3rd International Conference on Health Promotion in Sundsvall focusing on supportive environments. WHO develops health-promoting settings in hospitals, schools, workplace
	1992	The 'Health of the Nation' strategy for England published. Identifies five key target areas: coronary heart disease; accident; mental health; sexual health; cancers
		United Nations Conference on Environment and Development (the 'Earth Summit') held in Rio de Janeiro. Local authorities adopt Agenda 21 strategies which link the environment, sustainable development and health
	1993	'Working Together for Better Health' introduced a strategy for developing health alliances
		GP contract introduced a banding system for the payment of health promotion work

Table 4.1   *Cont'd*

	1995	National Environmental Health Action Plan
	1997	2nd Earth Summit in New York
		4th International Conference on Health Promotion in Jakarta highlights the importance of socio-economic development for health
		Appointment of a Minister for Public Health. 'The New NHS: modern, dependable' White Paper outlines plans to measure performance in six key areas: health improvement; fair access; effective delivery of appropriate health care; efficiency, patient/carer experience and health outcomes
		The establishment of health action zones (HAZ) to pilot good practice in local partnerships to reduce health inequalities
		The appointment of a 'Drug Czar' to oversee all developments related to drug education and prevention
	1998	'Our Healthier Nation' draft health strategy for England is published. Proposes 'contracts' for health between government, local communities and individuals; four national targets – for CHD and stroke, cancers, accidents and mental health; and three settings and population groups to be prioritized – schools and young people, workplaces and adults, neighbourhoods and older people
		Other national strategies published: 'Working Together for a Healthier Scotland', 'Better Health, Better Wales' and 'Fit for the Future' (Northern Ireland)
		Lottery funding is made available for local healthy living centres
		Acheson Report on public health
	1999	Primary care groups established. Role is to assess local health needs and commission appropriate services. All areas required to produce local health improvement programmes (HImPs) in consultation with local authorities and communities

By the 1970s there was an increasing recognition that health policy could not continue to be confined to clinical and medical services, which were both proving expensive and not improving the health status of the population. Health education and the prevention of disease represented a means of cutting costs and an ideology which could place the onus of responsibility on the individual.

The government document *Prevention and Health: Everybody's Business* (DHSS 1976) was published in 1976 and encapsulated a behavioural approach which saw health problems as the result of individual lifestyles.

'To a large extent though, it is clear that the weight of responsibility for his own health lies on the shoulders of the individual himself. The smoking-related diseases, alcoholism and other drug dependencies, obesity and its consequences, and the sexually transmitted diseases are among the preventable problems of our time and, in relation to all of these, the individual must decide for himself' (DHSS 1976).

The message of the document is that improving health depends on individuals changing the way they live in order to avoid 'lifestyle' diseases. A decade later in 1987 a similar message was put forward by the White Paper *Promoting Better Health* which suggested that the major killer diseases could be avoided if people took greater responsibility for their own health (DoH 1987). The 'Health of the Nation' strategy was also permeated by a philosophy of individualism despite the acknowledgement in the strategy that 'responsibilities for action are widely spread from individuals to government' (DoH 1992).

Alongside this government response, however, was the awareness that poor health was linked to poverty. In 1980 the Black Report commissioned by the Government showed how those in lower social classes had a far higher risk of dying prematurely than more advantaged groups (Townsend & Davidson 1982). The last 2 decades have thus seen a re-emergence of public health measures and a recognition of the need to address the social, economic and environmental determinants of health (see Fig. 4.1).

The World Health Organization has played a key part in proposing a broader agenda for health promotion. In 1977 the World Health Assembly at Alma Ata committed all member countries to the principles of *Health for all 2000* (HFA 2000) that there 'should be the attainment by all the people of the world by the year 2000 of a level of health that will permit them to lead a socially and

Figure 4.1 *The development of health promotion. From Bunton & Macdonald 1992.*

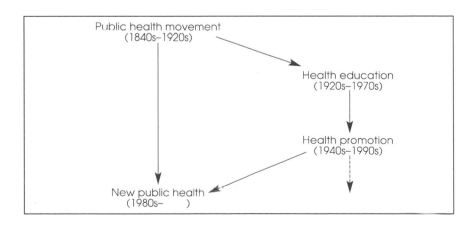

economically productive life.' The WHO made explicit five key principles for health promotion:

1. It involves the population as a whole in the context of their everyday life, rather than focusing on people at risk for specific diseases.
2. It is directed towards action on the causes or determinants of health to ensure that the total environment which is beyond the control of individuals is conducive to health.
3. It combines diverse, but complementary, methods or approaches including communication, education, legislation, fiscal measures, organizational change, community development and spontaneous local activities against health hazards.
4. It aims particularly at effective public participation supporting the principle of self-help movements and encouraging people to find their own ways of managing the health of their community.
5. While health promotion is basically an activity in the health and social fields and not a medical service, health professionals – particularly in primary health care – have an important role in nurturing and enabling health promotion (WHO 1977).

The context for the development of broad-based health strategies thus needed to be based on equity, community participation and intersectoral collaboration, The WHO also identified that improvement in lifestyles, environmental conditions and health care will have little effect if certain fundamental conditions are not met. These include:

- peace and freedom from the fear of war
- equal opportunity for all and social justice
- satisfaction of basic needs including food and income, safe water and sanitation, housing, secure work and a satisfying role in society
- political commitment and public support (WHO 1985).

The WHO launched a programme for health promotion in 1984, and conferences at Ottawa (1986), Adelaide (1988), Sundsvall (1991) and Jakarta (1997) have further outlined areas for action. The principles of health promotion are developed in the Ottawa Charter which outlines these areas as important:

1. building a healthy public policy
2. creating supportive environments
3. developing personal skills including information and coping strategies
4. strengthening community action including social support and networks
5. reorienting health services away from treatment and care and improving access to health services (WHO 1986).

The processes of mediation, advocacy and enablement were identified as ways in which health could be promoted. These processes are discussed further on page 86.

Defining health promotion

Disease prevention

In Chapter 1 we saw that there are many different meanings attached to the concept of health but the notion that health is the 'absence of disease' is a dominant one. Different perceptions about the nature of health and the factors contributing to it underpin interpretations of health promotion. The historical outline (pp. 74–76) has shown a shift from public health measures in the 19th century, through health education aimed at giving advice and information, to social and environmental measures in the later 20th century. One of the most important shifts has been from a focus on disease and treatment to health. Nevertheless the dominance of the medical model has meant that health promotion is frequently seen as the prevention of disease, often through targeting high-risk groups who have an increased likelihood of developing a specific disease.

Health education is often categorized as concerned with primary, secondary or tertiary prevention. Primary prevention seeks to avoid the onset of ill health by the detection of high-risk groups and the

 McKinlay (1979), in persuading us of the need to refocus upstream, tells a story:

'There I am standing by the shore of a swiftly flowing river and I hear the cry of a drowning man. So I jump into the river, put my arms around him, pull him to shore and apply artificial respiration. Just when he begins to breathe, there is another cry for help. So I jump into the river, reach him, pull him to shore, apply artificial respiration, and then just as he begins to breathe, another cry for help. So back in the river again, without end, goes the sequence. You know I am so busy jumping in, pulling them to shore, applying artificial respiration, that I have no time to see who the hell is upstream pushing them all in'.

The concept of refocusing upstream is a powerful and persuasive argument for health promotion. It can help us to reorient our thinking from a belief that medical care can, or will, solve most health problems towards prevention. You might like to discuss these fundamental questions with colleagues:

■ What examples can you think of in your own work of short-term problem-specific activity?
■ What would a reorientation upstream involve?
■ Who or what do you think is pushing people in?

provision of advice and counselling. Examples of primary prevention would include immunization and cervical cytology. Secondary prevention seeks to shorten episodes of illness and prevent the progression of ill health through early diagnosis and treatment. Examples include education about medication, advice on healthy eating for a diabetic and relaxation for cardiac patients. Tertiary prevention seeks to limit disability or complications arising from an irreversible condition. Examples include education about the use of a disability aid and rehabilitation.

For those working in a clinical setting, this is the usual interpretation of health promotion. It can differ little from the education of patients about the condition that brought them to the health service. Its aim is for patients to avoid a recurrence by following a treatment regime or some change in their lifestyle. Disease prevention does not, however, look beyond the risk factors or groups to the origins of ill health.

Health education

Until the mid-1980s the term 'health education' was most widely used to describe the work of practitioners such as nurses and doctors in promoting health. An awareness that individuals make health choices which can contribute to the development of disease led to the view that it was possible to inform people about the prevention of disease, to motivate them to change their behaviour, through persuasion and mass communication techniques, and to equip them through education with the skills for a healthy lifestyle. For some health educators, this means providing people with information about health and disease issues. 'Our Healthier Nation' (DoH 1999) includes the following health education responsibilities in its contract for health:

- (government and national players can) assess risks and communicate these risks clearly to the public
- ensure that the public and others have the information they need to improve their health
- (people can) take responsibility for their own health and make healthier choices about their lifestyle.

One of the paradoxes of health education and a prevailing professional dilemma is the degree of voluntarism or free choice. Health education is based on an expert authority model derived from both medicine and education. It is the health educator or doctor who decides if there is a health need and the adequacy of an individual's lifestyle, who decides the nature of the intervention and the most effective means of communication, who tries to ensure compliance, and who will decide if the intervention has 'worked'.

Health education may be defined as planned opportunities for people to learn about health and make changes in their behaviour. It includes:

- Raising awareness of health issues and factors contributing to ill health
- Providing information
- Motivating and persuading people to make changes in their lifestyle for their health
- Equipping people with the skills and confidence to make those changes.

How do you account for this narrow interpretation by many practitioners of their role in promoting health?

When we look at the practice of health education, we might be led to believe that health education is the *giving* of information and success in promoting health is when the client follows the advice.

For other health educators education is a means of *drawing out*. Clients are not 'empty vessels' who will rationally change their behaviour once provided with the relevant information, advice or guidance. After all, information about the risks to health from smoking has been known since 1963 and information about HIV transmission since 1986, yet people continue to smoke and not use condoms. These health educators seek neither to coerce nor to persuade, both because this is unlikely to be effective but also because it is unethical. The health educator is a facilitator and enabler rather than an expert. Rather than telling clients what to do, the health educator works with them to identify their needs and work towards an informed choice, even when this may lead to health-damaging behaviour.

John is a labourer on the roads. He is 47 and single and his social life revolves around the pub. He drinks a few pints at lunchtime with his sandwiches and usually four pints on the way home. He visits his GP with backache. The GP takes his blood pressure and finds it dangerously high. Do you:

1. Tell him that the recommended drinking limit for adult males is 28 units per week. Stress the damage to his heart and liver and that he risks a heart attack.
2. Discuss the reasons for his drinking behaviour and whether he sees it causing problems.
3. Prescribe medicine to lower his blood pressure and tell him to see the practice nurse in 2 weeks to see if his blood pressure has come down.

This scenario illustrates some of the key tensions in health education:

- Should health education be about telling people what is best for them?
- Are health educators failing in their role if they accept their clients' health damaging behaviour?
- Who should determine what constitutes a healthy life – practitioner or client?
- Should health behaviour and its effects be seen as a matter of individual choice?

These issues are discussed further in Chapter 6 on ethical issues (p. 113) and Chapter 11 'Supporting people to change' (p. 219).

The two strands of voluntarism and authoritarianism reflect the historical development of health education, as educationists and social scientists challenged the mainstream of preventive medicine by contesting the assumption that health education could, or indeed should, seek to bring about behaviour change through information or persuasion. Thus emerged the principle of self-empowerment which many argue is central to the practice of health education (Tones 1992). Empowerment is an approach which enables people to take charge of their lives including changing their behaviour if they so wish. It inevitably involves a reduction in professional dominance and control.

The range of approaches to health education are outlined and discussed in the following chapter. They range from the medical model, focusing on health surveillance and achieving behaviour change, to the educational model which relies on the exploration of attitudes and values. Alongside these are the approaches more closely aligned to health promotion, such as community development, which emphasizes the need to take collective action for health, and a social model which focuses on the need to influence decision makers at local and national level.

Health promotion

The WHO has moved the definition of health promotion away from prevention of specific diseases or the detection of risk groups towards the health and well-being of whole populations. Instead of experts and professionals diagnosing problems, the people themselves define health issues of relevance to them in their local community. Teachers, primary health-care workers, workplace managers, social and welfare workers can all be involved in promoting health. Instead of health being seen as the responsibility of individuals alone, the social factors determining health are taken into account, and health is viewed as a collective responsibility of

Consider these descriptions of the work of a nurse on an acute medical ward and a health promotion adviser working with young people. Would you consider them to be practising health education or health promotion? What criteria do you use to make your judgement?

■ 'Patient education for coronary care is carried out one to one with information booklets. The overall aim is to alleviate anxiety, promote recovery and educate about the cause of the attack to get the patient back to normal and even healthier. Patients may be given factual information about the working of the heart, be taught relaxation exercises and encouraged to talk about concerns such as sex after a heart attack. They will be educated about their medication, how to eat healthily, keeping their weight down and curbing their cholesterol intake, and ways to increase physical activity.'

■ 'Health education in schools passes on knowledge, allows for discussion and leads to understanding. It gives young people the freedom to choose and make health decisions and at the same time it asserts an appreciation and respect for the choices of others. The end result should lead to positive pleasure for the young person whilst enabling them to remain healthy and disease-free'.

A key difference between these two interventions is their aims. In the coronary care unit, the nurse is actively engaged in disease prevention – to prevent a further heart attack. In the school, the health promotion adviser aims to equip young people with the information and skills for a healthy lifestyle. In both cases, the health promoter aims for behaviour change, more obviously so in the coronary care unit. Both use similar educational methods of providing information, encouraging clients to reflect on their attitudes and experience, and providing opportunities to practise skills.

society which needs to be prioritized by organizations and government in their decision-making.

The terms health education and health promotion are often used interchangeably but whilst health promotion can be seen as an umbrella term incorporating aspects of health education, it is much broader in conception.

Health promotion incorporates all measures deliberately designed to promote health and handle disease ... A major feature of health promotion is undoubtedly the importance of 'healthy public policy' with its potential for achieving social change via legislation, fiscal, economic and other forms of 'environmental engineering.

(Tones 1990)

There are, as we saw in Chapter 2, a range of factors which influence people's health. Some are material–structural and some are behavioural. These need to be addressed other than by education alone. Health promotion thus involves public policy change and community action to enable people to make changes in their lives. A phrase first coined by Milio (1986) has come to encapsulate health promotion – 'making the healthy choice the easier choice'. It is, as we have seen, easy for practitioners to confine their health promotion role to offering information and advice on how to adopt a healthier lifestyle. However, for people to make such changes, the factors and situations which led them to adopt 'unhealthy' behaviours need to be addressed. People may smoke because of stress, even though they know it is bad for their health. Others may use an illegal drug because it is widely used by their peer group and is part of their social life. Equally, it is easier for some people to make healthy choices than it is for others. It is easier to eat a diet with fresh fruit and vegetables for people with reasonable incomes who have easy access to supermarkets or high street shopping. Some factors affecting individual health are outside individual control: inadequate housing, busy roads, lack of child care.

 Midwives at a local hospital were concerned that a high proportion of newborn infants were being taken home in cars or taxis in their mother's arms and not restrained in safety seats.

How can the healthy choice be made an easier choice?

The midwife could advise new mothers and provide leaflets on appropriate safety restraints but this puts the onus of responsibility on the parents. A baby seat loan scheme would help to make such seats more available when income is a barrier to purchase. As it is against the law for infants to travel in cars without being restrained, the need to comply with legislation or regulations may make the 'healthy choice' a necessary one.

A key feature which distinguishes health promotion from health education is that it involves environmental and political action. Health education is distinguished by the centrality accorded to autonomy and voluntarism. The underlying principles of health education include the promotion of self-esteem and non-coercion (French 1990). Whilst health educators may respect cultural norms and take account of the social and economic constraints which affect people's ability to make health choices, essentially people are facilitated to make their own informed choice about health behaviour. For those who believe that the roots of ill health lie in the social structure, this emphasis on choice is merely illusory. In Chapter 6 we shall explore further the limits to freedom of choice and how far an ethical principle such as the promotion of autonomy can govern our practice as health educators and health promoters. Conversely, adherents of health education might describe health promotion measures, such as legislation for the compulsory wearing of safety belts or smoking restrictions in public places, or the fluoridation of the water supply, as 'social engineering'. Such activities, by limiting individual choice, might be deemed unethical or undesirable.

'The new methods of health promotion are introducing new forms of social regulation which are not ostensibly oppressive or obviously controlling. In these, often innocuous-looking forms, they nevertheless enter and regulate our lives in new ways and bring with them new concerns for our civil liberties and rights' (Bunton 1992).

Think of some examples of social regulation aimed to promote health. Do you share this concern at the extension of health promotion into areas beyond 'health'?

An integrated definition of health promotion

In practice, health promotion encompasses different political orientations which can be characterized as the individual versus structural approaches. For some, health promotion is a narrow field of activity which seems to explain health status by reference to individual lifestyles and is a process largely determined by an expert. In its emphasis on personal responsibility it sees a minimal role for the state and, thus, has come to be associated with a conservative viewpoint. For others, including the World Health Organization, health promotion recognizes that health and wealth are inextricably linked, and seeks to address the root causes of ill health and problems of inequity using radical and challenging approaches.

It is not helpful to debate whether one form of activity is better or worse than the other: both are necessary. Health promotion may involve lobbying and political advocacy, but it may just as easily involve working with individuals and groups to enhance their knowledge and understanding of the factors affecting their health.

Many practitioners believe that their role is limited in achieving the social changes necessary to eliminate health inequalities or the community change necessary to provide social support. Yet there are ways in which individual practitioners working with clients can promote health over and beyond merely informing, advising or listening. The World Health Organization identify three ways in which practitioners can promote health through their work: advocacy, enablement and mediation.

Advocacy

■ **To what extent do you work 'on behalf of' clients or the public?**
■ **Do you regard advocacy as part of your health promotion role?**

Advocacy means representing the interests of disadvantaged groups and may mean speaking on their behalf or lobbying to influence policy. It can include any attempt to exert pressure on policy makers to recognize the nature of health disadvantage. For example, evidence on individual and community health needs should be collected showing the implications for health of social and political issues. People's knowledge and understanding of the factors which affect health should be increased and health promoters should work to empower people so they may argue their own right to health and negotiate changes in their personal environment.

Enablement

Health promotion should aim to reduce differences in current health status and ensure equal opportunities to enable all people to achieve their full health potential. Health promoters should work to increase knowledge and understanding, and individual coping strategies. In an attempt to improve access to health, health promoters should work with individuals and communities to identify needs and help to develop support networks in the neighbourhood. Enablement is an essential core skill for health promoters since it requires them to act as a catalyst and then stand aside, giving control to the community. (See Ch. 10 for further discussion of working with communities.)

Mediation

To what extent do you encourage participation and enable your clients to take more control over their health?

Health promotion requires coordination and cooperation by many agencies and sectors. Chapter 8 considers the nature and type of partnerships for health. Health promoters mediate between different interests by providing evidence and advice to local groups; by influencing local and national policy through lobbying, media campaigns and participation in working groups.

   In the definitions of health promotion so far, health promotion has been interpreted as a process of improving the health of individuals or community. It can also be seen as a set of values or principles. The World Health Organization identify these as empowerment, equity, collaboration and participation. These values should be incorporated in all health and welfare work for it to be health promoting (see Naidoo & Wills 1998).

Health promotion is thus an integrating approach to identifying and doing health work. Cribb & Dines (1993) argue that 'the central question is not what is the domain of health promotion but is this being done in a health promoting way? And this is a question that can be asked about any and every example of practice, not merely those which are clearly aimed at disease prevention or health education.'

To accept such a definition means there can be no boundaries to health promotion since any situation or event between client and practitioner has the potential to be health promoting.

 What would you define as health promoting aspects of your contact with clients?

You might have included:

■ Listening in an open way to the client's views and using as a starting point their knowledge, attitudes and beliefs
■ Taking opportunities to be positive about the client's achievements and abilities
■ Making links between the client's situation and those of others in the community
■ Providing information about informal support available in the community
■ Negotiating future action with the client to ensure that it is reasonable, appropriate and realistic.

Conclusion

Many health workers are strongly committed to health education and the promotion of health. However, this has often been manifested in one-to-one programmes limited to providing information. Many may be daunted by the broad definition of health promotion and feel that this broad approach is beyond their professional remit. Indeed, it would not be possible for any one worker or group to bring about the changes needed for a health-promoting society. It is important that we remind ourselves of the WHO view which describes the process of promoting health as not only involving political change and interagency collaboration, but also enabling people to take more control over their own health and equipping them with the means for well-being. Health promotion thus includes increasing individual knowledge about the functions of the body and ways of preventing illness, raising competence in using the health care system, and raising awareness about the political and environmental factors that influence health.

The number of teenage pregnancies is rising in the UK and is now the highest in Europe. The conception rate was 9.4 per 1000 girls under 16 in 1998. 8800 girls under 16 get pregnant each year. The number of girls attending family planning clinics has risen from 27 000 in 1993 to 61 000 in 1996.

Which of the following aims for a health promotion intervention around teenage pregnancy would come closest to your own?

■ Reduce teenage pregnancy rates.
■ Educate young people about the risks of under-age sex.
■ Support and advise young mothers.
■ Improve access to services and contraceptive advice.
■ Raise awareness of sexual health among teenagers.
■ Enable young people to make informed and confident choices about their sexual health.

Which of the following activities would you consider a priority for a health promotion intervention? Why?

■ Run a youth counselling drop-in service.
■ Work with teachers to develop a sex education curriculum.
■ Give talks at local schools.
■ Open a young people's session at the family planning clinic.
■ Write a leaflet on contraception.
■ Research the pattern and trends of teenage pregnancies in the area.
■ Set up a teenage mothers' group.
■ Set up an information stall on the local market.
■ Set up an interagency group with employers, housing, education and leisure services to discuss young people's needs.
■ Lobby the Health Authority to provide free condoms for all clubs and leisure centres.
■ Run a training course for doctors on counselling young people.

See the Health Education Authority publication *Reducing the rate of teenage conceptions: an overview of the effectiveness of interventions and programmes aimed at reducing unintended conceptions in young people* (HEA 1998).

Questions for further discussion

■ Is it useful to try to distinguish between health education and health promotion? Which term would you choose to describe your work in improving people's health?
■ How do you explain the emphasis on health promotion in contemporary health care work?

Summary

This chapter has looked at the origins of health promotion and shown how different interpretations arise from different origins. It has shown that health promotion is a broad term encompassing interventions which differ in aims and purpose and in the role accorded to the practitioner. It may be seen as a set of activities clearly intended to prevent disease and ill health, to educate people to a healthier lifestyle, or to address the wider social and environmental factors which influence people's health. It may also be seen as a set of principles to orient health work towards addressing inequality and promoting collaboration and participation. Health promoters thus need to be clear in their understanding of what health is, what aspect of health is being promoted and the ways in which health is affected by wider influences than individual behaviour.

Further reading

Beattie A, Gott M, Jones L, Sidell M (eds) 1993 Health and wellbeing: a reader. Macmillan/Open University, Basingstoke. *An excellent collection of articles to accompany the Open University course K258 'Health and Wellbeing'. The reader illustrates competing perspectives on health in wider debates about social planning and policy making.*

Bunton R, Macdonald G 1992 Health promotion: disciplines and diversity. Routledge, London. *An interesting collection of contributions which traces the theoretical roots of health promotion through the disciplines of psychology, sociology, education and epidemiology.*

Downie R S, Tannahill C, Tannahill A 1996 Health promotion; models and values, 2nd edn. Oxford Medical Publications, Oxford. *A useful introduction which outlines the debate about boundaries for health promotion.*

MacDonald T H 1998 Rethinking health promotion: a global approach. Routledge, London *A discussion of the relationship between biomedicine and health promotion. Not easy reading, but stimulating.*

Seedhouse D 1997 Health promotion: philosophy, prejudice and practice. Wiley, Chichester. *A stimulating, personal analysis of the conceptual roots of health promotion.*

References

Acheson D 1988 Public health in England, report of the Committee of Inquiry into the future development of the public health function. HMSO, London

Amos A 1993 In her own best interests: women and health education, a review of the last 50 years. Health Education Journal 52: 3

Blythe M 1986 A century of health education. Health and Hygiene 7: 105–115

Bunton R 1992 More than a woolly jumper: health promotion as social regulation. Critical Public Health 3: 4–11

Bunton R, Macdonald G 1992 Health promotion: disciplines and diversity. Routledge, London

Cohen Committee 1964 Health education, report of a joint committee of the Central and Scottish Health Services Councils. HMSO, London

Cribb A, Dines A 1993 What is health promotion? In: Dines A, Cribb A (eds) Health promotion: concepts and practice. Blackwell Scientific, Oxford

Department of Health (DoH) 1987 Promoting better health. HMSO, London

Department of Health (DoH) 1992 The health of the nation. HMSO, London

Department of Health (DoH) 1997 The new NHS: modern, dependable. Stationery Office, London

Department of Health (DoH) 1999 Saving Lives: our healthier nation (white paper). Stationery Office, London

Department of Health and Social Security (DHSS) 1976 Prevention and health; everybody's business. HMSO, London

French J 1990 Boundaries and horizons, the role of health education within health promotion. Health Education Journal 49: 7–10

Gott M, O'Brien M 1990 Attitudes and beliefs in health promotion. Nursing Standard 5(2): 30–32

Health Education Authority (HEA) 1998 Reducing the rate of teenage conceptions: an overview of the effectiveness of interventions and programmes aimed at reducing unintended conceptions in young people. HEA, London

McKinlay J B 1979 A case for refocussing upstream: the political economy of health. In: Jaco E G (ed) Patients, physicians and illness. Macmillan, Basingstoke

Milio N 1986 Promoting health through public policy. Canadian Public Health Association, Ottawa

Naidoo J, Wills J 1998 Practising health promotion: dilemmas and challenges. Baillière Tindall, London

Seedhouse D 1997 Health promotion: philosophy, prejudice and practice. Wiley, Chichester

Sutherland I 1987 Health education: half a policy. National Extension College, Cambridge

Tannahill A 1985 What is health promotion? Health Education Journal 44: 4

Tones K 1990 Why theorise: ideology in health education. Health Education Journal 49: 1

Tones K 1992 Empowerment and the promotion of health. Journal of the Institute of Health Education 30: 4

Tones K, Tilford S 1994 Health education: effectiveness, efficiency and equity. Chapman & Hall, London

Townsend P, Davidson N 1982 Inequalities in health: the Black report. Penguin, Harmondsworth

Welshman J 1997 Bringing beauty and brightness to the back streets: health education and public health in England and Wales 1890–1940. Health Education Journal 56(2): 199–209

Williams G 1984 Health promotion – caring concern or slick salesmanship. Journal of Medical Ethics 10(4): 191–195

Wilson-Barnett J 1993 The meaning of health promotion: a personal view. In: Wilson-Barnett J, Macleod Clark K (eds) Research in health promotion and nursing. Macmillan, Basingstoke

World Health Organization 1977 Health for all by the year 2000. WHO, Geneva

World Health Organization 1984 Health promotion: a discussion document on concepts and principles. WHO, Geneva

World Health Organization 1985 Targets for health for all. WHO, Geneva

World Health Organization 1986 Ottawa charter for health promotion. WHO, Geneva

5 *Models and approaches to health promotion*

OVERVIEW

The diversity in concepts of health, influences on health and ways of measuring health lead, not surprisingly, to a number of different approaches to health promotion. The previous chapter began to explore the concepts of health education and health promotion. In this chapter, five different approaches will be discussed:

- medical or preventive
- behaviour change
- educational
- empowerment
- social change.

These approaches will be examined in terms of their different aims, methods and means of evaluation. These approaches have different objectives:

- to prevent disease
- to ensure that people are well informed and able to make health choices
- to help people to acquire the skills and confidence to take greater control over their health
- to change policies and environments in order to facilitate healthy choices.

All of the approaches reflect different ways of working. Identifying the different approaches is primarily a descriptive process. The framework is descriptive – it does not indicate which approach is best nor why a practitioner might adopt one approach rather than another. Alongside these descriptions is emerging a theoretical framework for health promotion which provides a representation in the form of models. The last part of this chapter is an outline of the principal theoretical models of health promotion and a discussion of their usefulness in explaining health promotion practice.

It is common for a practitioner to think that theory has no place in health promotion and that action is determined by work role and organizational objectives rather than values or ideology. We have argued elsewhere that practitioners should be aware of the values implicit in the approach they adopt: 'In so doing, practitioners begin to clarify their view of the purpose of health promotion and which strategies are suggested by different aims. Otherwise practitioners merely respond to practice imperatives and their health promotion work is limited to narrow tasks' (Naidoo & Wills 1998, p. 3).

Models of health promotion are not guides to action but attempts to delineate a contested field of activity and to show how different priorities and strategies reflect different underlying values. They are useful in helping practitioners think through:

- aims
- implications of different strategies
- what would count as success
- own role as a practitioner.

The medical approach

Aims

This approach focuses on activity which aims to reduce morbidity and premature mortality. Activity is targeted towards whole populations or high-risk groups. This kind of health promotion seeks to increase medical interventions which will prevent ill health and premature death. This approach is frequently portrayed as having three levels of intervention:

- *Primary prevention* – prevention of the onset of disease through risk education, e.g. immunization, encouraging non-smoking.
- *Secondary prevention* – preventing the progression of disease, e.g. screening and other methods of early diagnosis.
- *Tertiary prevention* – reducing further disability and suffering in those already ill, preventing recurrence of an illness, e.g. rehabilitation, patient education, palliative care.

The medical approach to health promotion is popular because:

1. It has high status because it uses scientific methods, such as epidemiology (the study of the pattern of diseases in society).
2. In the short term, prevention and the early detection of disease is much cheaper than treatment of people who have become ill. Of course, in the long term, this may not be the case as people live longer and experience degenerative conditions and draw pensions for a longer period.
3. It is an expert-led, or top-down, type of intervention. This kind of activity reinforces the authority of medical and health

professionals who are recognized as having the expert knowledge needed to achieve the desired results.

4. There have been spectacular successes in public health as a result of using this approach, for example the worldwide eradication of smallpox as a result of the vaccination programme.

As we have seen in Chapter 1, the medical approach is conceptualized around the absence of disease. It does not seek to promote positive health and can be criticized for ignoring the social and environmental dimensions of health. In addition, the medical approach encourages dependency on medical knowledge and removes health decisions from the people concerned. Thus, health care workers are encouraged to persuade patients to cooperate and comply with treatment.

Public health medicine is the branch of medicine which specializes in prevention, and most day-to-day preventive work is carried out by the community health services which include health visitors and district nurses.

Methods

The principle of preventive services such as immunization and screening is that they are targeted to groups at risk from a particular condition. Whilst immunization requires a certain level of take-up for it to be effective, screening is offered to specific groups. For example, cervical screening every 3 years is offered to sexually active women aged 20–64.

For screening to be effective for the condition or disease:

■ The disease should have a long preclinical phase so that a screening test will not miss its signs
■ Earlier treatment should improve the outcomes
■ The test should be sensitive, i.e. it should detect all those with the disease
■ The test should be specific, i.e. it should detect *only* those with the disease
■ It should be cost-effective, i.e. the number of tests performed should yield a number of positive cases.

Preventive procedures need to be based on a sound rationale derived from epidemiological evidence. The medical approach also relies on having an infrastructure capable of delivering screening or an immunization programme. This includes trained personnel, equipment and laboratory facilities, information systems which determine who is eligible for the procedure and record uptake rates, and, in the case of immunization, a vaccine which is effective and safe. It can be seen then that the medical approach to health

Consider the example of amniocentesis – the testing of the amniotic fluid around a fetus to detect chromosomal abnormalities. Does this test meet the criteria for effective screening outlined above?

In most districts, amniocentesis is only offered to women over the age of 37 and those with a family history of chromosomal abnormality. Yet 90% of children with Down's syndrome are born to mothers under 37 simply because more women in this age group have babies. Amniocentesis is not a simple test. It carries a risk of miscarriage. It can also only be performed after 14–16 weeks of pregnancy when a possible termination is more difficult. It is less than 100% sensitive and therefore some women may go away falsely reassured. A termination and/or counselling is the only intervention available.

promotion can be a complex process, and may depend on the establishment of national programmes or guidelines.

Having screening or immunization facilities available is effective only if people can be persuaded to use them.

 What methods can you think of that are used to increase the uptake of preventive services?

National campaigns may be launched but the one-to-one advice given to patients by health care workers is generally accepted as being more effective. Increasing uptake may thus depend on training health workers, having an efficient call system and offering screening at a convenient community location, such as in a mobile van.

Evaluation

Evaluation of preventive procedures is based ultimately on a reduction in disease rates and associated mortality. This is a long-term process and a more popular measure capable of short-term evaluation is the increase in the percentage of the target population being screened or immunized.

Although there appears to be a close correlation between immunization uptake and a decline in disease rates, the example of whooping cough suggests some caution is needed. In 1974 80% of children were vaccinated against whooping cough. Following media publicity about the safety of the vaccine, immunization rates fell and did not reach 80% population coverage again until 1987. There were major whooping cough epidemics in 1977–1979 and 1981–1983, suggesting that immunization had contributed to the decline in notifications. However, the overall decline in mortality from whooping cough was occurring before the vaccine was introduced in 1957, suggesting that better nutrition, living conditions and medical care may also be significant.

The medical approach is not always successful. Consider the example of cervical screening. Whilst mortality has been reduced, the death rate in England remains amongst the worst in Western Europe. What could account for this?

You probably included some of the following:

- Inadequate training of laboratory staff in detecting cancerous cell changes
- Faults in the recall system
- A more virulent virus
- Inability to reach women most at risk
- Low take-up.

Behaviour change

Aims

This approach aims to encourage individuals to adopt healthy behaviours, which are seen as the key to improved health. Chapter 11 shows how making health-related decisions is a complex process and, unless a person is ready to take action, it is unlikely to be effective. As we saw in the previous chapter, seeking to influence or change health behaviour has long been part of health education.

The approach is popular because it views health as a property of individuals. It is then possible to assume that people can make real improvements to their health by choosing to change their lifestyle. It also assumes that if people do not take responsible action to look after themselves then they are to blame for the consequences.

Consider the reasons why people may not be able to put a healthy diet into practice. Reasons include:

- Lack of information
- Lack of cooking skills
- Lack of money
- Family preferences
- Lack of availability of healthy foods in local shop
- Lack of cooking facilities.

It is clear that there is a complex relationship between individual behaviour, and social and environmental factors. Behaviour may be a response to the conditions in which people live and the causes of these conditions (e.g. unemployment, poverty) are outside individual control.

Methods

The behaviour-change approach has been the bedrock of activity undertaken by the lead agencies for health promotion. Campaigns persuade people to desist from smoking, adopt a healthy diet and undertake regular exercise. This approach is targeted towards individuals, although mass means of communication may be used to reach them. It is most commonly an expert-led, top-down approach, which reinforces the divide between the expert who knows how to improve health and the general public who need education and advice. However, this is not inevitable. Interventions may be directed according to a client's stated needs when these have been identified.

Many health care workers educate their clients about health through the provision of information and one-to-one counselling. Patient education about a condition or medication may seek to ensure compliance, in other words, a behaviour change, or it may be more client directed and employ an educational approach.

Evaluation

Evaluating a health promotion intervention designed to change behaviour would appear to be a simple exercise. Has the health behaviour changed after the intervention? But there are two main problems: change may only become apparent over a long period, and it may be difficult to isolate any change as attributable to a health promotion intervention.

The Stanford Three Community Study began in the USA in 1972. It sought to evaluate a year-long heart disease prevention project in two trial communities in California. One community received an intensive mass-media campaign; the second community received, in addition, screening and face-to-face health education; a third community was a control study which received no intervention. Both trial communities showed an increased knowledge of the risk factors associated with heart disease. Behavioural changes such as reduction in smoking and in dietary cholesterol were greater in the community receiving screening and health education. This study and a similar project in North Karelia in Finland, have shown that it is possible to bring about behaviour change. But it is difficult to prove unequivocally that observed changes were due to the health education project and not other factors, or the effect of being part of a research project.

Source: Tones & Tilford (1994)

The educational approach

Aims

The purpose of this approach is to provide knowledge and information, and to develop the necessary skills so that people can make an informed choice about their health behaviour. The educational approach should be distinguished from a behaviour change approach in that it does not set out to persuade or motivate change in a particular direction. However, education *is* intended to have an outcome. This will be the client's voluntary choice and it may not be the one the health promoter would prefer.

The educational approach is based on a set of assumptions about the relationship between knowledge and behaviour: that by increasing knowledge, there will be a change in attitudes which may lead to changed behaviour. The goal of a client being able to make an informed choice may seem unambiguous and agreed upon. This ignores, however, not only the very real constraints that social and economic factors place on voluntary behaviour change, but also the complexities of health-related decision-making (see Ch. 11).

Methods

Psychological theories of learning state that learning involves three aspects:

- cognitive (information and understanding)
- affective (attitudes and feelings)
- behavioural (skills).

An educational approach to health promotion will provide information to help clients to make an informed choice about their health behaviour. This may be through the provision of leaflets and booklets, visual displays or one-to-one advice. It may also provide opportunities for clients to share and explore their attitudes to their own health. This may be through group discussion or one-to-one counselling. Educational programmes may also develop clients' decision-making skills through role plays or activities designed to explore options. Clients may take on roles or practise responses in 'real-life' situations. For example, clients taking part in an alcohol programme may role-play situations where they are offered a drink. Educational programmes are usually led by a teacher or facilitator, although the issues for discussion may be decided by the clients. Educational interventions require the practitioner to understand the principles of adult learning and the factors which help or hinder learning (Ewles & Simnett 1999, Rogers 1996).

Evaluation

Increases in knowledge are relatively easy to measure. Health education through mass-media campaigns, one-to-one education and classroom-based work have all shown success in increasing information about health issues, or the awareness of risk factors for a disease. Information alone is, however, insufficient to change behaviour and, as we shall see in Chapter 11, even the desire and ability to change behaviour is no guarantee that the individual will do so.

Empowerment

Aims

■ **What do you understand by the term 'empowerment'?**

■ **Can a practitioner empower a client?**

■ **Are there health promotion actions which can disempower someone?**

The World Health Organization defined health promotion as enabling people to gain control over their lives (WHO 1986). This approach helps people to identify their own concerns and gain the skills and confidence to act upon them. It is unique in being based on a 'bottom-up' strategy and calls for different skills from the health promoter (Kendall 1998). Instead of the expert role adopted by the other approaches, the health promoter becomes a facilitator whose role is to act as a catalyst, getting things going, and then to withdraw from the situation.

When we talk of empowerment, we need to distinguish between *self*-empowerment and *community* empowerment. Self-empowerment is used in some cases to describe those approaches to promoting health which are based on counselling and which use non-directive, client-centred approaches aimed at increasing people's control over their own lives. For people to be empowered they need to:

■ recognize and understand their powerlessness
■ feel strongly enough about their situation to want to change it
■ feel capable of changing the situation by having information, support and life skills.

Empowerment is also used to describe a way of working which increases people's power to change their 'social reality'. Chapter 10 includes a discussion of community development as a way of working which seeks to create active participating communities who are *empowered,* and able to challenge and change the world about them. This may or may not include political consciousness raising such as that advocated by the radical educationist Paulo Freire (1972).

Methods

The emphasis on empowerment is probably familiar to many nurses developing a care plan with a patient, and to teachers working to raise pupils' self-esteem and to many other health promoters. They may call this approach client-centred or use terms such as advocacy or self-care. The role of the health promoter is to help clients to identify their health concerns and areas for change.

Empowering older people though reminiscence

Reminiscence is an example of a communication strategy which encourages older people to tell their story and provides opportunities for them to say what kind of care they want. It shifts the balance of the relationship to the client or patient and helps build trust and understanding. In dementia care, older people can be encouraged to retrieve their past experience and maintain their personhood.

Community development is a similar way of working to empower groups of people by identifying their concerns and working with them to plan a programme of action to address these concerns. Some health promoters have a specific remit to undertake community development work; most do not. Community development work is time-consuming and most health promoters have clearly defined priorities which take up all their time. Funding for this kind of work is invariably insecure and short term. The communication, planning and organizational skills necessary for this approach may not be included in professional training. For many health promoters, relinquishing the expert role may be difficult and uncomfortable. Ways of working with communities are discussed more fully in Chapter 10.

 Examples of health promotion through community development are:

1. Community development workers working with tenants on a housing estate to improve play space
2. Health promotion specialists using a variety of methods to identify health needs of residents in a particular area
3. Setting up groups to meet specific needs, e.g. a girls' group at a youth centre
4. Multilingual linkworkers running health sessions for Asian women.

Evaluation

Evaluation of such activity is problematic, partly because the process of empowerment and networking is typically long term. This makes it difficult to be certain that any changes detected are due to the intervention and not some other factor. In addition, positive results of such an approach may appear to be vague and hard to specify, especially when compared to outcomes used by other approaches, such as targets or changes in behaviour which are capable of being quantified. Evaluation includes the extent to which specific aims have been met (outcome evaluation) and the degree to which the group has gelled, or been empowered as a result of the intervention (process evaluation).

Social change

Aims

This approach, which is sometimes referred to as radical health promotion, acknowledges the importance of the socio-economic environment in determining health. Its focus is at the policy or environmental level, and the aim is to bring about changes in the physical, social and economic environment which will have the effect of promoting health. This may be summed up in the phrase 'to make the healthy choice the easier choice'. A healthy choice is available, but to make it a realistic option for most people requires changes in its cost, availability or accessibility.

Several studies have shown that a healthy diet which includes fruit, vegetables, high-fibre foods and less fat and sugar, may cost up to a third more than the typical diet of a low income family (DoH Nutrition Task Force 1996). What should be the focus of health promotion interventions on healthy eating?

You may have included some of the following:

- Changes in pricing structures such as reducing the price of wholemeal bread compared to white bread
- Working with food manufacturers and distributors to promote food labelling, making it easier for customers to identify low-fat, low-sugar foods
- Farming subsidies which encourage the production of lean meat
- The provision of healthy food in workplaces and hospitals
- The reintroduction of nutritional standards for school meals which promote healthy food
- Widening the number and type of food outlets in local communities.

Methods

The social change or radical approach is targeted towards groups and populations, and involves a top-down method of working. Although there may be widespread consultation, the changes being sought are generally within organizations, and require commitment from the highest levels. Chapter 9 discusses public health work and how legislation has had an enormous impact on the nation's health. For such a policy to be successfully implemented, however, it has to be supported by a public who have been made aware of its importance.

For most health promotion workers, the scope for this type of activity will be more limited than for the traditional medical or behaviour change approaches. The necessary skills for working in this way, such as lobbying, policy planning, negotiating and implementation, may not be included in professional training. Working in such a way may be interpreted as beyond the brief of the job, too political or someone else's remit.

Evaluation

Evaluation of the social change approach includes outcomes such as legislative, organizational or regulatory changes which promote health, e.g. the provision of safe play areas, a ban on tobacco sponsorship and advertising or increased provision of no-smoking areas in public places.

The extent of partnership working, and the profile of health issues on common agendas may also be used to demonstrate a greater degree of commitment to social change for health. These outcomes are typically long-term, complex processes where it would be difficult to prove a link to particular health promotion interventions.

Are there parts of your work which are aimed at social change? Have you sought to influence policies and practices which affect health?

Organizational development, environmental health measures, economic or legislative activities and public policies on housing, education or the future of the NHS may all be examples of health promotion aimed at social change.

Practitioners may seek to address the root causes of ill health by developing health profiles, working in partnerships with other agencies, social commentary and research.

Table 5.1 uses the example of healthy eating to show how different approaches to health promotion will have different aims and use different methods. The health strategy for England 'Saving Lives' identifies the following as key areas for health promotion: accidents, coronary heart disease and stroke, mental illness, and cancers. Consider how health promotion interventions in one of these areas will be affected by working with the five identified approaches to health promotion: medical, behaviour change, educational, empowerment, social change.

- In each case what would working within this approach entail in terms of:
  - ❑ Aims or focus?
  - ❑ Methods?
  - ❑ Worker–client relationship?
- How would you evaluate your success using each approach?
- With which approach would you feel most comfortable?

Table 5.1 *Approaches to health promotion: the example of healthy eating*

Approach	Aims	Methods	Worker/client relationship
Medical	To identify those at risk from disease	Primary health care consultant, e.g. measurement of body mass index	Expert led Passive, conforming client
Behaviour change	To encourage individuals to take responsibility for their own health and choose healthier lifestyles	Persuasion through one-to-one advice Information, mass campaigns, e.g. 'Look After Your Heart' dietary messages	Expert led Dependent client Victim-blaming ideology
Educational	To increase knowledge and skills about healthy lifestyles	Information Exploration of attitudes through small group work Development of skills, e.g. women's health group	May be expert led May also involve client in negotiation of issue for discussion
Empower-ment	To work with clients or communities to meet their perceived needs	Advocacy Negotiation Networking Facilitation, e.g. food co-op, fat women's group	Health promoter is facilitator Client becomes empowered
Social change	To address inequalities in health based on class, race, gender, geography	Development of organizational policy, e.g. hospital catering policy Public health legislation, e.g. food labelling Lobbying Fiscal controls, e.g. subsidy to farmers to produce lean meat	Entails social regulation and is top-down

Models of health promotion

The above schema of different approaches to health promotion is primarily descriptive. It is what health promoters do, and it is possible to move in and out of different approaches depending on the situation. A more analytic means of identifying types of health promotion is to develop models of practice. All models, be they building models, diagrammatic maps or theoretical models, seek to represent reality in some way and try to show in a simplified form how different things connect. Thus a nursing model includes the essential components of practice – the client, goals, activities and outcomes. Models of health promotion serve different purposes – they are not a guide to action but may help to:

■ conceptualize or map the field of health promotion
■ interrogate and analyse existing practice
■ plan and chart the possibilities for interventions (Naidoo & Wills 1998).

Using a model can be helpful because it encourages you to think theoretically, and come up with new strategies and ways of working. It can also help you to prioritize and locate more or less desirable types of interventions.

There has been a proliferation of models in health promotion literature, with large areas of overlap but little consensus on terminology or underlying criteria. Thus we find that Beattie (1991) uses criteria of 'mode of intervention' (authoritative–negotiated) and 'focus of intervention' (individual–collective) to generate four models (see Fig. 5.2, p 106). Caplan & Holland (1990) use 'theories of knowledge' and 'theories of society' (see Fig. 5.1, p. 104). The terminology for models also varies. Ewles & Simnett (1999) describe a 'social change' approach to health promotion. French (1990) calls this 'politics of health' whilst Caplan & Holland (1990) distinguish between a radical model and a Marxist model. This can be extremely confusing for the reader. However, as Rawson (1992) points out, the debate about models of health promotion may be viewed as a healthy sign of an emerging occupation's concern to develop a sound theoretical basis for action.

The following two models derive from sociological and social policy frameworks. They adopt a structural analysis which draws attention to the material and social influences on health and the social structures which contribute to inequalities in health. They show how health promotion approaches are influenced by political ideology and different value positions about power, responsibility and autonomy.

1. Caplan & Holland (1990)

This model suggests that there are essentially four paradigms or ways of looking at health promotion. These paradigms can be generated from two dimensions (see Fig. 5.1). The first dimension is concerned with the nature of knowledge. Knowledge is seen as based along a continuum which ranges from subjective approaches to understanding through to objective approaches. Objective

Figure 5.1 *Four paradigms or perspectives of health promotion. Adapted from Caplan & Holland 1990.*

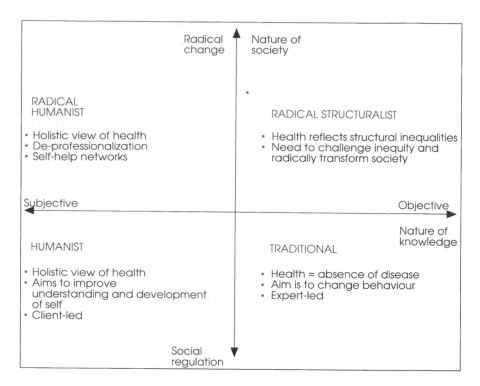

explanations deriving from science (e.g. health is the absence of disease) are only part of the picture. Emphasis may also be given to lay accounts and people's own unique interpretations of what their health means to them.

The second dimension relates to assumptions concerning the nature of society. These range from theories of radical change to theories of social regulation. When these two dimensions are put together it suggests four paradigms or perspectives of health promotion as illustrated in Figure 5.1.

Each quadrant represents a major approach to the understanding of health and the practice of health promotion. They are not necessarily exclusive but there will be situations when to hold one position or approach precludes the adoption of other approaches. Each quadrant incorporates different theoretical and philosophical assumptions about society, concepts of health and the principal sources of health problems.

a. **The traditional perspective** relates to the medical and behaviour-change approaches described earlier. Knowledge lies with the experts and the emphasis is on information giving to bring about behaviour change.

b. **The humanist perspective** relates to the educational approach. Individuals are enabled to use their personal resources and skills to maximize their chances of developing what they consider to be a healthy lifestyle.

c. **The radical humanist perspective** relates to the empowerment approach. Health promotion is concerned to raise consciousness and part of the emphasis is on the exploration of personal responses to health issues. Alongside this, individuals are encouraged to form social, organizational and economic networks.

d. **The radical structuralist perspective** holds that structural inequalities are the cause of many health problems, and the role of health promotion is to address the relationship between health and social inequalities.

The model is useful in showing that practice is the outcome of deeper social conflicts and values.

2. Beattie (1991)

Beattie offers a structural analysis of the health promotion repertoire of approaches. He suggests that there are four paradigms for health promotion (see Fig. 5.2). These are generated from the dimensions of mode of intervention which ranges from authoritative (top-down and expert-led) to negotiated (bottom-up and valuing individual autonomy). Much health promotion work involving advice and information is determined and led by practitioners. Equally, policy work may also be expert led, the priorities determined by epidemiological data. The other dimension relates to focus of intervention which ranges from a focus on the individual to a focus on the collective and the roots of ill health.

Beattie's typology generates four strategies for health promotion.

a. **Health persuasion.** These are interventions directed at individuals and led by professionals. An example is a primary health care worker encouraging a pregnant woman to stop smoking.

b. **Legislative action.** These are interventions led by professionals but intended to protect communities. An example is lobbying for a ban on tobacco advertising.

c. **Personal counselling.** These interventions are client led and focus on personal development. The health promoter is a facilitator rather than an expert. An example is a youth worker working with young people who helps them to identify their health needs and then works with them one-to-one or through group work to increase their confidence and skills.

d. **Community development.** These interventions, in a similar way to personal counselling, seek to empower or enhance the skills of a group or local community. An example is a community worker working with a local tenants' group to increase opportunities for further education and active leisure pursuits.

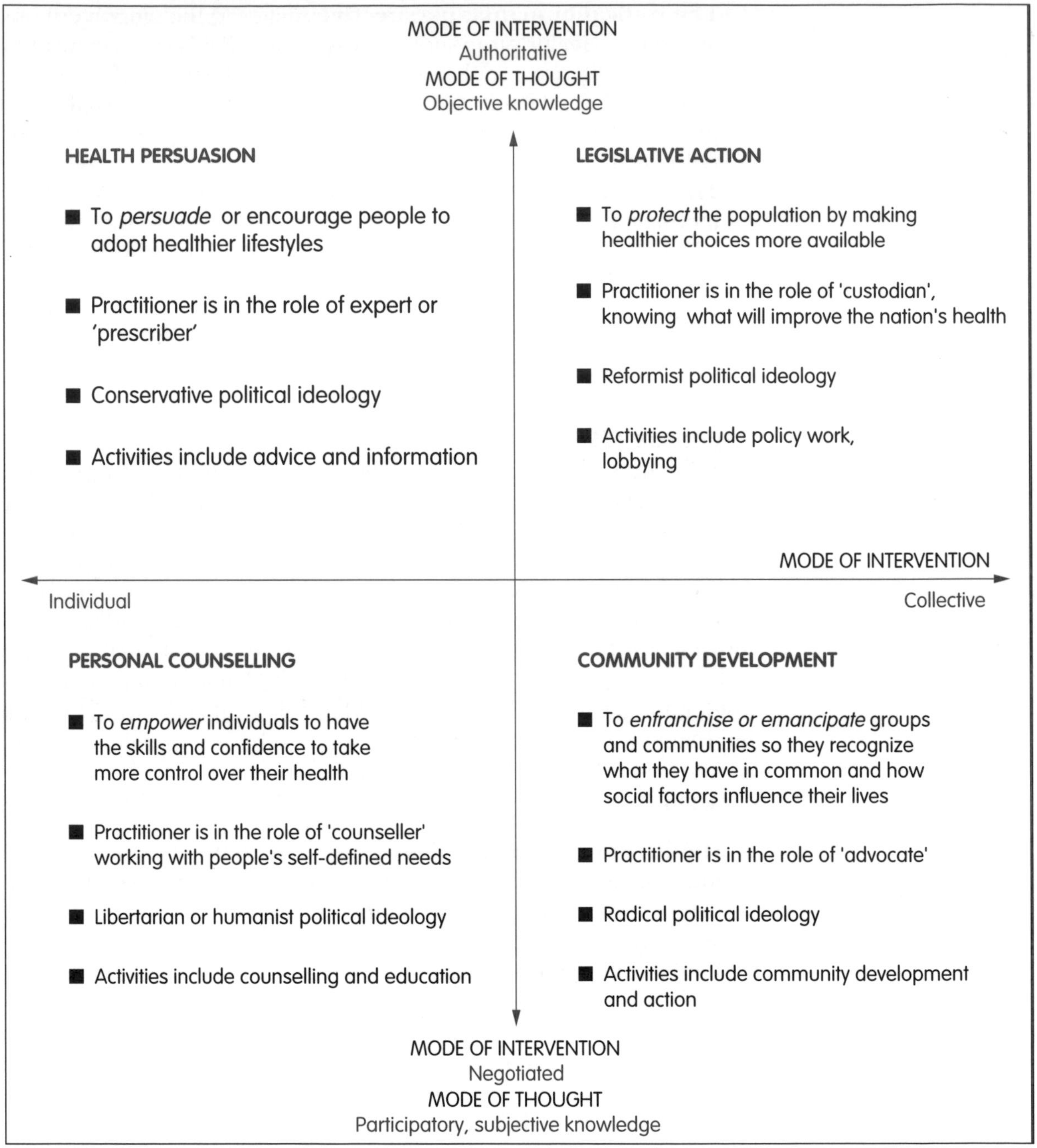

MODE OF INTERVENTION
Authoritative
MODE OF THOUGHT
Objective knowledge

HEALTH PERSUASION

■ To *persuade* or encourage people to adopt healthier lifestyles

■ Practitioner is in the role of expert or 'prescriber'

■ Conservative political ideology

■ Activities include advice and information

LEGISLATIVE ACTION

■ To *protect* the population by making healthier choices more available

■ Practitioner is in the role of 'custodian', knowing what will improve the nation's health

■ Reformist political ideology

■ Activities include policy work, lobbying

MODE OF INTERVENTION

Individual   Collective

PERSONAL COUNSELLING

■ To *empower* individuals to have the skills and confidence to take more control over their health

■ Practitioner is in the role of 'counseller' working with people's self-defined needs

■ Libertarian or humanist political ideology

■ Activities include counselling and education

COMMUNITY DEVELOPMENT

■ To *enfranchise or emancipate* groups and communities so they recognize what they have in common and how social factors influence their lives

■ Practitioner is in the role of 'advocate'

■ Radical political ideology

■ Activities include community development and action

MODE OF INTERVENTION
Negotiated
MODE OF THOUGHT
Participatory, subjective knowledge

Figure 5.2   *Using Beattie's model to analyze practice. Based on Beattie 1991, 1993.*

Figure 5.2 shows how Beattie's model can point up the following aspects:

■ goals and activities
■ client–practitioner relationship
■ political ideologies.

Each of the strategies above corresponds to a different political perspective. Thus conservative reformist perspectives see health promotion as attempting to correct or repair what is seen as a deficit in the conservative perspective, or an aspect of deprivation in the reformist perspective. These perspectives give rise to authoritative and prescriptive approaches. Libertarian and radical perspectives both see health promotion as seeking to empower or enfranchise individuals. The radical perspective, in addition, seeks to mobilize and emancipate communities. Each of these perspectives also casts the practitioner in a different role in relation to clients.

Beattie's model is a useful one for health promoters because it identifies a clear framework for deciding a strategy, and yet reminds them that the choice of these interventions is influenced by social and political perspectives.

3. Tannahill (Downie et al 1996)

This model of health promotion is widely accepted by health care workers. Tannahill talks of three overlapping spheres of activity: health education; health protection; and prevention.

Health education – communication to enhance well-being and prevent ill health through influencing knowledge and attitudes.

Prevention – reducing or avoiding the risk of diseases and ill health primarily through medical interventions.

Health protection – safeguarding population health through legislative, fiscal or social measures.

Tannahill's diagrammatic representation (Fig. 5.3) shows how these different approaches relate to each other in an all-inclusive process termed health promotion.

The model is primarily descriptive of what goes on in practice. It is useful for the health promoter to see the potential in other areas of activity, and to see the scope of health promotion. It does not, however, give any insight into why a practitioner may choose one approach over another. It suggests that all approaches are interrelated but, as we have seen, they reflect distinctive ways of looking at health issues.

Take one of the following programme objectives and using Beattie's model plot the different strategies which might be possible to reduce:

- Smoking in pregnant women
- Drinking in young people
- Accidents in older people.

Figure 5.3

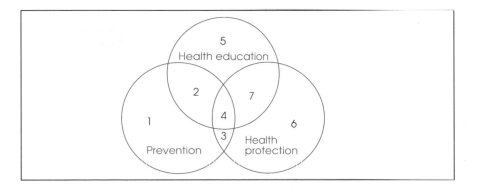

Figure 5.3 *Tannahill's model of health promotion. From Downie et al 1996.*

1. *Preventive services, e.g. immunization, cervical screening, hypertension case finding, developmental surveillance, use of nicotine chewing gum to aid smoking cessation.*
2. *Preventive health education, e.g. smoking cessation advice and information.*
3. *Preventive health protection, e.g. fluoridation of water.*
4. *Health education for preventive health protection, e.g. lobbying for seat-belt legislation.*
5. *Positive health education, e.g. lifeskills work with young people.*
6. *Positive health protection, e.g. workplace smoking policy.*
7. *Health education aimed at positive health protection, e.g. lobbying for a ban on tobacco advertising.*

4. Tones (Tones & Tilford 1994)

The following model claims to be an empowerment model which has as its cardinal principle the goal of enabling people to gain control over their own health. It prioritizes empowerment, which is seen as both the core value and the core strategy underpinning and defining the practice of health promotion.

Tones makes a simple equation that health promotion is an overall process of healthy public policy × health education (see Fig. 5.4).

Tones considers education to be the key to empowering both lay and professional people by raising consciousness of health issues. People are then more able to make choices and to create pressure for healthy public policies. We have seen how there is a distinction between self-empowerment and community empowerment. Tones argues that there is a reciprocal relationship between the two.

Figure 5.4 *The contribution of education to health promotion. Adapted from Tones & Tilford 1994.*

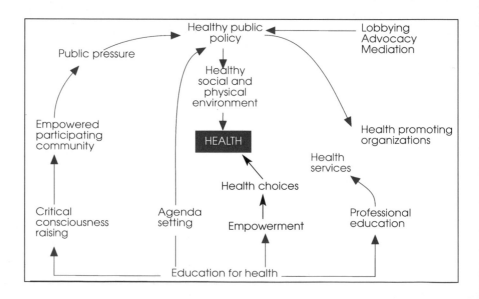

Changes in the social environment achieved through healthy public policies will facilitate the development of self-empowered individuals. People who have the skills to participate effectively in decision-making are better able to access resources and shape policy to meet their needs. The support of individuals is also necessary for implementing change. Empowerment, as opposed to prevention or a radical–political approach is the main aim of health promotion in Tones' model. Working for empowerment enhances individual autonomy and enables individuals, groups and communities to take more control over their lives.

Conclusion

A number of quite different activities are subsumed under the label 'health promotion'. Attempts to organize these activities into different categories have generated a plethora of models and typologies. The most obvious starting point is to describe the variety of current practice and this is the approach taken at the beginning of this chapter. However, there are limitations to this method and it may be criticized as being insufficiently analytical. Theorists who have taken this one step further have identified key criteria which serve to locate different forms of practice, both existing and potential. Adopting a more analytical approach enables judgements to be made about more and less desirable forms of practice, and opens up these judgements for debate. If health promotion is to progress as a discipline and an activity in its own right, a strong theoretical framework is necessary.

The search to clarify models and typologies of practice may appear to be academic and unrelated to the 'here and now' of your activities to promote health. However, we would argue that for practice to grow beyond a reactive response to demands made by others, practitioners need to have an idea of all available options. It is only when we can contemplate different ways of promoting health that we can make judgements as to what is possible and what is preferable. Recognizing that the two are not always synonymous may be frustrating in the short term, but must in the long term contribute towards the effectiveness and efficiency of health promotion.

Questions for further discussion

■ Which approach(es) to health promotion do you adopt in your work?
■ What are the most important reasons for adopting your approach(es)?
■ Which typology or model of health promotion do you find most helpful in providing a theoretical framework with which to analyze your health promotion activities?

The smoking rate among women on low income increases with:

- Greater disadvantage
- More children to care for
- Children in poorer health
- Caring alone
- Carrying extra responsibility for family members.

Using one of the models discussed earlier, map those health promotion interventions which you would regard as:

    a. Most appropriate for women smokers on a low income

    b. Most likely to be adopted

    c. Ones you would use.

- If the answers to a, b and c are different, what might account for this?
- What factors influence your choice of strategies (e.g. professional training, job remit, personal values, local priorities)?

Summary

This chapter has examined five different approaches to health promotion: the medical or preventive approach; the behaviour change or lifestyles approach; the educational approach; the empowerment and community development approach; and the social change or radical approach. In practice, the edges between them may be blurred. However, they do differ in significant ways. They encompass different assumptions concerning the nature of health society and change. The preferred methods of intervention, necessary skills and means of evaluation all differ. Many health promoters will find that the approach they adopt is dictated, in part at least, by their job role and functions. This chapter stresses the importance of examining your approach to health promotion and identifying any changes you may wish to make.

Further reading

Ewles L, Simnett I 1999 Promoting health: a practical guide, 4th edn. Baillière Tindall, Edinburgh. *Chapter 3 provides a short and straightforward guide to approaches to health promotion and identifies their aims and values.*

Naidoo J, Wills J 1998 Practising health promotion. Baillière Tindall, London. *Chapter 1 examines the body of health promotion theory, the key principles which inform practice and why their application may be difficult.*

Rawson D 1992 The growth of health promotion theory and its radical reconstruction. In: Bunton R, Macdonald G 1992 Health promotion: disciplines and diversity. Routledge, London. *A powerful argument for the importance of theory in developing health promotion practice. This chapter examines the multidisciplinary roots of health promotion theory and practice.*

Tones K, Tilford S 1994 Health education: effectiveness, efficiency and equity, 2nd edn. Chapman & Hall, London. *Chapter 1 explores the values underpinning three different models of health promotion: radical–political model; self-empowerment; and preventive model.*

References

Beattie A 1991 Knowledge and control in health promotion: a test case for social policy and social theory. In: Gabe J, Calnan M, Bury M (eds) The sociology of the health service. Routledge, London

Beattie A 1993 The changing boundaries of health. In: Beattie A, Gott M, Jones L, Sidell M (eds) Health and wellbeing: a reader. Macmillan/Open University, Basingstoke

Caplan R, Holland R 1990 Rethinking health education theory. Health Education Journal 49: 10–12

Department of Health (DoH) Nutrition Task Force 1996 Low income, food, nutrition and health: strategies for improvement. HMSO, London

Downie R S, Tannahill C, Tannahill A 1996 Health promotion: models and values, 2nd edn. Oxford Medical Publications, Oxford

Ewles, Simnett I 1999 Promoting health: a practical guide, 4th edn. Baillière Tindall, Edinburgh

Freire P 1972 Pedagogy of the oppressed. Penguin, Harmondsworth

French J 1990 Models of health education and promotion. Health Education Journal 49: 1

Kendall S (ed) 1998 Health and empowerment: research and practice. Arnold, Kendall

Naidoo J, Wills J 1998 Practising health promotion: dilemmas and challenges. Baillière Tindall, London

Rawson D 1992 The growth of health promotion theory and its rational reconstruction. In: Bunton R, Macdonald G (eds) Health promotion: disciplines and diversity. Routledge, London

Rogers A 1996 Teaching adults, 2nd edn. Open University, Buckingham

Tones K, Tilford S 1994 Health education; effectiveness, efficiency, equity, 2nd edn. Chapman & Hall London,

World Health Organization 1986 Ottawa charter for health promotion. WHO, Geneva

6 *Ethical issues in health promotion*

OVERVIEW

Health promotion involves working to improve people's health. This requires a series of value judgements: about what better health means for the individual and society; and about whether, when and how to make a health promotion intervention. This book has used the perspectives of social science to help you explore your role and aims in health promotion. In this chapter we consider some of the prevailing problems for a health promoter from a philosophical perspective. In particular, the chapter focuses on the limits to individual freedoms and how these are balanced against the health of the community. The chapter outlines the key ethical principles of beneficence (doing good), non-maleficence (doing no harm), justice, telling the truth and respect for people and their autonomy.

The need for a philosophy of health promotion

Debate in health promotion has centred on discussion of practice and some attempts to develop a theoretical base. However, according to Seedhouse (1988), there has been little discussion concerning the philosophy of health and yet it is an essential part of the way in which we understand the world.

Health promotion involves decisions and choices that affect other people which require judgements to be made about whether particular courses of action are right or wrong. There are no definite ways to behave. Health promotion is, according to Seedhouse (1988), 'a moral endeavour'. Philosophical debate helps to clarify what it is that one believes in most and how one wants to run one's life. It can and does help practitioners to reflect on the principles of practice, and thus to make practical judgements about whether to intervene and which strategies to adopt.

Philosophy has three main branches:

- Logic – the development of reasoned argument

- Epistemology – the debate and discussion of truths such as the meaning of health
- Ethics – the formal study of the principles on which moral rule and values are based.

Morals refer to those beliefs about how people 'ought' to behave. These debates about right and wrong, good and bad, and duty are part of everyday discourse. Is it wrong to tell a lie? Is it justified to kill another? Is it our duty to look after ageing parents? Judgement about the morality of these actions may derive from our personal values and moral beliefs which derive from: religion, culture, ideology, professional codes of practice or social etiquette, the law, or our life experience. The function of ethical theory is not to provide answers but to inform these judgements and help people work out whether certain courses of action are right or wrong, and whether one ought to take a certain action.

Most ethical theories fall into two types – deontological and consequential. Deontology comes from the Greek word *deonto* meaning duty. Deontologists hold that we have a *duty* to act in accordance with certain universal moral rules. Consequential ethics are based on the premise that whether an action is right or wrong depends on its end result.

Duty and codes of practice

Deontologists hold that there are universal moral rules that it is our duty to follow. Many of the philosophical discussions about the nature of duty are based on the theories of Immanuel Kant. The essence of Kant's thinking is encapsulated in the categorical imperative which can help us to discover, through reason, if a rule or moral principle exists (Kant 1909).

The major features of Kant's theory are:

1. Act as if your action in each circumstance is to become law for everyone, yourself included, in the future. In other words, if everyone always behaved this way, would the overall effect be good? If it would, then this is the rule to apply in all similar situations. The biblical 'Do unto others as you would they do unto you' becomes a universal moral imperative.
2. Always treat human beings as 'ends in themselves' and never merely as 'means'. A moral rule then is one that respects all people.

Deontological theories make decision-making apparently easy because, as long as we obey the rules, then we must be doing the right thing, regardless of the consequences.

This example centres on the duty to respect life and highlights some of the difficulties that can arise from carrying out this duty.

There is in medical care a commonly accepted doctrine of 'acts and omissions' which states that if a person fails to perform an action that would prevent negative consequences he or she is morally less blameworthy than if he or she performed an action that resulted in the same consequence.

In 1992 Dr Nigel Cox was convicted of murdering his patient Lilian Boyes who was suffering a lingering and painful death. Dr Cox administered a lethal dose of potassium chloride. This was regarded as active killing, although the General Medical Council decided not to strike Dr Cox off the medical register.

In 1992 medical staff stopped feeding Tony Bland, a young man crushed into a permanent vegetative state by the Hillsborough football disaster. This action was regarded as withholding life-saving treatment and morally acceptable.

Both acts had brought about the same consequence – the death of a patient. Is there a moral distinction, in your view, between killing and letting die? Must human life be preserved regardless of its quality?

Many health care workers have codes of practice which set out guidelines for the fulfilment of duties. For example, doctors take the Hippocratic oath which requires them as a first principle to avoid doing harm. The 1992 code of practice from the UK Central Council for Nursing, Midwifery and Health Visiting states the duty to respect life, the duty to care, and the duty to do no harm. Kant would have added 'the duty to be truthful in all declarations is a sacred, unconditional command of reason, and not to be limited by any expediency' (Kant 1909). The Society of Health Education and Promotion Specialists includes these principles in its code of conduct:

Practitioners have a
- duty to care
- duty to be fair
- duty to respect personal and group rights
- duty to avoid harm
- duty to respect confidentiality
- duty to report (SHEPS 1997).

Consequentialism and utilitarianism: the individual and the common good

The other classical school of ethics is known as consequentialism of which utilitarianism is its best-known branch. Consequentialism differs from deontological theories because it is concerned with ends and not only means. The utilitarian principle is that a person should always act in such a way that will produce more good or benefits than disadvantages. Utilitarians such as John Stuart Mill and Jeremy Bentham aimed for the greatest good or pleasure for the greatest number of people. Utilitarians can thus respond to all moral dilemmas by reviewing the facts and weighing up the consequences of alternative courses of action. This can, of course, prove difficult. What exactly is a good end? How does one predict whether an outcome will be favourable? One of the main problems with utilitarianism is that, if the aim of all actions is to achieve the greatest good, does this justify harm or injustice to a few if society benefits? Smoking restrictions offer an example where the health of society takes precedence over the right of the individual to smoke.

This raises key philosophical and political questions about freedom and its limits. Should the interests of the majority always take precedence over those of the individual? In Chapter 4 we saw that some writers have expressed concern over 'social engineering' in health promotion and think that government intervention has risked becoming government intrusion. Many interventions are justified as being in the interests of a 'healthy society'; yet they may not have been requested or desired.

 Consider these examples of possible healthy public policies and whether, in your view, they are ethical.

- Fluoridation of tap water
- Subsidy of lead-free petrol
- Ban on smoking in public places
- Complete ban on drinking and driving
- Compulsory testing of all visitors to the UK for HIV infection
- Ban on the use of mobile phones in cars
- Government subsidy of childminding places
- Reintroduction of nutritional standards for all school meals

Ethical principles

Ethical principles can help to clarify the decisions that have to be taken at work. Sometimes decisions may be guided by trying to do the best for the most number of people; at other times they may be guided by an overriding concern for people's right to determine their own lives; and sometimes decisions may be guided by other ethical principles or a professional code of conduct.

There are four widely accepted ethical principles (Beauchamp & Childress 1995):

- respect for autonomy (a respect for the rights of individuals and their right to determine their lives)

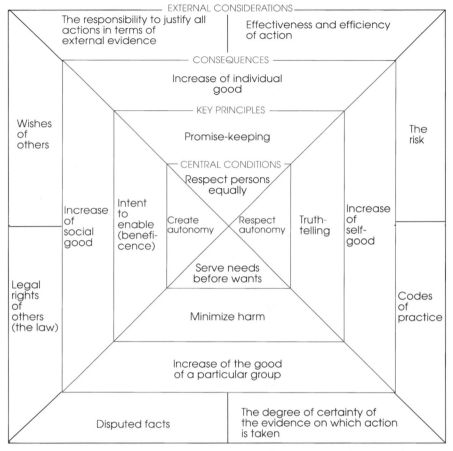

Figure 6.1 *The ethical grid (from Seedhouse 1988). The limit to the use of the grid is that it should be used honestly to seek to enable the enhancing potentials of people.*

■ beneficence (doing good)
■ non-maleficence (doing no harm)
■ justice (being fair and equitable).

These principles provide a framework for consistent moral decision-making. However, situations rarely involve a single option, but can encapsulate increasingly complex and sometimes conflicting choices between these principles. Seedhouse (1988) has developed these principles into an ethical grid which helps provide health promoters with an easy-to-follow guide on which to ground their work on moral principles (see Fig. 6.1).

The ethical grid
This provides a tool for practitioners, helping them to question basic principles and values, and be clear about what they mean and intend to do. The grid suggests ways in which practitioners can

work through proposed actions. In any situation we should be asking ourselves:

1. **Central conditions in working for health**
   - Am I creating autonomy in my clients, enabling them to direct their own lives?
   - Am I respecting the autonomy of my clients whether or not I approve of their chosen direction?
   - Am I respecting all people as equal?
   - Do I work with people on the basis of needs first?

2. **Key principles in working for health**
   - Am I doing good and avoiding harm?
   - Am I telling the truth and keeping promises?

3. **Consequences of ways of working for health**
   - Will my action increase the individual good?
   - Will it increase the good of a particular group?
   - Will it increase the good of society?
   - Will I be acting for the good of myself?

4. **External considerations in working for health**
   - Are there any legal implications?
   - Is there a risk attached to the intervention?
   - Is the intervention the most effective and efficient action to take?
   - How certain is the evidence on which this intervention is based?
   - What are the views and wishes of those involved?
   - Can I justify my actions in terms of all this evidence?

Health promotion involves working to improve people's health. This requires a series of value judgements: about what health means

In the USA a charity has offered young women addicted to heroin or crack cocaine and who have frequent pregnancies resulting in abortions, stillbirths or addicted babies, a sum of money to be sterilized.

Use Seedhouse's ethical grid to consider whether or not such action is morally justified.

You probably concluded that offering money as an inducement for sterilization is a coercive measure that does not respect the autonomy of the individual. Although it may give women greater control over their reproduction, having more money may result in increased drug use. Sterilization is an irreversible procedure about which women need to be fully and freely informed. This action is not, then, one which increases morality. It is a quick-fix solution which fails to deal with the root causes of drug addiction.

In the following scenarios, decide what ethical issues are involved and what action you would take and why.

1. You are nursing a 50-year-old who has chronic obstructive lung disease. The patient has smoked 40 cigarettes a day since he was 17. He has become very distressed by advice to stop smoking.
2. A vocal group of residents has asked for your support in a campaign against drug-taking and prostitution in your area. A local agency, working on harm minimization strategies with young people, has also requested your support.
3. A child has recently died from glue sniffing at a local secondary school. The community police officer is keen to visit all local schools to show a video depicting a group of children who sniff glue and get into all kinds of trouble.
4. As part of a local mental health strategy, a general practice has introduced questionnaires to detect early indicators of mental health problems, at all its clinics. A middle-aged, single, unemployed man regularly attends the diabetic clinic. His questionnaire indicates that he has sleep disturbance and high levels of anxiety.

for the individual and society and about whether, when and how to intervene.

Autonomy

Autonomy derives from the Greek word *autonomous* meaning self-rule. It refers to people's capacity to choose freely for themselves and be able to direct their own life. Since people do not exist in isolation from each other, there will be restrictions on individual autonomy and autonomous people have a sense of responsibility: they cannot do entirely as they like. Thus, people do not have complete freedom of choice. The limits to an individual's autonomy are when that individual's action affects others in a negative way. Beyond this, traditional notions of liberal individualism see autonomy as essential to all human beings. It is only constrained by:

■ reason and the ability to make rational choices
■ the ability to understand one's environment
■ the ability to act on one's environment.

In addition, a person needs to be free from pressures such as fear and want, and have the personal and social circumstances to make any chosen action possible.

Autonomy must, therefore, be thought of not as an absolute but as attainable, to a greater or lesser extent. Not everyone has autonomy. When people's capacity for rationality is affected in some way, decisions are often taken on their behalf on the basis that 'they do not know what's best for them'. Thus people with learning difficulties or mental illness, young children and older people with mental confusion are often assumed to be unable to make a rational choice. It was not until the 20th century that women were deemed able to make a rational choice in a democratic vote. The Children Act of 1989 first recognized the rights and capacity of children to have a say in their care.

The rights of young people with severe learning difficulties to determine their sexual health is a contested area:

■ **Should young people with severe learning difficulties have sexual relationships?**
■ **Should they decide whether or not to use contraception?**
■ **Should they decide if they wish to have children?**

In recent years, the courts have ruled that a young woman with learning disabilities should be sterilized to avoid the possible trauma of pregnancy and childbirth or abortion, for which it was considered she would not be prepared. It was also deemed in the best interests of a possible child who would not be able to be brought up by the young woman.

In these situations, what do we mean by autonomy? In part, we must mean respecting our clients as persons and helping them to cope with the consequences of their choices. Seedhouse (1988) makes a distinction between creating autonomy and respecting autonomy, which he regards as the central conditions when working for health.

Creating autonomy is making an effort to improve the quality of a person's autonomy by trying to enhance what that person is able to do. In health promotion work, this is often called empowerment. It may involve information to enable clients to make choices or developing the clients' skills in analyzing situations and making decisions through increasing self-awareness and assertiveness. As we have stated elsewhere in this book, it is of prime importance in health promotion practice to recognize the limits to individual autonomy, and that social and economic circumstances can constrain individual health choices. Health promoters must avoid victim blaming and seeing people as solely responsible for their own ill health.

Respecting autonomy is agreeing to the wishes of the individual and respecting a person's chosen direction, whether or not it is approved. Creating and respecting autonomy are closely related. People cannot express a free wish if they are not aware of the possibilities open to them and thus it may, in some circumstances, be ethically justifiable not to respond to a client's expressed wishes but to attempt to open up other options.

Respecting clients' autonomy can be difficult for health promoters. There is often a tendency to give advice, to offer information or to persuade clients to change their behaviour. The challenge is to accept a role of partner and enabler rather than expert and controller. Ewles & Simnett (1999) identify three common ways in which health promoters hinder rather than respect their clients' autonomy:

■ by imposing their own solutions to the clients' problems
■ by instructing clients on what to do because they take too long to work it out for themselves
■ by dismissing the client's ideas without providing an adequate explanation or the opportunity to try them out.

Think of some examples from your work when you have attempted to *create* autonomy in your clients so that they are able to express their wishes and wants.

At what point did you decide that the client is autonomous and to *respect* his or her wishes?

Chapter 10 explores a community development way of working which aims to empower people with regard to their own health agenda. It explores this dilemma of control and autonomy, and to what extent community development workers impose, collaborate with, or genuinely facilitate local or community health needs. Chapter 11 looks at ways practitioners support individuals to change and whether such approaches are intent on empowering individuals or merely getting them to change.

Perhaps the starkest example of the ethical problems associated with respecting autonomy is that which confronts the health worker when a patient or client chooses not to follow advice or treatment which is known to be beneficial. It would seem straightforward that this is the client's right and the health worker should respect the client's autonomy in choosing such a decision, if the client is properly informed and understands any risks involved. However, the health worker is committed to 'doing good' and may feel it is her duty to persuade the client. This is particularly so if the client's decision has implications for other people. Certainly this is paternalistic and putting the health worker's need to do good above the client's wish for autonomy. Yet, by not seeking to persuade or motivate the client, the practitioner may, by omission, be doing harm.

Respecting autonomy involves respecting another person's rights and dignity such that a person reaches a maximum level of

A patient who has undergone heart bypass surgery continues to smoke after the operation.

■ Is it justifiable to refuse further treatment?
■ What factors do you take into account in making your judgement?

This extract suggests the following:
'a doctor who takes seriously his self-imposed and professional obligation to benefit his patient ought to treat the patient if that is what the patient on reflection wants him to do, if some treatment is available which will provide net benefit to the patient ... Of course that in no way prevents the doctor from advising that the most effective way of regaining and maintaining health is to alter one's lifestyle in the relevant way. But coercion will generally be contraindicated by the requirement to respect people's autonomy, and withdrawal of care from those who reject one's advice will generally be contraindicated by a doctor's personally and professionally undertaken duty of care, or obligation of beneficence' (Gillon 1990, p. 34).

fulfilment as a human being. In the context of health promotion and health care this means that the relationship with patients or clients is based on a respect for them as people, and with individual rights. It follows that we must then see them as 'whole people' – with physical, social, emotional and spiritual needs – as fundamentally equal and also as unique individuals.

Rights in relation to health care are usually taken to include:

■ the right to information
■ the right to privacy and confidentiality
■ the right to appropriate care and treatment.

Parents, pupils or staff of a school may wish to know of the presence of an HIV-positive child or member of staff, either out of concern about a possible health risk to themselves or their child, or because they believe a sharing of such information would enable them to provide better care and support for the child.

Should this information be disclosed?
This situation raises issues about the right to information and the right to privacy. Most authorities would emphasize respect for the individual's right to privacy. As there is no health risk attached to the presence of an HIV-positive person if good hygiene is routinely applied, there is no harm in keeping HIV status confidential. Indeed, the possible harm to the individual that might arise in the case of disclosure, from possible discrimination or isolation, outweighs these understandable concerns.

Health workers are often placed in the position of deciding whether to inform patients or relatives of an adverse prognosis. Although the patients' right to information is usually considered paramount, there are occasions when the health workers' duty of beneficence – to do good and avoid harm – may outweigh this right.

Beneficence and non-maleficence

Frankena (1963) suggests that beneficence means doing or promoting good as well as preventing, removing and avoiding evil or harm. The common good is often put before individual good. The wearing of a seat belt may halve the risk of death to the driver but the odds that a particular individual will ever benefit are not great, as few people will be killed on the roads. Rose (1981) termed this the 'prevention paradox', according to which a measure that brings large benefits to the community offers little to each participating individual. The alternative to a mass approach is to focus on risk groups but this may stigmatize certain groups (Naidoo & Wills 1998).

 Immunization is effective only if a high level of immunity is achieved in the population. Is it ethical for individuals to be persuaded to take up a vaccine if its safety is in doubt?

After considering a response to this dilemma, note the example of congenital rubella syndrome.

Rubella vaccine is given to children of both sexes as part of the two-stage (15 months and 4 years) measles, mumps and rubella (MMR) combined immunization programme. Unless 90% of children are immunized, girls who are not vaccinated are likely to reach child-bearing age without a natural immunity. Before MMR, when the vaccine was given only to girls at puberty, this situation would have been unlikely.

The intent to promote the health of the community may thus have adverse consequences for a small minority of women.

 What is the nature of 'goodness' in health promotion work?

For the health promoter doing good may be said to be improving the health and well-being of individuals or groups. Traditional preventive health education may be regarded as a protective beneficence which prevents harm in the long term. A dilemma arises for the practitioner when the outcome or consequence of an action which is deemed 'good' for the health of the community may involve harm for the individual. Immunization, regarded as a key element in preventive health education, poses this sort of dilemma.

In such circumstances the duty to care has to be extended to include the concept of informed consent. The individual must be informed, and understand the information and implications of any action which is taken to be beneficial. In this way the health worker can be said to be avoiding harm.

In the field of drug education, harm minimization is increasingly adopted as a way of working. This is perhaps more realistic than the encompassing principle of doing no harm. The health care worker recognizes that clients may not wish to change their behaviour, and therefore seeks to encourage a safer way of life and reduce its harm. Drug workers may give clients clean needles, condoms, and provide information about emergency first aid to reduce the risks of HIV infection or accidents.

The example of screening illustrates the complexities of ethical decision-making and how attempting to follow the key ethical principles of doing good and avoiding harm is not a simple process. Most preventive services are offered with an explicit promise that they will do some good and an implicit understanding that they will do no harm. Yet what is the nature of that good? Screening, for example, only tells people that they are healthy at the present time. A negative result does not mean that illness will not develop the following year. Screening cannot promise a good outcome. Early detection can mean more effective or less radical treatment in some cases, but there may be no medical benefit and no treatment

 Consider these points in relation to a screening process with which you are familiar. Do you conclude that screening is of benefit, avoids harm and respects all persons equally?

1. Screening is never wholly routine and inclusive. It is targeted to identified risk groups and therefore excludes certain categories of people, usually on the grounds of age.
2. Screening is spaced because of economic considerations and therefore people may develop the disease in the intervening period.
3. The screening process may foster anxieties.
4. The screening process may be uncomfortable or painful.
5. The call and recall procedures may be poorly handled and the informing of results may take some time.
6. Laboratory protocols may not be rigorous enough, leading to the need for repeat tests.
7. Screening uses high-sensitivity methods which can result in a high number of false positive results. These people will be subjected to unnecessary worry and distress, and in some cases treatment.
8. Screening uses methods which are less than 100% specific – therefore some people will go away falsely reassured.

available. This used to be the case with HIV infection. However, combination therapies may present or delay illness in some people with HIV.

Ethically, screening represents the tension between beneficence and non-maleficence. It is seen as good but is not without harm. Stoate (1989) has argued that poorly conducted screening can cause psychological harm from, for example, receiving false positive results. Duncan (1990) argues that screening highlights the importance of informed consent, and clients being aware of the benefits and disadvantages. Unfortunately, the pressure to ensure adequate take-up and to demonstrate success of a service means screening is often 'sold' to the public and they are not fully informed. Duncan concludes that health promoters must ask:

- Are we enabling our clients' participation in screening?
- Are we helping to put this episode and any resulting advice in the context of their lives?
- Are we selling what is on offer in such a way that it is quite clear what is being sold? (Duncan 1990).

Justice

Philosophers suggest three versions of justice:

- the fair distribution of scarce resources
- respect for individual and group rights
- following morally acceptable laws.

Thus, justice requires that people are treated equally. But what is meant by equal? Does it mean according to equal need? Or according to merit? Or according to equal contribution? Or ensuring non-discriminatory practices?

For example, the equal distribution of resources can mean different things. It could mean that resources should be distributed equally in mathematical terms. Or should they be distributed according to how much was contributed – thus those that have and can put in most get out most? Or should we apply the Marxist adage 'From each according to his ability, to each according to his needs'? The NHS was established on the basis of free medical care to all those who need it. In an era of scarce resources, demand far exceeds supply. Need is an obvious criterion for distributing care but it is not sufficient. Tudor Hart, whose inverse care law was described in Chapter 2, observed that those who needed health care most received least (Tudor Hart 1971). As we shall see in Chapter 17 although we may use some objective measurement for the assessment of individual health needs, such as the ability to self-care or to perform certain tasks, this does not overcome the subjective value judgement that is involved in making these decisions. In recent years, health economists have tried to establish some other sort of objective and measurable criteria to compare competing claims – possibly the relative financial costs of treatment or an assessment made on QALYs, which are described in Chapter 3.

Justice and resource distribution

Families of children with Down's syndrome have claimed that the National Health Service withheld life-saving surgery. Research by the Down's Syndrome Association reveals medical prejudice and defeatism, leading in some instances to denial of pain relief and surgery. A BMA spokesperson stated '(patients) should all be treated as individuals, not on the basis of some classification'.

Source: *The Observer*, 22 February 1998, page 5

Issues of justice are glaringly evident in health promotion. We read earlier the evidence of wide differences in health status between different groups in society. Whilst health promoters may be unable to alter society's inequities they may, nevertheless, be able to work on programmes which acknowledge that people's abilities to achieve health differ, which avoid victim blaming and which tackle discriminatory practices.

Being fair to everyone might seem to suggest adopting public health measures which iron out differences in resources, health care or environmental quality. Yet any kind of state intervention means addressing the issue of individual rights versus the common good. For instance, would it be just that top wage earners should pay 50% income tax to finance public spending on health and welfare? The following chapter examines different political perspectives on health promotion, and the fundamental differences between right and left of the political spectrum towards health and welfare.

Telling the truth

The process of health education and information-giving in health promotion also involves complex ethical decisions. Seedhouse (1988) identifies truth-telling and promise-keeping as principles which the health promoter should hold on to when deliberating a course of action. As we saw earlier, the individual's right to information and the health promoter's duty to tell the truth may conflict with the duty of beneficence.

Practitioners want people to make healthy choices. When convinced of the 'good' of an action, practitioners may seek to persuade, perhaps through raising clients' anxiety or selecting the information or evidence. Yet ethical health promotion also includes a commitment to enhancing autonomy. As we saw in Chapter 4, the essential nature of health promotion is that it is based on a principle of voluntarism. It should neither seek to coerce or persuade, but to facilitate an informed choice.

Is it ethical to carry out opportunistic health education in primary health care?

Consider the example of a patient who goes to her GP with back pain. The doctor takes the opportunity for some health education, and takes the patient's blood pressure and family history. The patient had neither sought this nor was she made aware beforehand of the implications should raised blood pressure be found. The patient has not freely chosen to have her blood pressure checked in this way. Although she gave her consent, it might not be regarded as fully informed.

Campbell (1990) suggests that persuasion is acceptable only if a true picture of various aspects is presented. All education, he argues, involves some persuasion, and it is too simplistic to suggest that a desire to empower and create autonomy rules out persuasion. This means, however, that the health promoter must ensure that clients *seek* advice and help, and are not persuaded against their will. Yet many health promoters would argue that the only way to balance this need to empower people *and* facilitate healthier choices is to make this easier through policy decisions and frameworks (see Chapter 9). This takes us back to the argument that healthy public policy prioritizes the public good over individual freedom of choice and may not even be mandated by public opinion.

There may also be debate about the point at which enough information has been collected to justify legislative or coercive means of health promotion. Government bans on beef on the bone and unpasteurized green-top milk are examples where government action has been criticized for removing choice and leading to negative effects on employment and economic activity. Yet government inaction in the field of regulation and labelling of genetically modified food has also been criticized for removing people's right to make decisions based on information.

In the following chapter we will explore how information about what is deemed 'healthy' is often influenced by political decisions and vested interests.

There is also an increasing trend towards sponsorship for health promotion activities. This ranges from health research sponsored by a tobacco company trust to the sponsorship of health information by drug companies, sanitary wear manufacturers or a local health food shop. Is sponsorship compatible with health promotion? The code

Because the knowledge base of health promotion is changing, there are few areas where recommendations can be made on a factual basis. Kemm (1991) has described health promotion as lacking rigour and based on 'best available opinion'. It is possible to think of numerous examples in recent years where information on the risks or benefits of certain behaviours has changed.

■ The contraceptive pill is now contraindicated for a wider group of women.
■ The importance of reducing saturated fat for those with normal cholesterol levels is disputed.
■ Potatoes are no longer thought to be fattening but a good bulk food and source of fibre.
■ Moderate amounts of alcohol are now thought to have a beneficial effect on the heart.

Should the public be made aware of debates over the evidence for health promotion advice? Should interventions be employed when the evidence for their effectiveness is in doubt?

of practice of the Society of Health Education/Promotion Specialists (1997) suggests that sponsorship is acceptable when it comes from enterprises compatible with health promotion principles and practices, and when the acceptance of income does not divert the practitioners from meeting more demonstrable health needs.

Which of the following would you find acceptable?

■ A curriculum pack for schools on puberty, sponsored by a sanitary wear manufacturer
■ A leaflet on safer sex sponsored by the London Rubber Company manufacturers of condoms
■ A research project on healthy lifestyles supported by a tobacco company trust
■ An education project for convicted drink-drivers sponsored by a brewery group
■ An information handbook on local support services which includes advertisements for local businesses

Conclusion

Do practitioners whose work involves decisions affecting the lives of others engage in a moral deliberation about the best course of action? In general, most combine features of utility and deontology.

They respect autonomy, try to be honest and fair, and avoid victim blaming. At the same time they try to achieve the best overall solution to any given situation. Yet situations can involve complex layers of decision-making involving many ethical dilemmas. Screening, for example, a frequently unchallenged linchpin of preventive health promotion, raises key issues about its benefits for an individual versus the increase of the social good, as well as questions about the extent to which screening is honestly presented. Before we can make any sort of ethical judgement we need to be clear about the values and principles which underpin our actions. If we return to the questions asked earlier in this chapter, what do we mean by doing good and avoiding harm? At what point should we switch from creating autonomy to respecting autonomy? What does justice and equity mean in health promotion practice?

Tools to enable clear thinking around ethical issues, such as the SHEPS (1997) code of practice or Seedhouse's (1988) ethical grid provide a way to clarify decision-making and make the process more transparent. But dilemmas remain, and following different principles (each of which is sound and desirable) may lead to contradictory courses of action. Whilst there may never be absolute answers in ethical decision-making, a way forward is to be clear about which principles and duties you value most, and to encourage an open debate about ethical principles and how these translate into health promotion practice.

Take a health promotion programme with which you are familiar. To what extent does this programme incorporate the following principles of practice (SHEPS 1997)?

- The promotion of self-esteem and autonomy
- The attempt to counter prejudice and discrimination
- The recognition of and action focused on the social, economic and environmental determinants of health
- Empowerment to enable the exercise of informed choice and influence
- Sustainability (positive impact on both present and future generations)
- Accurate and appropriate information flow between public, professionals and local and national agencies
- Health-promoting processes and methods

Questions for further discussion

- Should we 'sell' health?
- Should there be more legislation to promote health?

Summary

Health promoters need to be clear that what they do involves certain values and principles about what is 'good' health and health promotion. Beneficence, justice and respect for persons and their autonomy are fundamental ethical principles in health promotion. Their application in practice, however, is often problematic. Every situation or potential intervention involves a judgement not only of its possible effectiveness but of its morality – whether it is 'right' or 'wrong'. In this chapter we have defined these key ethical principles and considered how they are manifested in common dilemmas for the health promotion practitioner.

Further reading

Doxiadis S (ed) 1987 Ethical dilemmas in health promotion. Wiley, Chichester. *Contains theoretical chapters which examine the conflict between autonomy and the common good, and then considers practical problems such as the value of health legislation, health economics and paternalism in disease prevention. A final section covers ethical aspects of reproductive medicine, screening programmes and mass communication in health education.*

Doxiadis S (ed) 1990 Ethics in health promotion. Wiley, Chichester. *Ethical issues in health education are the focus of this book which looks at the ethics of health persuasion and legislation. A final section covers the ethical dilemmas of HIV and AIDS prevention, nutrition education and mental health promotion.*

Downie R S, Tannahill C, Tannahill A 1996 Health promotion: models and values. Oxford Medical Publications, Oxford. *Chapters 10 and 11 consider the nature of autonomy and justice and the value base for health promotion activities. The book sets out to answer the questions: 'What is health promotion for and why is it worthwhile?'*

Gillon R 1985 Philosophical medical ethics. Wiley, Chichester. *An accessible introduction to ethics in medicine with numerous case studies.*

Rumbold G 1993 Ethics in nursing practice, 2nd edn. Baillière Tindall, London. *An introduction to ethics and ethical theories and principles. It discusses how these relate to the work of health care workers.*

Seedhouse D 1988 Ethics: the heart of health care. Wiley, Chichester. *An excellent guide for health promotion practitioners which uses accessible case studies to show how working for health is inextricably bound up with ethics. The ethical grid provides a practical framework to be applied in day-to-day work.*

References

Beauchamp T L, Childress J F 1995 Principles of biomedical ethics. Oxford University Press, Oxford

Campbell A V 1990 Education or indoctrination? The issue of autonomy in health education. In: Doxiadis S (ed) Ethics in health promotion. Wiley, Chichester, pp 15–27

Doxiadis S (ed) 1990 Ethics in health promotion. Wiley, Chichester

Duncan P 1990 To screen or not to screen: a question of ethics. Health Education Journal 49: 120–122

Ewles L, Simnett I 1999 Promoting health: a practical guide, 4th edn. Baillière Tindall, Edinburgh

Frankena W K 1963 Ethics. Prentice Hall, Englewood Cliffs, NJ

Gillon R 1990 Health education: the ambiguity of the medical role. In: Doxiadis S (ed) Ethics in health promotion. Wiley, Chichester, pp 29–41

Kant I 1909 On the supposed right to tell lies from benevolent motives. Cited in: Rumbold G 1991 Ethics in nursing and midwifery practice. Distance Learning Centre, South Bank University, London

Kemm J 1991 Health education and the problem of knowledge. Health Promotion International 6(4): 261–269

Naidoo J, Wills J 1998 Practising health promotion: dilemmas and challenges. Baillière Tindall, London

Rose G 1981 Strategy of prevention: lessons from cardiovascular disease. British Medical Journal 282: 1847–1851

Seedhouse D 1988 Ethics: the heart of health care. Wiley, Chichester

Society of Health Education and Promotion Specialists 1997 Principles of practice and code of professional conduct for health education and promotion specialists. SHEPS

Stoate H G 1989 Can health screening damage your health. Journal of Royal College of General Practitioners 39: 193–195

Tudor Hart J 1971 The inverse care law. Lancet 1: 405

United Kingdom Central Council for Nursing, Midwifery and Health Visiting (UKCC) 1992 Code of Professional conduct for the nurse, midwife and health visitor. UKCC, London

7 *The politics of health promotion*

OVERVIEW

Politics and health promotion are often thought of as separate activities. However, different approaches to health promotion reflect different political positions. This chapter outlines the diversity of social and political philosophies, which helps us to understand how health promotion has developed in the social and political context of the late 20th century. Understanding our own values helps us to see the logical consequences for health promotion. The political dimensions of health promotion in relation to its organization, its methods and the content of health promotion activity are then explored.

What is politics?

Politics is most often thought of as relating to party politics but we shall use a broader definition of the term in this chapter. Politics may be defined as the study of the distribution and effects of power in society. Power itself may be defined in different ways. Power includes not only material or physical resources, but also psychological and cultural aspects, which may be equally effective in limiting or channelling people.

No-one is totally devoid of power and no-one is all powerful. But within a highly stratified society, such as the UK, different groups of people typically will possess different amounts of power. Although we live in a democratic society with one person one vote, power is unequally distributed. Gender, race, age, social class, wealth and disability structure power relationships between groups of people, and this has effects on health, as discussed in Chapter 2. Structural factors such as class and gender affect power relationships in an institutionalized and patterned manner. In general, people in the lower social classes and women have less control over their own lives, and the lives of others compared to men in higher social classes. But it is impossible to predict the power relationships between people. This is due both to the complexity of the interrelationship between different factors, and also to personal power or charisma which exists in the relationships between actual people. People in subordinate positions may have the opportunity and skills to exercise a greater degree of power or influence than could be anticipated. Hence the well-known phenomenon of the receptionist or secretary who is said to 'run the office'.

Political ideologies

One of the arenas in which power relationships are manifest is social policy, which may be defined as planned government activities designed to maintain, integrate and regulate society. This includes both welfare and economic policies, ranging from national legislation to local policy developments within local authorities. Government policies are determined according to its beliefs and ideas – its ideological position. Different political positions give rise to certain types of policy interventions. Analysts have identified many different frameworks (Bunton 1992, George & Wilding 1994, Lee & Raban 1988). In general, ideological positions are identified along a spectrum ranging from those advocating a free market economy with minimal state intervention to those advocating a planned economy with maximum state intervention. Conservatives or socialists who advocate a mixed economy and a welfare state occupy the middle of the spectrum (see Table 7.1).

Views on health and health promotion reflect a complex mix of values and beliefs which, in turn, reflect different political ideologies. These ideas and values will lead to us having different explanations for, and responses to, social and health problems. For example, the sedentary condition of the population may be seen as a consequence of individual laziness or the lack of an integrated transport policy which would encourage people to walk and cycle. Key beliefs on which people differ concern:

- the extent of personal responsibility
- the role of government legislation and intervention
- legitimate means to encourage choices and decisions
- the nature of society and the extent to which people are connected to each other.

On the right of the political spectrum there is a belief in individual self-determination and an antipathy to government intervention which not only restricts freedom, but also inhibits enterprise. Conservatism sees inequality as inevitable but advocates a paternalistic state which safeguards the most vulnerable. It was a Conservative politician, Beveridge, who first mooted the idea of a welfare state and the need for government to tackle the five giants of 'want, disease, ignorance, squalor and idleness'. Socialism is

Table 7.1 *A typology of welfare ideologies*

(Political left)   (Political right)

Political ideology	Marxism	Fabian socialism	Conservatism	Liberalism/new right
Role of state	Collectivist	Collectivist	Reluctant collectivists	Anti-collectivist
View of economy	Planned economy	Mixed economy	Mixed economy	Free market Market liberals
View of society	Present class society characterized by class conflict will be superseded by socialism characterized by 'from each according to their ability; to each according to their need'	Equality of opportunity, economic and political freedom is safeguarded by the State The State should enable individual self-fulfilment and social justice through redistribution	Inequality is inevitable but there should be equality of opportunity The State's role is to provide for the vulnerable and needy, but individual freedom of choice must be protected	Inequalities in wealth are inevitable Market forces ensure people's needs are met in a satisfactory manner
View of health care	Universal and free State provision	Universal and free State provision to promote social cohesion and redistribution plus individual provision if desired	Paternalistic State should provide a safety net of health care provision, alongside individual responsibility	Individual responsibility and freedom of choice Needs are best met through the free market Consumerism
Core values	Equality Collective responsibility Freedom from material want	Equality Collective responsibility Humanitarianism Social harmony Social justice	Individualism Freedom Responsibility Authority	Individualism Freedom Choice Competition

based on a belief in equality and fellowship, or a sense of responsibility for others. The government has a distinct role to play in redistributing material resources and promoting a sense of community. Marxism embraces the values of equality, collective responsibility and freedom from want. To achieve these goals requires revolutionary change and the transformation of the capitalist state to a Marxist state. The Marxist state has a key role in planning the economy to meet needs.

Following the Second World War, British policy favoured a middle point in the spectrum. All political parties were united by a consensus that the Welfare State was a desirable goal and that a certain amount of state intervention was necessary. From a 'one nation' Tory point of view, state intervention was necessary to curb the worst excesses of capitalism, which left some people without means of support. For example, if capitalist recession leads to mass unemployment, it is legitimate to intervene to protect the unemployed from destitution. Without this intervention, the system becomes unstable. From a socialist perspective, the Welfare State is a means of gradually reforming the State from within. The Welfare State is a means of redistributing wealth, and incremental reforms are capable of transforming the State from an instrument of capitalism to an instrument of socialism.

This consensus was disrupted by the economic recession and fiscal crisis of the mid-1970s. The burgeoning costs of welfare, triggered by the changing demographic structure of the population and mass unemployment, gave rise to government concern, and set the scene for the ascendency of a new political ideology. The new right or Thatcherism became the dominant ideology in the 1980s. The new right is characterized by a more laissez-faire attitude favouring no state intervention in the economy. It is argued that the State needs to retreat from its commitment to welfare. The Welfare State is seen as having undesirable effects, such as raising the level of expectations beyond what can be provided. Universal provision for all denies individual choices and is an ineffective means of meeting needs. In addition, the Welfare State transforms people into dependents and saps their independence. The free market is seen as a more desirable means for meeting welfare needs. The free market protects individual choice, and will lead to a more rational provision of goods and services, as only those things for which there is a demonstrable need will be produced. Competition will reduce wastage and inefficiencies in the system.

The new right combines this economic liberal or laissez-faire attitude with a conservative authoritarianism which prioritizes the need for strong moral values and authority invested in the power of the State. This combination means that, at the same time as government is retreating from economic intervention, it is engaged in extending state power over the everyday lives of the population.

Thus health is something we can all choose and the market is the mechanism through which health – a commodity supposedly available to all – can be 'purchased'.

Consider the social policy interventions referred to in these newspaper headlines about particular government policies. What values are being reflected?

■ Patients become consumers with the right to choose
■ Hospitals forced into competitive tendering to provide services for health districts
■ New moves to force absent fathers to provide for their children
■ Minister calls for parents to be responsible for crimes committed by their children
■ Ban on tobacco advertising and sponsorship announced
■ Lower benefits for lone parents to encourage women to work
■ Health checks for everyone over 75

In 1997 a Labour Government was elected in the UK. This government eschewed old-style socialism in favour of a 'New Labour' philosophy, characterized by a strong sense of social responsibility and concept of community. Instead of the retreat of government from its role in welfare, New Labour promotes an active, protective role for the State in creating individual opportunities. England's 'Our Healthier Nation' strategy proposes a contract between individuals, communities and government, where each has defined responsibilities. Chapter 8 explores in more detail the idea of working in partnerships to promote health. The New Right's simplistic assertion that health and ill health lie in the hands of the individual have been replaced by a broader explanation for health and ill health which locates root causes in social conditions such as income levels, employment opportunities, quality of housing and the environment.

The political context affects all areas of government policy including health. The central proposition of this chapter is that health promotion takes place in the policy area and is, therefore, inescapably, a political activity. The next sections will examine the evidence for this proposition, looking first at the structure and organization of health promotion, then at its methods, and finally at the content of health promotion.

The politics of health promotion structures and organization

Health promotion has enjoyed varying levels of government support throughout the 20th century. The box on page 138 gives a brief history of political ideologies and their impact on health promotion.

In most recent times, health education and promotion was enthusiastically supported in the mid 1970s and again in the beginning of the 1990s. The Department of Health and Social Security (DHSS) report, Prevention and Health: Everybody's Business, was published in 1976, and was followed by other reports which examined health promotion in relation to specific topics such as heart disease and alcohol (DHSS 1981a, 1981b). The priority accorded to health promotion has been directly related to the state of the economy. With the economic crisis of the mid-1970s, health promotion came to be viewed as a means of cost cutting. If people could be prevented from becoming ill, health service costs could be

 A brief history of health promotion in the UK

1800–1900 Public health movement
Arose out of a conservative tradition of reluctant collectivism, that the State had to intervene to ensure national efficiency, economic advantage and social stability

1900–1940 Health education
A liberal laissez-faire agenda which allowed voluntary organizations to provide preventive health education

1940–1970s Rise of prevention
A broadly conservative ideology with the emphasis on individual responsibility for health with information and advice being provided by health professionals; this was coupled with state intervention to provide a safety net for the most vulnerable

1980s The rise of the individual
Despite calls for a coherent national programme to tackle widespread inequalities in health and the WHO Ottawa Charter, New Right ideology dominates the health service; individual freedom is emphasized

1990s The rise of the market
Emphasis is on public accountability to the consumer in services and the need to consult lay views
Collaboration is advocated as means of efficiency and to reduce demands on the health service
Despite an environmental consciousness this is not seen as an agenda for government action

1997 onwards The rise of social responsibility and the New Public Health
Acknowledgment of the link between poverty and ill health
Emphasis on public participation in care and services, and the development of social capital
Promotion of the New Public Health

reduced and economic productivity increased. In the 1990s with an ageing population and technological advances there were great demands on health care. Health promotion was again seen as a way of preventing ill health and a cheaper form of provision than care.

Whilst health promotion is seen as 'everybody's business', certain groups and organizational settings have been identified as the base for health promotion. In the 19th century, public health was the key function of local councils who regulated and legislated to control what were seen as the causes of disease – poor sanitation, food hygiene and waste disposal. In the late 20th century UK, the National Health Service (NHS) has come to be regarded as the natural home for health promotion.

In 1974 a reorganization separated environmental health (located in local authorities) from community health and health promotion (located in the NHS). Health promotion has been a 'Cinderella' service subordinated to health care provision and the medical model. The siting of health promotion within the NHS has made it more difficult to influence other factors which affect health, such as housing, education, transport and leisure facilities. A major reorganization took place during the period 1989–1991. The NHS and Community Care Act 1991 established an internal market within the NHS with purchaser health authorities and provider NHS trusts established as separate organizations. These reforms reflected the view of the government that it was necessary to not only control health service costs but also health service professionals through managed competition. The Conservative Government's view that people are consumers of services and that a market would lead to greater efficiency and more choice was also reflected in these reforms. Specialist health promotion departments providing training, resources, media liaison and support for projects were mostly located in trusts. A small proportion adopted a more strategic health assessment and planning role within purchasing authorities and some divided to retain a foothold in both providing and purchasing organizations (French & Milner 1997).

In 1997 the new Labour Government created a Minister for Public Health whose responsibility it is to coordinate health policy across different sectors and highlight the health impact of different policies. Chapter 11 on public health work examines the relationship between health promotion and public health in more detail.

The Labour Government introduced new reforms of the NHS in a White Paper 'The New NHS – Modern, Dependable' in 1997 (DoH 1997). The new NHS reforms are intended to replace the competitive ethos and wasteful duplication which characterized the internal market with integrated care led by primary care groups (PCGs). PCGs are groups of GPs and community nurses who are responsible for commissioning, and possibly providing, health care

The following example shows how 'joined-up policy-making' by different agencies can contribute in a coordinated way to the aim of suicide reduction.

Socio-economic policies
- New Deal employment policy to reduce joblessness
- Social Exclusion Unit to promote social integration

Environmental policies
- Public housing to reduce homelessness
- Integrated transport policy to reduce isolation

Lifestyle policies
- Healthy Living Centres to promote exercise and healthy lifestyles amongst disadvantaged and vulnerable groups
- Reducing access to means of suicide through, for example, blister packs and catalytic converters

Service provision policies
- Training for primary care staff
- Funding for voluntary mental health agencies

What could joined-up policies contribute to the aims of:
1. coronary heart disease prevention?
2. cancer prevention?

Consider the following health topics. How do they rank in terms of importance to health? Which are the most politically 'sensitive'? Which have been the subject of health education and promotion campaigns?

- Coronary heart disease
- Poverty
- Homelessness
- Asthma
- Unemployment
- Accidents
- Mental ill health
- Poor housing

services for their local population. PCGs along with health authorities, NHS trusts and local authorities will contribute to local 3-year health-improvement programmes (HImPs). Health promotion is thus implicit in the new reforms but it is unlikely to get a greater share of the budget. These reforms reflect the wish of the Government for more 'bottom-up' services and a greater focus on public health rather than acute services.

Each of the United Kingdom countries has a national lead body for health promotion. In England, this role is taken by the Health

Development Agency which is responsible to the Department of Health and which commissions research and health promotion interventions. A similar role is taken by the Health Education Board for Scotland, the Northern Ireland Health Promotion Agency and the Welsh Assembly.

Health promotion activities are structured by the prevailing policy framework which has the effect of legitimizing certain approaches and excluding others. Until 1997 the New Right political ideology was paramount. The combination of free market economics with authoritarianism favoured medical preventive approaches and those which focus on individual lifestyles. Health promotion was seen as a means to prevent morbidity and mortality from specified diseases. Education and advice were the key strategies. Primary care practitioners would identify individuals at risk from a database of the practice population and carry out lifestyle interventions.

The New Labour ideology sees a highly interventionist role for government. The emphasis is on local collaborative planning by groups of key stakeholders to determine health priorities. The NHS is not seen as 'uniquely placed' to deliver health promotion. There is a greater belief in a social model of health which recognizes the impact of social inequalities on health. Health promotion activities are less centred on education and information and more on changing policies and conditions to enable people to make healthier choices.

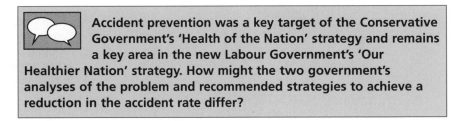

Accident prevention was a key target of the Conservative Government's 'Health of the Nation' strategy and remains a key area in the new Labour Government's 'Our Healthier Nation' strategy. How might the two government's analyses of the problem and recommended strategies to achieve a reduction in the accident rate differ?

The politics of health promotion methods

The methods used in health promotion are often viewed as a technical choice. Health promotion specialists are seen as possessing the expertise to decide what methods will prove most effective given the circumstances. However, we shall argue that methods imply political perspectives, and that the choice of which methods to use is not a politically neutral decision.

Health promotion has at its disposal a large repertoire of methods. These are discussed in greater detail in Section 2. Beattie's typology of health promotion described on pages 105–106 classifies health promotion models according to two dimensions, the focus of intervention and the mode of intervention (Beattie 1991). Health promotion methods may be similarly classified (see Fig. 7.1). Figure

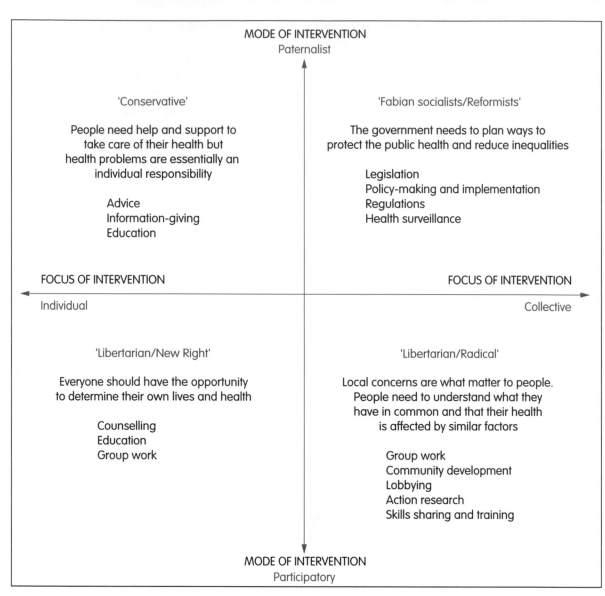

Figure 7.1   *Health promotion methods and political philosophies. Adapted from Beattie (1991, 1993).*

7.1 is not an exhaustive list of the repertoire of health promotion methods but it does indicate the range of methods used in health promotion. We shall consider each cell in turn, identifying the methods used and tracing their political implications. Social policy, similarly, is divided between paternalist ('top-down') and participatory ('bottom-up') approaches and between an emphasis on individualized or collective problems and solutions (Beattie 1993).

The individual paternalist approach (Conservative)
Methods focused on the individual send a clear message about individual responsibility for health. Such methods rely on the belief

that individuals can make significant changes in their lifestyle or environment. The focus on the individual also implies that everyone has equal resources and means of complying with health promotion messages. This may be viewed as ineffective, or incorrect, and there has been much criticism of these methods in these terms, as 'victim-blaming' and misconceived (Naidoo 1986). However, such a viewpoint is also politically inspired, which may go some way to explaining its endurance in the face of professional criticism.

By ignoring structural factors which affect the life chances and perceptions of different groups of people, the fact that people's personal identity is bound up with their membership of such groups is obscured.

**Write down 10 words which describe yourself.
How many of the following did you include? Which of the features are used to divide people into different social groups?**

- Gender
- Age
- Class
- Occupation
- Education
- Ethnic origin
- Family relationships
- Appearance
- Character
- Sexuality

People are seen as separate from others and their environment. Individualism is firmly entrenched in liberalism and the new right. The notion of individual free choice is a central tenet of both the free-market economy and liberal political ideology. By contrast, socialism and Marxism prioritize the collectivity, people united by circumstances into groups with opposing interests.

The individual participatory approach (Libertarian/New Right)

The individual negotiated cell includes methods such as counselling, education and group work. These methods envisage a different, and more equal, relationship between the health promoter and the client than those derived from the individual paternalist cell. The health promotion intervention is to be negotiated between both parties, taking into account people's beliefs, attitudes and knowledge. The client is an active partner in the process and the end goal is enhanced client autonomy. Many professional groups have shifted

What criticisms can be offered of this approach in terms of promoting the nation's health?

their practice in recent years and tried to become more client-centred. Many health promoters feel more comfortable using these methods.

It may be argued that individually negotiated methods are most used and valued by the relatively privileged and healthy sections of society. Those with the greatest need are least likely to be able to access this kind of health promotion intervention.

The collective participatory approach (Libertarian/Radical)

Methods which focus on the collectivity are more likely to be allied to socialist or Marxist political ideologies. The emphasis here is on understanding the processes which shape health outcomes, and assisting people to develop the skills to challenge these processes. The spectrum of political beliefs may range from a sense of responsibility to others to a sense of sharing the same experience as one's neighbour. Freire (1972) described this process of identifying and naming the problem and recognizing it as a shared experience of oppression as conscientization or critical consciousness raising.

Methods of health promotion seek to redistribute power by empowering disadvantaged groups through such means as action research, skills sharing and training and lobbying.

In the late 1990s there has been a renewed interest in community programmes and an increasing recognition that engaging local people and training and supporting volunteers and networkers is an effective means of promoting health. The Jakarta Declaration stated that health promotion is a means of building 'social capital' with the ultimate goal being 'to increase health expectancy and to narrow the gap in health expectancy between countries and groups' (Health Promotion International 1997, p. 261).

'Health promotion needs to be involved in helping to repair the social fabric of society by building "social capital": communities with a high level of social capital are characterised by high levels of trust, positive social norms and many overlapping and diverse horizontal networks for communication and exchange of information, ideas and practical help.' (Gillies 1997, p. 15).

- What could account for this interest in social capital?
- What particular political beliefs does it reflect?
- Does it suggest that health promotion is a political undertaking?

The collective paternalist approach (Fabian socialists/Reformists)

The collective paternalist methods of working may be located in either the Marxist or new right political ideologies, depending on the underlying values and purposes of such methods. For Marxists, the collectivity is structured into opposing classes by social stratification variables. Appropriate action uses methods such as the active redistribution of power in favour of the disadvantaged, which is also advocated by socialist groups. Examples of this range from proposals for equal pay across the NHS to welfare-oriented policies such as proposals to improve housing, increase maternity benefits, or to provide universal free school meals. All of these measures are supported by research as effective means of improving health and reducing health inequalities (Townsend et al 1988).

On the other hand, the New Right represents the collectivity as the sum total of many individuals, each with different and competing interests. Appropriate intervention is then designed to protect individual rights, which may only be superseded to protect the common good or the wider body politic. For example, immunization is an imposition on individual freedom but may be supported because it helps protect the health of the whole community. The tension between individual freedom and

---

 The methods adopted by practitioners in response to particular issues reflect political values about:

- humanity – the rights of people
- responsibility – whether health is in the hands of the individual or a result of particular social patterns which are reproduced and maintained by social policies
- the role of the practitioner – whether practitioners should hold power in the form of professional expertise or whether knowledge should be defined and shared by people themselves
- the role of government – whether the State should take an active role in protecting its citizens' health or whether responsibility for health should lie with the individual.

Consider the following methods which might be adopted to support HIV prevention with vulnerable young people:

- enhancing self-esteem
- peer education
- educational media campaign
- young people's sexual health clinic run by nurses
- funding for a telephone helpline run by a voluntary self-help group
- easier and more open access to condoms
- more opportunities for young people to gain work experience and skills
- creation of hostels and sheltered housing for homeless young people.

What political values are being reflected in each approach?

community well-being may explain why immunization remains voluntary in the UK, whereas in other countries, including the USA, child immunization is a prerequisite of school enrolment.

This discussion has presented the view that the methods chosen to promote health are not politically neutral. Certain methods fit into, maintain and reproduce the ideological assumptions of certain political perspectives. However, it is important not to overstate this view. Methods and ideology are not deterministically linked in a cause and effect manner. A variety of methods across all four cells may be used by health workers who espouse a particular political viewpoint. There may be convincing reasons for adopting an eclectic methodology to promote health. But it is a fallacy to assume that methods are a technically neutral aspect of the health promoter's activity.

The politics of health promotion content

The previous sections have examined the view that the structure, organization and methods used in health promotion have a political dimension. It is sometimes argued that, although the process of promoting health is a political activity, the content of health promotion is neutral. Our position is that health promotion content is inevitably political. The framing of suitable agendas and the construction of what information is relevant are not value-neutral activities. On the contrary, they imply certain political values.

 What are health promotion priorities for the 21st century?

The Jakarta Conference (WHO 1997) identified the following priorities for worldwide health:
- urbanization
- demography (ageing population and population growth)
- chronic disease
- sedentary lifestyle
- resistance to antibiotics
- substance misuse
- violence (domestic, civil and international warfare)
- communicable disease
- environmental degradation
- globalization.

Perhaps the clearest example of the political nature of health promotion is the ongoing debate surrounding inequalities in health. Whilst there is a wealth of research evidence linking poverty and disadvantage with ill health (Acheson 1998, Benzeval et al 1995), different governments have reacted differently. For 18 years a

Conservative Government refused to recognize the evidence on social inequalities and health.

>
> In 1980 the Government released a limited number of copies of the Black Report on health inequalities over a bank holiday weekend. The recommendations of the Black Report included government investment and spending on housing, pre-school child care, child benefits, maternity grants and free school meals in order to reduce inequalities in health.
>
> How could you explain government action in the light of what the report contained?

Accepting the evidence, and the desirability of a healthy population, would have led the Government to adopt a policy of active intervention to reduce inequalities (similar to the socialist position in Fig. 7.1). By denying the evidence, a non-interventionist policy could be adopted which argued that the free market is the best means of meeting health needs. The 1992 'Health of the Nation' strategy did not even acknowledge health inequalities as an issue, referring only to 'variations in health status between different socio-economic groups within the population' (DoH 1992, p. 121).

By contrast, the Labour Government elected in 1997 acknowledges the link between social inequalities and disadvantage and health, although the strategy for health in England (DoH 1999) does not include targets to reduce health inequalities. Whilst there is little disagreement that major causes of disability and premature death, such as the key topics identified in 'Saving Lives: Our Healthier Nation' (CHD, cancers, accidents and mental health) deserve attention, there is disagreement concerning other known causes of ill health, such as poor housing, unemployment or low income.

Should issues such as poverty and unemployment be part of an agenda for health promotion?

Illegal drug use and drink driving have both been the subject of major government mass-media campaigns in the last decade. Why do you think these particular topics have been chosen?

The content of health promotion interventions is also affected by its media image and by concerns for proven effectiveness and evidence. If a health topic is constructed so that it mixes with other topics of central concern, such as maintaining law and order, it is more likely to receive recognition and funding.

Increasingly, practitioners are called upon to base their work on evidence. The rise of evidence-based practice can be clearly linked to New Right ideas about the accountability of practitioners and services to the 'consumer'. In health promotion, research is said to have identified certain risk factors for disease, and the health worker's role is to impart this knowledge to clients in an accessible way. This view of scientific neutrality has been criticized by social scientists (Chalmers 1982, Kuhn 1962), who point out that science is a social activity like any other, subject to similar constraints. Health-related research does not take place in ivory towers. Researchers

Funded health promotion research

- In 1989 Margaret Thatcher vetoed a proposed survey of people's sexual habits as part of the HEA's HIV/AIDS prevention strategy because she thought it intruded too much in people's personal affairs.
- Many health promotion researchers have accepted money from the tobacco industry's Health Promotion Trust in order to carry out their research.
- The British Nutrition Foundation, which funds research into diet and health, is sponsored by major food producers.

have to bid for funds, and provide findings which are acceptable to funders and the academic community.

The process of research is therefore not immune to political considerations. What evidence filters through to the general public as the scientific consensus on health topics is also the result of political processes. The very idea of scientific consensus in social science is debatable. There is no issue where there is 100% agreement of the 'scientific facts'. There are still scientists (albeit funded by the tobacco industry) who claim the causal link between cigarette smoking and lung cancer is unproven (FOREST 1981) and who contest the evidence that passive smoking is a health hazard (Huber et al 1993). And there are researchers who dispute the links between saturated fats and CHD (Le Fanu 1994).

The BSE crisis in the UK during the 1990s showed clearly how the meat industry, scientific experts, consumer groups and the government all have different interests in the presentation of information about BSE. This case study (summarized in the box on page 149) shows how the 'evidence' may be disputed, and how different groups have different evidence thresholds which they find persuasive in arguing for a policy response.

Being political

We have seen how health promotion arises from and reinforces political values and beliefs and takes place in a political context. Health promoters hold values and beliefs which are underpinned by established sets of ideas of ideologies. Many health promoters are engaged in practice which accords (more or less) with their personal values. The medical model of health provides a clear role for practitioners because it recognizes their expertise. It also gives a clear role for individuals to act to protect their own health. Some health promoters may find that their professional role at times comes into conflict with their political beliefs and values. A belief in

> **Bovine spongiform encephalopathy (BSE) crisis**
>
> | | |
> |---|---|
> | 1986 | Bovine spongiform encephalopathy (BSE) also known as 'mad cow disease' is first identified. |
> | 1989 | The specified bovine offals (SBO) ban is introduced to ensure potentially infective material from cows is excluded from the human food chain. |
> | December 1995 | The first deaths of young people from new-variant Creutzfeldt–Jakob disease, a fatal brain condition linked to eating contaminated beef, are reported. The Health Secretary and the Chief Medical Officer declare beef to be safe. Scientists state that beef products may carry a risk of contamination from BSE which could be transmitted to humans. The Meat and Livestock Commission take out advertisements in newspapers quoting the Chief Medical Officer's views that beef is safe. Oldham and Humberside Local Education Authority drop beef from their school menus. A BBC radio helpline advises callers to avoid certain beef products. The National Consumer Council suggests tighter controls in abattoirs to reduce the risk of infection. |
> | 1996 | British beef is banned worldwide, with a devastating effect on British farmers and the cattle industry. |
> | Late 1997 | New scientific research shows beef sold on the bone may carry a risk to humans of contamination from BSE. The Government immediately bans the sale of beef on the bone. Farmers blockade ports to halt the import of Irish beef. An enquiry is set up. |
> | 1998 | Since 1995 a total of 27 people have died from new-variant Creutzfeldt–Jakob disease. Scientists announce that sheep may carry a disease similar to BSE which theoretically could be transmitted to humans. |
>
> Source: Katz & Peberdy (1997)

collective health goals and the need to empower people to be involved and take control over factors influencing their health may be at odds with a health promotion role bound by corporate contracts and the need to show clear outcomes.

The development of a critical understanding around health issues, in order to identify options and priorities, is thus a primary task for health promoters. This requires an open, sharing and egalitarian relationship between health promoters and the public. Health promoters need to be clear about what they are doing and why. Health promotion is often described in terms of activities and these change in the light of political changes and consequent government priorities. If health promotion is to be secure and well funded it has 'never been more important to be clear, well-focused and tactical' (Jones & Adams 1997, p. 157).

The following activity is designed to help radical health promoters identify where they could make changes in their practice.

 The following are suggestions for developing radical health promotion practice. How many do you think are feasible for you? Be clear and honest about your own political standpoint.

- Develop an equal relationship with clients, where beliefs and values are respected, and information shared
- Try to ensure real community involvement in policies and decision-making
- Try to address health as a collective issue, making explicit the facts about health inequalities and supporting collective action around health issues
- Vet the health education materials you use to ensure they do not reproduce stereotypes or assumptions about gender, class, race, disability, age or sexuality
- Engage in action research in which researchers and researched are partners
- Develop a support network with like-minded health workers, where perspectives can be shared and issues discussed
- Be honest to yourself and others about the limitations of your work role.

Adapted from Adams & Slavin (1985) and O'Neill (1989)

Conclusion

There is often resistance to the idea that health promotion is a political activity. Accepting the premise that politics is involved in health promotion may be experienced as muddying the waters, for it transforms a situation of relative certainty to one of uncertainty. It is no longer sufficient to rely on professional training to ensure effective health promotion. A whole range of different considerations needs to be taken into account, some of which threaten and call into question the whole notion of professional expertise.

However uncomfortable the process may be, an awareness of the political nature of health promotion is vital to its effectiveness (O'Neill 1989). Accepting the status quo is not an apolitical position but a deeply political one. What exists is not inevitable, but the result of complex forces and historical processes. Things might be otherwise. Health promotion is centrally concerned with a vision of better health for all. This vision may be informed by scientific knowledge and technical know-how, but its overall shape is determined by personal values and beliefs. Part of the task of health promoters is to uncover and hold up to scrutiny their values and beliefs. It is hoped that this and the previous chapter (Ch. 6 on ethics) will help health promoters in this task.

The following statements reflect particular political philosophies. Can you identify these political philosophies? Which statements do you agree with?

1. There should be a system of economic and social support for the needy.
2. Energy and enterprise should be rewarded, not stifled by high taxation.
3. All people in a society have a commitment and responsibility to others.
4. Inequality is an inevitable result of the differences between people.
5. High levels of benefits make people dependent on support.
6. No group – business or labour – should be allowed to become too powerful.
7. There is no such thing as class in the modern UK.
8. People should be able to choose the type and level of health care or education they wish.
9. Certain services are essential and should be run by the State.
10. Macro politics is of less significance than issues, particularly those affecting local communities.
11. Businesses and services should be accountable to the people using them.
12. People cannot be equal, but everyone should have the same chances.

Questions for further discussion

■ To what extent may health promotion be said to be a political activity?

■ How could an understanding of politics help the health promoter develop more effective practice?

■ How have your political values and beliefs affected your practice?

Summary

This chapter has examined the political implications of health promotion structure, organization, methods and content. The central proposition is that health promotion is a political activity, and that to attempt to deny this lessens one's understanding and the possibility of effective action. It has been demonstrated that mainstream health promotion activity is predicated on certain political values. The new Labour Government elected in 1997 signalled a shift in these core values. Previous Conservative Governments had emphasized a non-interventionist role focused on individual advice and information giving. The new Labour Government has highlighted the social origins of health and expressed a need and a willingness to act across sectors and boundaries to address the fundamental causes of ill health – unemployment, low income, poor housing and environments. The role of the practitioner is still crucial, although it could be argued that the practitioner's function needs to expand to include client advocacy and empowerment with more emphasis on networking and collaborative working across sectors and professions. Whether this shift in practice can occur, given increasing demands on health care services, is problematic. Many practitioners may feel that the broad political framework is now more supportive of health promotion. However, the task of practising in accordance with one's political beliefs remains a challenge.

Further reading

Bunton R 1992 Health promotion as social policy. In: Bunton R, Macdonald G (eds) Health promotion: disciplines and diversity. Routledge, London. *A useful discussion of health promotion as social policy, identifying different political perspectives. It uses alcohol policies as a case study to explore the issues.*
George V, Wilding P 1994 Welfare and ideology. Harvester Wheatsheaf, Hemel Hempstead. *A readable account of the ideological and political debates of the 1990s. The book explores major schools of thought concerning the Welfare State.*

References

Acheson D 1998 Independent inquiry into inequalities in health: a report. Stationery Office, London

Adams L, Slavin H 1985 Checklist for personal action. Radical Health Promotion 2: 47

Beattie A 1991 Knowledge and control in health promotion: a test case for social policy and social theory. In: Gabe J, Calnan M, Bury M (eds) The sociology of the health service. Routledge, London, pp 162–201

Beattie A 1993 The changing boundaries of health. In: Beattie A, Gott M, Jones L, Sidell M (eds) Health and wellbeing: a reader. Macmillan/Open University, Basingstoke

Benzeval M, Judge K, Whitehead M (eds) 1995 Tackling inequalities in health. King's Fund, London

Bunton R 1992 Health promotion as social policy. In: Bunton R, Macdonald G (eds) Health promotion: disciplines and diversity. Routledge, London, pp 129–152

Chalmers A 1982 What is this thing called science? Open University Press, Milton Keynes

Department of Health (DoH) 1991 NHS and Community Care Act. HMSO, London

Department of Health (DoH) 1992 The health of the nation. HMSO, London

Department of Health (DoH) 1997 The new NHS: modern, dependable. White Paper. Stationery Office, London

Department of Health (DoH) 1999 Saving Lives: our healthier nation (white paper). Stationery Office, London

Department of Health and Social Security (DHSS) 1976 Prevention and health: everybody's business. HMSO, London

Department of Health and Social Security (DHSS) 1981a Prevention and health: avoiding heart attacks. HMSO, London

Department of Health and Social Security (DHSS) 1981b Drinking sensibly. HMSO, London

Freedom Organization for the Right to Enjoy Smoking Tobacco (FOREST) 1981 Newsletter No. 4. FOREST, London

Freire P 1972 Pedagogy of the oppressed. Penguin, Harmondsworth

French J, Milner S 1997 A survey of health promotion services in relation to purchasing and providing arrangements in England, Scotland and Northern Ireland. North Cumbria Health Development Unit, Carlisle

George V, Wilding P 1994 Welfare and ideology. Harvester Wheatsheaf, Hemel Hempstead

Gillies P 1997 Social capital: recognising the value of society. Healthlines 45: 15–16

Health Promotion International 1997 The Jakarta Declaration on Leading Health Promotion into the 21st Century. Health Promotion International 12(4): 261–264

Huber G L, Brockie R E, Mahajan V K 1993 Passive smoking: how great a hazard? FOREST Information Sheet No. 5. FOREST, London

Jones L, Adams L 1997 The politics of health promotion. In: Jones L, Sidell M (eds) The challenge of promoting health: exploration and action. Macmillan/Open University, Basingstoke, Hants

Katz J, Peberdy A (eds) 1997 Promoting health: knowledge and practice. Macmillan/Open University, Basingstoke, Hants

Kuhn T 1962 The structure of scientific revolutions. University of Chicago Press, Chicago

Le Fanu J (ed) 1994 Preventionitis: the exaggerated claims of health promotion. Social Affairs Unit, London

Lee P, Raban C 1988 Welfare and ideology. In: Loney M et al (eds) Social policy and social welfare. Open University Press, Milton Keynes, pp 18–32

Naidoo J 1986 Limits to individualism. In: Rodmell S, Watt A (eds) The politics of health education. Routledge and Kegan Paul, London, pp 17–37

O'Neill M 1989 The political dimension of health promotion work. In: Martin C J, McQueen D V (eds) Readings for a new public health. Edinburgh University Press, Edinburgh, pp 222–234

Townsend P, Davidson N, Whitehead M 1988 Inequalities in health: the Black Report and The Health Divide. Penguin, Harmondsworth

World Health Organization 1997 New players for a new era: leading health promotion into the 21st century. 4th International Conference on Health Promotion, Jakarta, Indonesia 21–25 July 1997. Conference Report. World Health Organization, Geneva/Ministry of Health, Indonesia

Strategies and Methods

This section addresses some of the practice issues for health promoters. The strategies and methods adopted pose particular dilemmas. How can health promoters work with communities and what are the strengths and limitations of a community development approach? What influences health behaviour and how can we help people to change? Is it effective to use the mass media? How can a population perspective be adopted in health promotion work?

8 *Partnerships for health – working together*

Key points

- Definitions of partnerships for health and ways of working together
- Characteristics of successful teams
- Main stakeholders in the promotion of health

OVERVIEW

In Chapter 4 we explored the shift in health promotion towards a broad view of health encompassing social and environmental factors. Improving health cannot, therefore, be the sole responsibility of the National Health Service (NHS). The health strategy for England 'Saving Lives: Our Healthier Nation' (DoH 1999) has called for 'a three-way partnership for better health. Under this contract, the Government, local communities and individuals will join in partnership to improve all our health'. Partners include the Government, health authorities, local authorities, business, voluntary bodies and individuals. The World Health Organization calls this process intersectoral collaboration.

Definitions

There are many different terms that are used to describe the ways that people work together to promote health. Although these are often used interchangeably it is possible to distinguish between them:

- **Partnership** refers to joint action between partners (national and local agencies and the public). It implies the equal sharing of power.
- **Service agreements and contracts** between partners set out mutual responsibilities for improving health.
- **Multiagency** refers to organizations that belong to the same sector such as health, social services, or education who are all statutory providers of public services.
- **Intersectoral** goes beyond any one sector and may include public, private (business and commerce) and voluntary groups.
- **Inter- or multidisciplinary working** is sometimes used to describe joint working of people with different roles or functions within the same organization or across sectors.

- **Joint planning** – organizations within or across sectors agree objectives, and meet regularly to develop and implement a joint plan.
- **Teams** usually have a common task and are made up of people chosen because they have relevant expertise. They may be multidisciplinary such as a primary health care team or a team who work in the same organization or they may be interagency such as an HIV team or child protection team.

 Think of a task you currently undertake which involves working with others in a team or where you share care with someone else.

- Who is or should be members of the team and why have they been chosen?
- Does everyone understand their role and those of the other members?
- Is everyone committed to the task and the methods to be used?
- How frequently do you meet to plan and review the task?
- Does the team discuss its own progress and development?
- Who leads the team and why?

You may not work in an established team or project but nevertheless work with other people in promoting health.

- Are there any ways you could develop stronger links with other staff in your own or other organizations?
- Are there opportunities for joint planning, target setting or joint aims and objectives?

Policy background

Collaboration is a familiar term in health promotion and it has long been recognized that it requires the active participation of a wide range of agencies at national and local level. The World Health Organization concluded that medical services have only a limited contribution to make towards health improvement and therefore intersectoral cooperation is of key importance: 'Health For All requires the co-ordinated action of all sectors concerned. The health authorities can only deal with part of the problems to be solved and multisectoral co-operation is the only way of effectively ensuring the prerequisites for health, promoting health policies and reducing the risks in the physical, economic and social environment' (WHO 1985). The WHO's new targets for the 21st century contain a specific target on mobilizing partners for health.

The 'Health of the Nation' strategy for England proposed the creation of healthy alliances defined as 'in effect, a partnership of individuals and organisations formed to enable people to increase their influence over the factors that affect their health and wellbeing – physically, mentally, socially and environmentally' (DoH 1993). The draft health strategy 'Our Healthier Nation' (DoH 1998a) proposed a contract for health (Table 8.1). In the white paper, *Saving Lives* (DoH 1999) contracts were proposed for each of the priority areas.

Alliances are not new. Ewles (1998) cites the example of the 1959 chest X-ray campaign in Liverpool to detect TB and lung cancer. The campaign was undertaken by the Corporation and The Regional

Table 8.1 *A contract for health*

Government and national players can:	Local players and communities can:	People can:
Provide national coordination and leadership	Provide leadership for local health strategies by developing and implementing Health Improvement Programmes	Take responsibility for their own health and make healthier choices about their lifestyle
Ensure that policy-making across Government takes full account of health and is well informed by research and the best expertise available	Work in partnerships to improve the health of local people and tackle the root causes of ill health	Ensure their own actions do not harm the health of others
Work with other countries for international cooperation to improve health	Plan and provide high quality services to everyone who needs them	Take opportunities to better their lives and their families' lives, through education, training and employment
Assess risks and communicate those risks clearly to the public		
Ensure that the public and others have the information they need to improve their health		
Regulate and legislate where necessary		
Tackle the root causes of ill health		

Source: DoH (1998a, p. 30)

Hospital Board, and involved health visitors, volunteers, public health inspectors, the local press, radio and television and the Automobile Association. Nearly 500 000 people came forward for X-rays which, at today's prices, would cost a million pounds.

In the 1970s health authorities, local authorities and voluntary organizations attempted to plan together services for client groups for whom both local and health authorities had an interest such as older people and the mentally ill. Joint Finance was an allocation of funds specifically earmarked for projects jointly agreed between the participating organizations. The NHS and Community Care Act 1990 requires local and health authorities to publish joint plans and commission appropriate services for the care of vulnerable groups. More recently, local health improvement programmes require consultation and agreement between health and social services and lay representatives in assessing local needs and setting local priorities (DoH 1998b).

These attempts at collaboration are primarily operational – ways to ensure the better use of scarce resources in service provision. The development of a national health strategy has given a major impetus to strategic planning across sectors. In addition, there are the numerous partnerships and networks that exist to plan and coordinate health promotion in particular settings and around particular health issues. Examples of such collaboration include: North Yorkshire Rural Initiative to reduce the suicide rate in the county's farmers, Derbyshire Welfare Rights Project to offer welfare advice through GPs surgeries, the Cycle Friendly Employers' Project in Cambridge, and collaborative schemes to address the needs of black and ethnic minority groups, young people in care or older people (see, for example, Bloxam 1996).

The Healthy Cities Project began in the UK in 1986 following publication of the 'Health For All' targets. More than 70 local authorities and 50 health authorities as well as voluntary organizations and academic institutions are involved.

The key characteristics of Healthy Cities programmes are that they:

■ involve collaboration of diverse groups
■ are based on a principle of community participation with priorities identified by the community themselves
■ set up structures to encourage collaboration.

In 1998 the government launched an initial 11 Health Action Zones. These are partnerships of health authorities, local authorities, unions, business and community agencies which aim to tackle health issues and reduce inequalities in the most deprived areas. Some of the first proposals include:

'Healthy Sheffield' was launched in 1987 as a joint initiative between the City Council, Community Health Council, Racial Equality Council, Family Health Services Authority (FHSA), Health Authority, Polytechnic and Voluntary Action Sheffield. Its aims were to improve the health of the people in Sheffield and reduce health inequalities. In order to achieve these aims 'Healthy Sheffield' has sought to extend the partner agencies to all major organizations, and voluntary and community groups, many of whom had not identified their part in health promotion. It now includes both 'old' and 'new' universities, the Chamber of Commerce and the Trades Council. As its members expand, it has set up a support team whose role is to introduce the concepts and values of 'Healthy Sheffield' to prospective partners helping them to embrace a holistic and social approach to health, and to clarify their own priorities in relation to health and the service they provide.

Another essential element for enabling change was the development of a range of demonstration projects and programmes to show what is possible in health promotion. Initially 'Healthy Sheffield' found it difficult to progress beyond generalities when trying to apply HFA targets to Sheffield. An approach was then chosen which concentrates on the health needs of the main groups of people in the city and identifies priority targets for each group. This formed the structure for a major 'Our City, Our Health' consultation exercise. This involved the training of over 200 facilitators to seek the views of their own colleagues and others. The consultation has been a political and educational process resulting in a document made accessible and readable for the community (Halliday & Adams 1992, Healthy Sheffield 1990).

- joint management of budgets by health authorities and social services to encourage better coordination of services
- 'one stop' primary care centres
- healthy living centres (see Ch. 13).

At the local level, many practitioners work in teams or with others to plan and coordinate individual client care. There is an increasing emphasis on working more widely and developing strategic health promotion responses to issues raised by client care.

Advantages of working together

Collaboration is a difficult challenge but, put simply, it creates 'additionality'. It brings together strengths and weaknesses, and makes something that exceeds the sum of the parts. Conventional wisdom favours group rather than individual decisions and phrases

The following practitioners wish to extend their role beyond individual client care. With which partners might they work?

■ A mental health nurse concerned about the high rate of suicide in clients with mental health problems
■ A ward nurse concerned about the fracture rate in older women
■ A residential care worker concerned about the inability of most residents to get out of a chair unaided.

such as 'two heads are better than one' reflect the view that better decisions are often made by people working together.

The advantages can be summarized as:

■ It brings together organizations and groups who would not normally see themselves as having a role in promoting health, and thus means that health is addressed holistically and not solely in a treatment-oriented setting.
■ It increases these organizations' knowledge and understanding of each other, helping to clarify roles and overcome rivalry.
■ Collaborative service planning is based on a comprehensive picture of local needs. This will help to eliminate gaps.
■ It ensures accurate targeting of services based on wider consultation, and a pooling of knowledge and awareness of community needs.
■ Working in a partnership may lead to more effective use of resources by, for example, joint commissioning of services. It can also avoid administrative duplication by partners working together on service specifications.
■ It ensures that the public are given the same, not conflicting, messages.
■ The root causes of ill health may be tackled, not just symptoms, and awareness can be raised of the determinants of ill health.

The experience of some collaborative projects, health strategy groups and 'Healthy Cities' initiatives have not all been unqualified successes. Such partnerships may fall apart, become 'talking shops' or achieve little. Not surprisingly, these are not fully documented but there are some general barriers that can arise:

■ lack of commitment at a senior level
■ differences in outlook
■ professional rivalry especially if there are differences in status
■ imbalance in the contributions to resourcing the alliance; voluntary organizations, for example, are not able to contribute to the costs of intersectoral collaboration
■ exclusion of new partners

- lack of appropriate skills
- lack of shared, achievable goals
- lack of understanding of different organizational cultures and the constraints of other organizations
- different geographical boundaries, for example between local authority and health authority
- lack of real achievement.

Many of these factors may also be relevant to interprofessional working. Beattie (1994) highlights two particular obstacles:

- competing professional rationales about values and ways of working
- interpersonal relations which, like partnerships in private lives, rest on friendship and trust.

In your experience of working in a team or partnership, how important have been the elements of different professional values and interpersonal relationships?

Individuals and groups who work together will have perceptions of the other's role and may not understand the ways in which their organization works. This example illustrates the changing views of a health education coordinator from a local education authority and a youth worker from a drug project.

'We did have concerns about the reliability of the advice which might be given and the informal ways of working. We were worried what might be said that could be thought to be the Authority viewpoint. We were reassured by the response from young people who had not previously had the trust and confidence to express their needs.'
(Local education authority coordinator working
with a voluntary drug project)

'At first we found the LEA very bureaucratic and hierarchical. Making the appropriate contacts was difficult. They seemed suspicious of our methods and our professionalism. Budget considerations and the corporate view seemed dominant. The success of the local drug education strategy has been because of individual effort and constant contact with those involved.'
(Drug project worker)

Characteristics of successful joint working

Health promotion requires good teamwork and coordination both with colleagues in your own department, but also with other disciplines and professions. In large organizations like health authorities or local authorities, it is especially important that there is good communication and coordination between departments because it is not always possible to have informal contacts or networking. Joint working does not happen easily and crossing professional lines is a difficult process perhaps involving rivalry, competing interests, and different models of health or different ways of working. In addition, people may feel their own jobs to be threatened by joint working.

When people refer to a 'good team', they usually mean a partnership in which the members work well together towards the same end and complement each other. An ideal team has certain essential characteristics:

■ A common task or purpose
■ Members are selected because they have specific expertise
■ Members know their own roles and those of other members
■ Members support each other in the task
■ Members complement each other in their skills and personalities
■ Members have a commitment to accomplishing the task
■ There is a leader who will coordinate and take responsibility
■ The team may have a base.

In addition, there are general skills of working with other people that contribute to a successful partnership. These skills include communication, participation in meetings, managing paperwork and time, and being and working in a group (Naidoo & Wills 1998).

'The Health of the Nation' handbook (DoH 1993) on health alliances identifies the following general factors as important:

■ Members must have sufficient time to devote to interagency activity, otherwise it gets relegated by pressing and immediate professional concerns.
■ A coordinator may help to maintain commitment and to identify potential resources.
■ Members must have sufficient status and authority in their own organization to influence decisions, otherwise collaboration becomes only a networking process.
■ There must be a shared vision and concept of health. Achieving this must be one of the first tasks of a healthy alliance. Most health authorities have a disease-related focus and most local authorities emphasize a behavioural approach. Some localities such as Sheffield explicitly state that their philosophy is that of a social model of health principally committed to reducing inequalities in health.
■ There must be shared goals and targets for promoting health. Some agencies may not be clear about their potential contribution or have their own objectives, interests and capacities. It is not uncommon for groups to spend years formulating operational targets which are relevant to local needs, realistic and compatible with the interests and business objectives of the individual partner agencies.

■ There must be support for collaboration and a mechanism for getting things done. Tangible results encourage people to keep working together.
■ It is important to demonstrate achievements. This may include monitoring the process of the alliance including levels of commitment and participation, and levels of activity. It may also measure outcomes and the achievement of original objectives.

Thompson & Stachenko (1994) identify the following factors which facilitate partnerships for health:

■ a partnership-building process
■ networks to stimulate and support change
■ material resources to support the process
■ a dedicated central coordinating body or person
■ a communication plan.

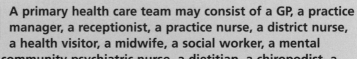 **A primary health care team may consist of a GP, a practice manager, a receptionist, a practice nurse, a district nurse, a health visitor, a midwife, a social worker, a mental health or community psychiatric nurse, a dietitian, a chiropodist, a physiotherapist, a counsellor and an interpreter.**

Consider some of the potential difficulties of these professions working together in a team:

1. There is no common task. All relate to the same registered population but activities range from episodes of illness in individuals, the care of the chronically ill and preventive activities for the whole population.
2. The membership will thus vary with the task. For example, a GP and district nurse may be the only members involved in the care of an elderly diabetic, whereas most of the above would be involved in the organization of a well woman clinic.
3. There are boundary problems. Jobs frequently overlap and there are aspects of social and personal care that would seem to be part of all members' occupational remit.
4. There may be status problems. Within a primary health care team there are members who differ widely in the extent of their training, salary levels, degree of occupational autonomy and power.
5. Members have different employers, which may result in different objectives. GPs are independent contractors who employ some team members, whereas others are employed by local or health authorities.

Key stakeholders

As we have seen earlier in this chapter, the wider policy environment and local structures as well as personality and skills

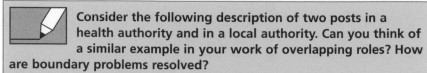

Consider the following description of two posts in a health authority and in a local authority. Can you think of a similar example in your work of overlapping roles? How are boundary problems resolved?

Many local education authorities have advisors whose role is to support and encourage programmes of health education in schools and colleges, particularly in relation to sexual health and substance use. Most health promotion departments have a designated worker for schools whose role would be similar in its objectives. The different employers influence the nature of the work undertaken and its perspective. The local education authority health education coordinator is concerned with educational management and whole curriculum issues, whereas the health promotion officer has a specific brief for health programmes. Health promotion services normally have a budget to support work in schools. LEA advisors have few resources and need to generate income by tendering their services. There is also a considerable difference in salary scales between the two posts, though not necessarily any difference in experience or training undertaken. Because health education is frequently squeezed out of school education, health education specialists have to work to raise awareness and market their services.

The health education coordinator and the health promotion officer are employed in similar jobs. They may be healthy collaborators or healthy (or unhealthy) competitors.

(For more information see Scriven 1995.)

will determine which people and organizations contribute to a partnership for health. The following will be key stakeholders in promoting health:

- government departments
- health authorities and health trusts
- the Health Education Authority and national lead agencies
- the primary health care team
- professions allied to medicine
- local authorities
- community groups and voluntary organizations
- business sector and major employers
- mass media.

How do you find out what people think of your service?

The public, who are the target of much health promotion, are a key stakeholder and means of accessing their views are varied. Community involvement is an important issue in partnerships (see Ch. 9).

Figure 8.1 indicates the most important agencies of health promotion.

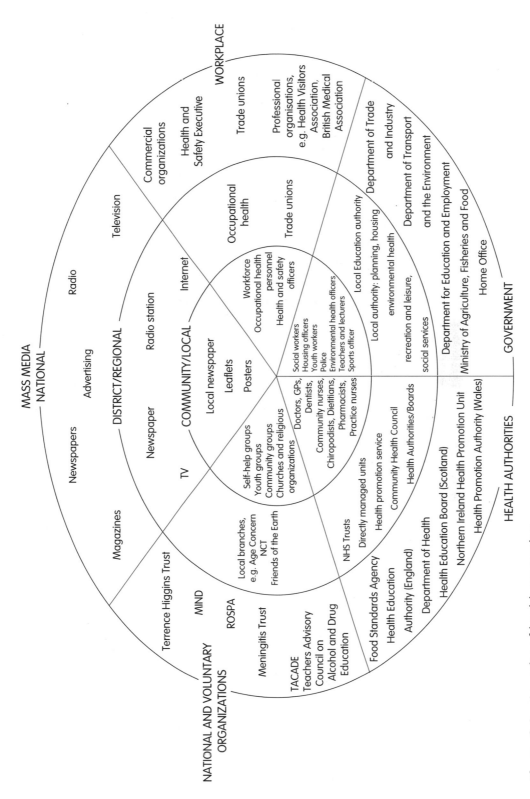

Figure 8.1 *Agencies of health promotion.*

Any account of the current structure and organization of health promotion services is in danger of becoming out of date in the near future. However, a brief description is included to outline the opportunities for health partnerships for each organization.

Government departments

'Our Healthier Nation', the health strategy for England, recognizes the need for a range of government departments to work together to promote health. The appointment of a Minister for Public Health is intended to ensure coordination of health policy across government, and is supported by an interdepartmental Cabinet Committee. Health impact assessments will ensure that the health consequences of a range of policies will be considered during their development stage. The Government is also committed to integrated or 'joined-up' policy making.

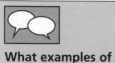

What examples of policy can you think of that have an impact on health?

Health authorities and health trusts

There are currently eight NHS Management Executive regional offices whose role is mainly confined to staffing and the supervision of contracts.

The NHS and Community Care Act 1990 divided health authorities into 'purchasers' or 'commissioners' and 'providers'. The purchasing authority has responsibility for determining health needs and commissioning services from provider units (often health trusts). Health authorities (HAs) are the main commissioning agencies of health care. HAs have to assess the health needs of their population and then agree service agreements with provider units, which may be hospitals or community services within the HA, self-governing hospitals, or other health authorities (see Table 8.2). The HA can purchase services outside the health service and is increasingly working with other agencies to deliver essential services. They also have to be responsive to their 'clients'. Chapter 14 looks at the ways in which HAs are having to use a wide range of research techniques and 'intelligence gathering' in order to build a picture of needs in their community.

Service agreements for health promotion may include requirements to:

- provide a certain standard of health education and promotion in patient care such as ensuring a smoke-free environment
- promote the health of NHS employees such as the provision of healthy catering
- define the coordinating and support role of a provider, usually the health promotion service
- use health needs assessment, to encourage the active participation of users and other members of the community in the planning of services, and to observe equal opportunities

Table 8.2
Commissioning and provider agencies

Commissioning agencies	
NHS Executive regional offices	Assess the need for health care
Health authorities	Develop service agreements
Primary care groups	Monitor the health of the population
Providers	
Directly managed units	
NHS trusts (acute, community, ambulance, primary care)	Provide services to their own or other districts
Private sector	
Voluntary sector	
Local authorities	

- establish a district register of people with diabetes and ensure that they have access to an education programme
- record major risk factors for coronary heart disease in patients' notes
- designate a member of staff in each health centre to offer smoking cessation advice.

(See Killoran 1992)

The government White Paper 'The New NHS' (DoH 1998b) has identified health improvement programmes as the key strategic mechanism for meeting the health needs of each locality. HAs are charged with the lead role but have a statutory duty of partnership with local authorities. Primary care groups (PCGs) based around clusters of GP practices will act in support of the HA in commissioning services including health promotion (Ch. 16 provides more details on this).

The Director of Public Health is a relatively new role established in 1988 following the publication of the Acheson report on public health in England (Acheson 1988). The role is far broader than the previous District Medical officer or, before that, the Medical Officers of Health who were employed by the local authority. The Director of Public Health is charged with assessing overall health needs, collaborating with other agencies in the promotion of health and prevention of disease, and producing an annual report on the state of public health locally.

Hospital nurses

Nurses in clinical practice are involved with the assessment and care of individual patients. Their health promotion role has been largely confined to patient education about the diagnosis and treatment procedures patients may expect. It is increasingly recognized that nursing needs to move beyond its traditional function of caring for the sick and take on a health promotion role. The emphasis is on a holistic model of health, and a client-centred approach is seen as the appropriate way of working. The values central to health promotion – collaboration, public participation and empowerment – do not sit easily with hospital care (Latter 1996). Chapter 16 looks at ways in which nurses can extend their work beyond individual patient care, e.g. setting up of health-promoting policies in hospital, patient participation schemes, carer groups, and working with other agencies, such as social services and voluntary groups.

Health promotion services

Health promotion departments are part of the health authority and are usually accountable to the Director of Public Health. They vary widely in size, from a handful to 50 staff, and will consist of health promotion specialists and several support and clerical staff. They have the lead role in initiating, coordinating, and supporting health education and health promotion activity. Health promotion units may have commissioning or providing functions, or a dual role. Commissioning activities include:

- assessing local health needs
- contributing to the operational and strategic plans of the HA
- reviewing service agreements to ensure that they seek to *promote* health
- coordinating the plans and services of different agencies.

    Provider activities include:

- managing health promotion programmes on specific issues such as HIV/AIDS, smoking or coronary heart disease
- providing advice and consultancy to the public and policy makers
- providing training, support, and advice to all health promoters and agencies who provide health promotion.

Community health councils

Community health councils (CHCs) were set up under the 1974 NHS reorganization to give a stronger voice to the views of the community on health services. CHCs have representatives from voluntary groups, local authorities and community groups. They act as a lobby group and will also participate in the NHS planning process. Their future is uncertain.

The HEA and national lead agencies

The HEA is part of the NHS and is designated a 'special' health authority with the task of leading and supporting health education in England. In Scotland, the Health Education Board carries out this function. In Wales, it is the Welsh Assembly and in Northern Ireland it is the Northern Ireland Health Promotion Unit.

 The role of the HEA (to be known as Health Development Agency) is:

- To maintain an evidence base for public health and health improvement
- To provide advice on targeting health promotion and narrowing the health gap

The primary health care team

Community nurses

Health promotion is a priority in the role of community nurses, and is written into the job specification of health visitors and school nurses (Health Visitors Association 1987). Their work is to promote the health of their clients as well as specific care and monitoring tasks. Because community nurses visit people in their own homes, they are able to build a strong relationship with their clients over a period of time. This enables them to carry out much one-to-one education, and counselling and opportunistic health education. Some nurses are also involved with supporting community and voluntary groups working in health-related areas.

Community nurses are part of the primary health care team and should work closely with other community nurses, GPs and social workers. The planning of health promotion may not always be coordinated or prioritized, however, as individual health care workers concentrate on their own case load. While health promotion is integral to the work of the service, this is commonly according to an individualistic model. The wide range of socio-economic influences on people's health status also needs to be taken into account. The potential for health promotion is discussed further in the section on primary health care in Chapter 16.

Health visitors

Health visitors have a duty to visit all mothers and new infants. Their public health role is expanding. Health visitors may run antenatal classes and postnatal support groups in addition to carrying out health checks for the under-fives and providing support, education and advice for parents. Health visitors will often build up a community profile of their area and this provides useful information on health needs.

District nurses

District nurses visit people with chronic sickness or disability at home. Much of their work is with older people, and they carry out opportunistic health education as well as liaising between people living in the community and other relevant health and welfare workers.

Mental health nurses

Mental health or community psychiatric nurses visit people who are mentally ill and ensure that they are coping. Increasingly, they are expected to be involved in the education of individuals and groups at risk of developing mental health problems. They may work with workplaces in developing stress and mental health policies, support self-help groups and train other practitioners in the early identification of problems.

School nurses

School nurses are part of the community nursing service but their role varies enormously. Originally, it was to focus on the detection and treatment of poor hygiene, infestations and malnutrition. A major part of their current role is routine health surveillance and screening. In addition, they may support children with chronic diseases, offer guidance and advice and be involved in classroom education (Farrow 1996). 'Saving Lives: Our Healthier Nation' (DoH 1999, p. 134) suggests that they will provide 'a safety net for children'.

Midwives

Hospital midwives are involved in the delivery of babies and antenatal education. Community midwives visit all new mothers in their area, and provide support and education as well as monitoring the health of mothers and babies.

> Midwives are in an ideal position to extend support to expectant and new families and to provide a service which helps parents to access information and use it effectively to nurture the health of their family. However, they also have an important role in bringing public attention to those issues which are beyond the scope of individuals to change, such as social and environmental obstacles.
>
> (Crafter 1997, p. 3)

General practitioners

General practice has traditionally been a private and personal consultation between doctor and patient. Health promotion consisted of opportunistic advice or information. GPs are essentially independent practitioners, their contracts administered by health authorities. The government White Paper 'Promoting Better Health'

(DHSS 1987), however, emphasized the role of GPs in prevention and the monitoring of chronic illness and revised contracts to provide additional payments to GPs to carry out preventive work. GPs are now required to lead the new primary care groups with a responsibility to commission services for a defined locality. Further details of these arrangements are included in Chapter 16.

This is an example of collaboration on an exercise project 'Prescription for Exercise' between health promotion, leisure services and a GP practice.

Clients at risk of coronary heart disease, at a check-up may be offered, if appropriate, a prescription for exercise. This gives information on types of recommended activities and a list of leisure centres. The 'prescription' can be handed in at a centre and the client can take part in activities at reduced cost. The referring GP will monitor the patient at intervals of 1 and 3 months.

Practice nurses

Practice nurses are directly employed by GPs. It is a relatively new profession but the numbers had increased to over 15 000 by 1993 (British Journal of General Practice 1997). Their health promotion role has been largely confined to lifestyle advice and health checks. The effectiveness of these activities is discussed in Chapter 16.

The Pioneer Health Centre was started in the 1930s by two doctors concerned at the health of the poor in South London. It came to be known as the 'Peckham experiment' because it tried to address health in a holistic way. The Health Centre incorporated a fitness club, theatre, gym, swimming pool, billiards table, children's nursery, a cafeteria serving healthy, cheap food, a library and medical consulting rooms. For one shilling (5p) a week per family, all the Centre could be used. In 1938, 600 families belonged. It closed during the Second World War, reopening in 1946 when it added a nursery school, youth club, marriage advisory service, Citizen's Advice Bureau and child guidance. It closed in 1950 because it did not fit into the structure of the emerging National Health Service. There have been recent attempts to revive the Centre which is to be renamed Pulse Health and Leisure – a partnership between Southwark Council and Lambeth, Lewisham and Southwark Health Authority and with £3.2 million of lottery money. Its aim is 'to provide a unique leisure, health and fitness resource that encourages local people to invest in their own health and well-being'. The new partnership thus puts the responsibility for health squarely with the individual.

Professions allied to medicine

Dentists

There is an increasing emphasis on prevention in dentistry particularly with children. Dentists receive a capitation fee per child and so have an interest in keeping that child's teeth healthy and free from treatment. Many practices employ a hygienist who will give advice on dental health. Health authorities also have a community dental service which may offer dental health promotion to schools and residential homes.

 Pharmacists

There are nearly 12 000 community pharmacists in the UK, which thus provide an ideal and easily accessible location for the provision of opportunistic health promotion advice. Pharmacists have always offered education about medication and patient counselling when prescription medicines are required. The priority accorded to health promotion is now much higher. Pharmacists may offer education about specific health issues when products are purchased. For example, pharmacists are active in raising awareness about skin cancer. There are also opportunities for opportunistic health advice. The client purchasing a laxative may be invited to discuss diet and sources of fibre.

There have been several pharmacy-based campaigns. The DUMP scheme encourages the public to return unwanted medicines. 'Health Care in the High Street' is a joint initiative by the Health Education Authority, the Family Planning Association, the National Pharmaceutical Society and the Royal Pharmaceutical Society of Great Britain. It aims to develop the community pharmacy as an information centre for general health advice.

Pharmacists have not necessarily been trained in health promotion or communication skills. They may receive special payments for health promotion work but the pharmacist is not generally seen by the public as a source of health advice apart from on medication (MarPlan 1982). *Promoting Better Health* (DHSS 1987) and a Nuffield Report on the future of pharmacists (Nuffield Foundation 1986) both suggested an extension of their role and closer links with other professionals, particularly in the primary health care team, so that pharmacists work with their clients' health not their illness, and with the person not the person's condition.

Many other professions allied to medicine such as chiropodists, physiotherapists, radiographers and dietitians have a part to play in health promotion, and particularly patient education. The expanded role of the community pharmacist is used above as an example.

Local authorities

Local authorities include county, district, borough and metropolitan authorities which provide a range of services for local communities. Local authority officers are accountable to elected councillors who represent the local community.

Some authorities are major providers of housing. Most are major employers. Individual departments also have key roles in the promotion of health: social services, recreation and leisure, planning and housing. The responsibility local authorities have for transport provides the opportunity for initiatives on accident prevention and environmental schemes, such as park and ride, bicycle lanes or home zones. Local authorities are also charged with the responsibility of producing Local Agenda 21 strategies on sustainable development. They have a statutory duty to promote the economic, social and environmental well-being of people in their area and to work in partnership with local people, businesses and voluntary organizations.

 Environmental health

The role of environmental health is particularly wide-ranging, encompassing statutory powers relating to food hygiene and pollution (both of noise and air) to specialist work on safety in the workplace and places of entertainment. Because environmental health officers have wide-ranging statutory powers, their work in health promotion is mainly advice on legislation and enabling people to fulfil those regulations. Their work may thus involve offering training courses or one-to-one advice in establishments.

Social services

The shift towards care in the community under the 1990 NHS and Community Care Act has increased the role of social services in promoting the health of older people, people with mental health problems, those with learning difficulties and people with a disability. The new legislation requires social service departments to work with health authorities to provide individualized care programmes for people in need, and also people with AIDS or drug or alcohol problems.

Social service departments already have a statutory responsibility for child protection and, under the Children Act 1989, a responsibility to provide a health-promoting environment for young people in its care. 'Social services could not be expected to provide mass health promotion in the way that primary health care may aim to do. But, since they work with many of the most vulnerable, frail

Joint discharge policies

Part of a community care plan by social services and a health authority has the objective that older people should be kept in their own homes as long as is desired and is appropriate. The departments agree a care management service which includes an agreed procedure on discharge from hospital.

and socially disadvantaged people in society, they have a potentially strategic role in any overall health promotion strategy' (Jones & Bloomfield 1996, p. 95).

This strategic role relates to:

■ prevention and early interventions especially in relation to family support, and home care for older people
■ building health partnerships which acknowledge the interrelatedness of social and health care goals
■ health education.

Residential care workers

'Health promotion in the continuing care of older people is frequently undervalued and unrecognised' (UKCC 1997). Yet care workers in residential settings have a key health promotion role where improved fitness and nutrition can minimize illness and dependency. They also have a role in positive mental health promotion and empowering older people to have a degree of control over their lives. The protection of health is also important in relation to safety and the prevention of falls and pressure sores. Residential care workers liaise with GPs, social workers, physiotherapists, chiropodists and catering staff.

Local education authorities

The LEA has responsibility for health promotion in schools, colleges and youth clubs. Over 6 million young people between the ages of 5 and 19 are in education. Over 3 million teenagers attend a youth club. Education is therefore a key setting for health promotion. There have been many recent changes in the management of education which have devolved budgets directly to schools and given governors greater powers. Governors are responsible for the provision of sexual health education. The introduction of the National Curriculum in schools in 1989 has meant that health education is often squeezed out of an overcrowded timetable. This process has been exacerbated by the disbanding of LEA specialist advisors for health education. On the other hand, there is far greater recognition of the importance of health education and many schools have a designated teacher coordinator. The opportunities for health promotion in schools are discussed more fully in Chapter 14.

A similar problem occurs in further education colleges where the huge increase in student numbers and vocational courses in recent years has meant a squeeze on pastoral time and non-vocational studies. The only health education for this age group is often advice or counselling provided by a counselling service.

Personal and social education has always been central to the work of the youth service. Increasingly, educational activity is offered alongside the traditional games and sports. Youth workers may also be involved with outreach work, drop-in advice centres and peer education (Jackson 1996).

Community groups and voluntary organizations

Fieldgrass (1992) estimates there are at least 300 000 voluntary organizations. These range from large organizations with paid staff and budgets to small groups run by volunteers. Many have an interest in health, ranging from MIND (the National Association for Mental Health) or Age Concern, to agencies such as the Alzheimer's Society concerned with particular conditions, to established projects staffed by paid workers in fields such as substance use, for example Turning Point.

Voluntary organizations act as service providers and self-help groups, as pressure groups and as sources of education and information. They are involved in statutory structures such as joint consultative committees and community health councils, and in planning and consultation exercises, such as the Community Care Plan of the health authority and local authority.

Voluntary organizations are important in providing specialized information, and being close to the community and harder-to-reach groups. They can reflect people's experience of a service and give an indicator of other needs, acting as a catalyst for change.

The development of the commissioner/provider role in the NHS and moves towards a mixture of health and social care services will necessitate good relations between statutory and voluntary sectors. However, the precarious funding of many voluntary organizations which need to be engaged in a constant search for grants can make long-term planning difficult and lead to low morale.

Business sector and major employers

In the workplace, trade unions may have an active role in health promotion. However, membership of unions has declined dramatically in the last decade. Traditionally, unions have protected rather than promoted their members' health, and have been more

Sickle cell service

The Brent Sickle Cell and Thalassaemia Centre provides an example of mutual respect and effective collaboration between statutory and voluntary sectors.

This service was set up in 1980 for those affected by sickle cell disorders. It includes the screening of babies and adults, genetic and general counselling, and health promotion advice on nutrition and welfare issues. The centre is part of health service provision. However, it is based in a small, easily accessible hospital and operates an open-door policy with no appointments. It is so sensitive to the needs of the local community and works so closely with the volunteer parents support group that it is often seen as a black voluntary organization. Its workers regard this as an achievement and a breaking down of barriers.

The centre relies on networking between volunteers, patients and health professionals and overlapping roles. Thus counselling is carried out by nurses, health visitors and volunteers. The local support group meets in the centre and uses its facilities.

Source: Fieldgrass (1992)

concerned with safety factors and environmental hazards than the general work environment. Similarly, but for different reasons, employers and managers have been concerned with safety conditions and the efficient working of staff rather than promoting their health. The potential and limitations are discussed further in the section on workplace health promotion in Chapter 13.

Large employers will have an occupational health scheme which may provide health checks and assessment of fitness to work, and health promotion advice as well as first aid. The service may be involved in developing policies to protect the health of employees (e.g. smoking, alcohol, safe working practices and stress management).

Mass media

Health promotion messages are presented in a variety of media including print or visual media produced by health promoters themselves, newspaper features or news, magazine advice columns, or health pages, radio phone-ins, and fictional television programmes. As Chapter 12 outlines, the role of health promoters in using the media and making it part of a 'health partnership' is still limited. This is despite the traditional use of advertising-type campaigns to present simple behavioural messages.

Conclusion

Intersectoral collaboration is one of the key principles outlined by the WHO if 'Health For All' is to be achieved. Partnership working is also key to the UK health strategies. It is not sufficient alone, however, to reduce inequalities or reorient health services, or catalyze and persuade communities to actively participate in their own health decisions. Chapter 9 goes on to look at community development approaches to health promotion and the consultation, training, support and resources that are necessary if there is to be a local health-oriented programme. The Ottawa Charter described the key processes and methods for health promotion as enablement, mediation and advocacy (see Ch. 4). Working together in partnership for health calls, in particular, upon practitioners' mediation skills.

Question for further discussion

- ■ What are the prospects and problems of working with others to promote health in your work?

Summary

This chapter has explored different examples of partnerships for health and ways in which health promotion practitioners can work together. It discussed the conditions that are necessary for effective collaboration, concluding that coordination and a greater understanding of other workers' roles would greatly enhance intersectoral collaboration. It then outlined the role and potential of the main agencies that promote health.

Further reading

Department of Health (DoH) 1993 Working together for better health. HMSO, London. *A handbook produced as part of the 'Health of the Nation' strategy. It summarizes the reasons for working together, how to organize a healthy alliance, whom to involve, and provides many case studies which set out the benefits for those involved.*

Funnell R, Oldfield K, Speller V 1995 Towards healthier alliances. Health Education Authority, London. *Guidelines on evaluating alliances and how partners can monitor progress.*

Scriven A (ed) 1998 Alliances in health promotion: theory and practice. Macmillan, Basingstoke. *The first book to analyze the theoretical issues relating to collaboration. It also includes a number of case studies of health promotion partnerships.*

Scriven A, Orme J 1996 (eds) Health promotion: professional perspectives. Macmillan/Open University, Basingstoke. *A useful insight into what health promotion means in different settings. Interesting accounts of practice will help to increase understanding for collaborative partnerships.*

References

Acheson D 1988 Public health in England, report of the Committee of Inquiry into the future development of the public health function. HMSO, London

Beattie A 1994 Healthy alliances or dangerous liaisons? The challenge of working together in health promotion. In: Leathard A (ed) Going interprofessional: working together for health and welfare. Routledge, London

Bloxham S 1996 A case study of inter-agency collaboration in the education and promotion of young people's sexual health. Health Education Journal 55: 389–403

British Journal of General Practice 1997 Who should give lifestyle advice in general practice and what factors influence attendance at health promotion clinics? Survey of patient views. British Journal of General Practice (Dec): 669–679

Children Act 1989 HMSO, London

Crafter H 1997 Health promotion in midwifery. Arnold, London

Department of Health (DoH) 1992 The health of the nation. HMSO, London

Department of Health (DoH) 1993 Working together for better health. HMSO, London

Department of Health (DoH) 1998a Our healthier nation. Stationery Office, London

Department of Health (DoH) 1998b The new NHS: modern, dependable. Stationery Office, London

Department of Health (DoH) 1999 Saving Lives: our healthier nation. Stationery Office, London

Department of Health and Social Security (DHSS) 1987 Promoting better health. HMSO, London

Ewles L 1998 Working in alliances: an inside story. In: Scriven A (ed) Alliances in health promotion. Macmillan, Basingstoke

Farrow S 1996 The role of the school nurse in promoting health. In: Scriven A, Orme J (eds) Health promotion: professional perspectives. Macmillan/Open University, Basingstoke

Fieldgrass J 1992 Partnerships in health promotion. Health Education Authority, London

Halliday M, Adams L 1992 Healthy Sheffield; the consultation experiment. Health Education Journal 51: 1

Health Visitors Association (HVA) 1987 Health visiting and school nursing reviewed. HVA, London

Healthy Sheffield 1990 Health promotion strategic plan 1990–1993. Sheffield Health

Jackson M 1996 Health promotion in a youth work setting. In: Scriven A, Orme J (eds) Health promotion: professional perspectives. Macmillan/Open University, Basingstoke

Jones L, Bloomfield J 1996 Promoting health through social services. In: Scriven A, Orme J (eds) Health promotion: professional perspectives. Macmillan/Open University, Basingstoke

Killoran A 1992 Putting health into contracts. HEA, London

Latter S 1996 The potential for health promotion in hospital nursing practice. In: Scriven A, Orme J (eds) Health promotion: professional perspectives. Macmillan/Open University, Basingstoke

MarPlan 1982 Survey of public attitudes and knowledge carried out on behalf of the National Pharmaceutical Association. NPA, London

Naidoo J, Wills J 1998 Practising health promotion: dilemmas and challenges. Baillière Tindall, London

NHS and Community Care Act 1990 HMSO, London

Nuffield Foundation 1986 Pharmacy: the report of a committee of inquiry appointed by the Nuffield Foundation. Nuffield, London

Scriven A 1995 Health alliances between specialist NHS health promotion units and LEAs/schools: the results of a national audit. Health Education Journal 54: 176–185

Thompson P R, Stachenko S 1994 Building and mobilising partnerships for health: a national strategy. Health Promotion International 9(3): 211–215

United Kingdom Council for Nursing, Midwifery and Health Visiting (UKCC) 1997 The nursing and health visiting contribution to the continuing care of older people. UKCC, London

World Health Organization 1985 Targets for health for all. WHO Regional Office for Europe, Copenhagen

9 *Public health work*

OVERVIEW

Public health – the promotion of the health of the population – depends on many factors which are the remit of government, such as transport, housing, income and the quality of the environment, food, air and water. Public health is therefore much broader than medicine. Public health came to the fore in the UK in the 19th century. The need for a healthy workforce and a concern for national efficiency, coupled with fears that the mass migration to the towns would lead to cholera and typhoid epidemics, led to the widespread adoption of public health measures. Recognition of the limits to clinical medicine has sparked off a renewed interest in public health. This is defined more broadly now as strategies to bring about health-promoting social, economic and physical environments.

Public health is characterized by several factors:

- a concern for the health of the whole population
- a concern for prevention of illness and disease
- a recognition of the many social factors which contribute to health.

This chapter explores the ways in which practitioners can help to change social conditions so that people have access to services, facilities and environments which protect their health. It is apparent that there is considerable overlap between the concepts 'public health' and 'health promotion'. This chapter provides a summary of recent developments in public health and flags up its relationship to health promotion.

Introduction

Historically, public health has been driven by social policy as much as by medicine. The early public health movement in the 19th century used a medical scientific model to explain the disease process whilst employing social policy interventions to prevent its occurrence. During the 20th century these two arms of public health became separated, with public health increasingly dominated by medicine. For example, a medical training has been seen as essential for the practice of public health. It is only very recently that, coming full circle, the medical dominance and ownership of public health has been challenged, and once again an emphasis placed on broader social interventions to promote the public health. The Labour Government elected in 1997 created a new post, Minister for Public Health, and there is also an ongoing investigation into the most appropriate kind of training for public health practitioners (DoH 1998).

Defining public health work

How would you define public health?

How does this differ from:
■ health care work?
■ social care work?

Identify some examples where local activities have led to changes which promote health.

Working for the public health means contributing at all levels to the task of making people and the environment healthier. Whilst action at governmental level is required to address many environmental factors, such as levels of air or water pollution, local activities can influence the local environment.

The following are all examples of public health work:

■ A community nurse compiles a local health profile.
■ A self-help group for people with disabilities lobbies the government to introduce comprehensive anti-discrimination legislation.
■ An environmental health officer sets up a local Heartbeat Award scheme to encourage caterers to produce healthier meals.
■ A child accident prevention liaison group is established to lead a local strategy. Members include health promotion specialists, community nurses, the police, teachers, environmental health officers, parents and representatives from local organizations e.g. ROSPA (Royal Society for the Prevention of Accidents).
■ A group of residents living in a council estate lobbies the local authority for better lighting and the instalment of CCTV to reduce people's fear of crime.

Public health work includes raising the profile of health issues in a community or in society, drawing attention to and carrying out research. Working in your own organization to create health awareness or working collaboratively with others to identify shared projects is also public health work. Public health work therefore includes research, partnership and intersectoral collaboration, and advocacy, as well as lobbying for policy changes. Many health practitioners may have some aspect of public health working as part of their role.

Public health has been defined as both a *resource* and an *activity* (Taylor et al 1998). Public health as a resource includes the gathering of health information and statistics (epidemiology) to underpin decisions and interventions which impact on health status. Epidemiology has a long history and high credibility. There is now a concern to broaden out the basis of epidemiology to include lay views and priorities and to acknowledge the effect of social factors on health (Naidoo & Wills 1998). Public health action refers to activities taken by agencies, organizations, professionals, communities, families and individuals which promote health.

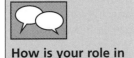

How is your role in public health defined?

The old public health

It is now well known that improvements in health in recent times owe more to public health measures than to clinical medicine (McKeown 1979). The 19th century saw the rise of the Sanitary Reform Movement and a wave of public health reforms, prompted by concerns about the spread of disease in overcrowded industrial slums. Many of the 19th century reformers attributed the unrest, crime and 'moral depravity' among the poor to their overcrowded and squalid conditions. The reforms owed little to the benevolence of the middle classes and much to an awareness that a competitive work and fighting force to match the strong nations of Europe would need an improvement in the health of the nation. Edwin Chadwick's *Report on the Sanitary Condition of the Labouring Population* (1842) was clear that the poor did not have the power to change their conditions:

> The individual labourer has little or no power over the internal structure and economy of the dwelling which has fallen to his lot. If the water be not laid on in the other houses in the street, or if it be unprovided with proper receptacles for refuse, it is not in the power of any individual workman who may perceive the advantages of such accommodations to procure them . . .

In the 19th century then, protecting and promoting the public health was clearly seen as the task of local government. Reforms focused on providing clean water, waste and sewage disposal, food hygiene and housing – what we would now regard as environmental issues. The Report of the Royal Sanitary Commission (1871) stated that 'the community will first learn, and then demand, their right to protection from preventable diseases and death, in return for the rates levied on them by a local authority'.

The old public health

1842 Edwin Chadwick's *Report on the sanitary condition of the labouring population of England* is published.
1843 The Royal Commission on the Health of Towns is established.
1844 The Health of Towns Association is founded.
1845 Final report from the Royal Commission on the Health of Towns is published.
1848 Public Health Act for England and Wales requires local authorities to provide clean water supplies and hygienic sewage disposal systems, and introduces the appointment of medical officers of health for towns.
1854 John Snow controls a cholera outbreak in London by removing a contaminated local water supply.
1866 Sanitary Act – local authorities had to inspect their district.
1868 Housing Act – local authorities could ensure owners kept their properties in good repair.
1871 Local Government Board (which became the Ministry of Health in 1919) was established.
1872 Public Health Act makes medical officers of health for each district mandatory.
1875 Public Health Act consolidates earlier legislation and the tone changes from *allowing* to *requiring* local authorities to take public health measures.
1906 Education Act established the provision of school dinners.
1907 Education Act establishes the school medical service. Notification of Births Act and the development of health visiting is encouraged.

The 19th century thus saw a wealth of legislation and regulations to promote health. In this century some examples of public health legislation have been the Clean Air Act 1956 to reduce air pollution and respiratory diseases, the Health and Safety at Work Act 1974 which requires all employers to secure the health, safety and welfare at work of all employees, the Housing (Homeless Persons) Act 1977 which places a duty on local authorities to house homeless persons, and the Water Bill 1988 to ensure privatized water suppliers conform to health standards. In addition, European Union regulations in many areas, including public health, for example health and safety at work, also apply to the UK.

In general, though, there has been a reluctance to socially regulate for health. For example, the thrust of measures to promote healthy eating has been informing and educating the public. Regulatory measures, such as the Food Standards Agency, focus on issues of food safety. Government action for the public health, if required, must be justified:

Why do you think there is a reluctance towards 'social engineering'?

Individuals taking action for themselves and their families are central . . . Communities working together can offer real help. And there is a vital role for Government too.

(DoH 1999, p. v)

The story of John Snow who stopped the cholera epidemic in Soho in 1854 by removing the handle of the Broad Street water pump illustrates the importance of the epidemiological (plotting and monitoring the incidence and prevalence of disease) approach in public health (Fig. 9.1). Previously, people had believed that bad air (miasma) from the rubbish and waste in the slums was responsible for the spread of disease. Snow's successful action demonstrated that cholera was a water borne disease which could be prevented by the provision of clean water supplies.

By the late 19th century sanitary reform was replaced by sanitary science based on germ theory, which located the causes of disease with individuals rather than their living conditions. Public health began to focus on preventive measures such as immunization and became the preserve of doctors, although it was still the responsibility of local government.

The decline of infectious diseases and the rise of new diseases (such as coronary heart disease and cancer) linked to lifestyles

Figure 9.1 *A portion of Snow's map of the spread of cholera in Soho. Purple bars represent the number of fatal cases in each house. The position of the Broad Street pump from which all the victims had obtained water is also marked.*

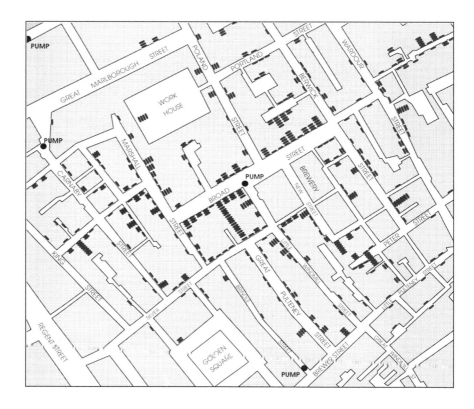

contributed to the low profile of public health in the mid-20th century. For most of the 20th century, public health continued to be the remit of local government, where the medical officers for health and environmental health officers were based. In 1975 community physicians employed by health authorities replaced the medical officers for health who had been employed by local authorities. Public health came to be seen as a medical speciality, and one which was marginalized and poorly funded. Public health was increasingly identified as the control of communicable diseases. Although the mid-1970s saw the separation of public health medicine from broader views of public health, there continued to be a steady stream of research reports which highlighted the role of social inequalities in producing ill health (Benzeval et al 1995, DoH 1996, Drever & Whitehead 1997, Townsend et al 1988). The broader view of public health became politically unpopular, but never disappeared.

The new public health

The 1980s saw a revival of interest in the concept of public health and a reframing and broadening of its boundaries. The strategies of developing health-promoting policies and working in partnerships with communities, which were used to make Liverpool a healthy city, came to be called the new public health (Ashton & Seymour 1988). The new public health drew on the World Health Organization (WHO) programme which set targets for healthy environments in its 'Health for All' European Region targets (WHO 1985). The Ottawa Charter identified healthy public policy as a central plank for health promotion. One of the aims of health promotion is to 'focus attention on public health issues, such as pollution, occupational hazards, housing and settlements' (WHO 1986). The Ottawa Charter identified the following fundamental resources for health: peace, shelter, education, food, income, a stable ecosystem, sustainable resources, social justice and equity.

The Adelaide Conference defined healthy public policy as 'an explicit concern for health and equity in all areas of policy and an explicit accountability for health impacts' (WHO 1988, p. 1). The main aim of healthy public policy is to create a supportive environment which enables people to live healthy lives, or to make the healthy choice the easy choice. The Sundsvall Conference concentrated on the global, interlinked nature of environmental change to promote health (WHO 1992). The Jakarta Declaration (WHO 1997) focused on the interlinked nature of social, economic and political development for health.

Whereas the 19th century view of public health was dominated by the role of the physical environment on health, the new public health is ecological in perspective. Economic, environmental and social factors all interconnect. When they are adequate, equitable and in balance with each other, populations are healthy.

In 1988 a commission of inquiry reported on public health in England. Known as the Acheson report after its chairman, Sir Donald Acheson, then Chief Medical Officer at the Department of Health, it defined public health as 'the science and art of preventing disease, prolonging life and promoting health through the organized efforts of society'. The report recommended a new post to replace the old District Medical Officer – a Director of Public Health. It is, however, local authorities and not the health service who have been most active in their support for public health and have supported legislation to produce a more health-promoting environment. Regulations, fiscal measures, policies and voluntary codes of practice may all be used to provide the population with the opportunities to make the healthier choice the easier choice. This might mean working towards no smoking in the workplace, the production of leaner meat and the introduction of alcohol labelling and warnings. What has been called the 'new public health' also means statutory and voluntary agencies working together to assess the implications for health in all public policies – agriculture, energy, transport, defence, economic development, employment, housing, education and leisure.

 Milio's pioneering work In Canada and North America (1986) has analyzed the effect on health of various public sectors and shown how alternative policy decisions could enhance health.

■ Can you think of examples for a healthy public energy policy?
■ Or transport?
■ Or agriculture?

The Labour Government elected in 1997 is committed to reviving the concept and function of public health. It is no longer solely a function of the NHS or local authorities. The new post of Minister for Public Health recognizes that the work of all government departments may impact on health and seeks to promote an integrated approach. The health strategy for England (DoH 1999) cites the Welfare to Work programme, the Housing Capital Receipts Initiative, the Integrated National Transport policy, and the Sport for All programme as policies which contribute to health.

Public health may involve confrontation with powerful vested interests.

The 1997 White Paper on the NHS (DoH 1997) introduced primary care groups (PCGs) and health improvement programmes (HImPs). PCGs are groups of GPs and community nurses

Food Standards Agency

An example of this is the proposal for an independent Food Standards Agency (FSA) to oversee the quality of food and to protect the public health. Proposals for the FSA, to be funded in part by the food industry, were met with scepticism: 'In the public's eyes the actual – and perceived – independence of the FSA will probably hinge less on such issues as remit and principles and more on its funding, its commissioners and staff' (Longfield 1998, p. 4). The FSA was not included in the legislative programme for 1999 but is likely to be set up in the year 2000.

responsible for working with social services and lay representatives to commission services for their population. Chapter 16 looks at these developments in more detail. Health authorities have a duty to consult with local authorities, NHS trusts and primary care groups, and to produce 3-year HImPs which identify local health priorities and strategies. 11 pilot health action zones (HAZs) were announced in 1998 with a second wave in 1999. HAZs are funded projects which seek to implement innovative strategies to promote health in deprived localities. These proposals all aim to increase partnership working and the participation of local communities to identify and meet health needs. Whereas in Victorian times public health was a function of benevolent government, the new public health is espoused as part of a broader project to revitalize democratic principles and government. Accountability for the public health lies with the public, not the medical profession. Public health is 'technically expert, but rooted in functioning democracies at both central and local levels' (Alderslade 1998, p. 550).

Public health has lacked prominence in the activities and publications commemorating 50 years of the NHS. The Victorians would be surprised at this and the limited role of local government. A recent White Paper 'Modern local government: in touch with the people' (Department of Environment, Transport and Regions 1998) may strengthen its public health role through a new duty to promote economic, social and environmental well-being of local residents. Local authorities must also consult and engage with their communities in producing a community plan which will make explicit links with regeneration, environmental policies and health improvement programmes to tackle public health.

The rise of the environmental movement and Green politics has been influential in raising the profile of public health, through the concepts of globalization and sustainability. The globalization of economic activities means that nation states no longer control those activities which affect physical and social environments. For example, pollution from the industrialized western countries leads to worldwide climate change, and the international money market affects employment patterns worldwide. More directly, the World Bank and International Monetary Fund, through their management of developing countries' debts, have been accused of stifling social, economic and health development in these countries (Townsend 1997).

Sustainable development has been defined as 'development that meets the needs of the present without compromising the ability of future generations to meet their own needs' (World Commission on Environment and Development 1987). The United Nations Rio Earth Summit on the Environment and Development in 1992 launched Agenda 21, which sets out a programme of action for sustainable development into the 21st century, addressing environmental, social and economic aspects of development. The Rio Declaration states that: 'Human beings are at the centre of concerns for sustainable development. They are entitled to a healthy productive life in harmony with nature' (United Nations 1992).

Agenda 21 commits governments to the following objectives on health:

■ meeting the basic essentials for health, e.g. safe food and water, sanitation and housing
■ controlling communicable diseases
■ protecting vulnerable groups, such as children
■ reducing the health risks caused by pollution, excessive energy consumption and waste.

Local Agenda 21, which developed as a result of the Rio Summit, is a comprehensive action plan for local development which aims to bring together local government, business, voluntary and community sectors to assess and meet local needs in a way which is sustainable.

 'Think globally, act locally'.

How might health promoters put this into practice?
Sustainable transport policies which seek to reduce dependency on private car use is an example of thinking globally, acting locally. By reducing harmful car emissions and congested roads, the environment is protected. At the same time, people can be encouraged to walk or cycle, benefiting their health.

Local authorities are responsible for consulting to produce 5-year transport plans which will:

■ cover all forms of transport
■ coordinate and improve local transport
■ set out strategies for promoting walking and cycling

- promote green transport plans for journeys to work, school and other places
- include measures to reduce social exclusion and address the needs of different groups in society
- set out proposals for implementation, including bus and freight quality partnerships, traffic management and traffic calming, proposals for road-user charging and private non-residential parking charges.

Hospitals in particular have been singled out as organizations which should be taking the lead in producing green transport plans. Hospitals will then be sending the right message to their communities on acting responsibly on health issues.

It can be seen then that many different agencies and movements bring their own priorities and agendas to public health. The new public health is therefore a hybrid creature. In the UK, the renaissance of the public health is linked to the election of the New Labour Government in 1997.

 The new public health

1974   Lalonde Report 'A new perspective on the health of Canadians' identifies the environment as crucial for health.
1985   The World Health Organization launches its 'Health for All' programme.
1986   The World Health Organization publishes the Ottawa Charter for health promotion.
1987   The Public Health Alliance is created.
1988   Acheson Report establishes the post of Director of Public Health within the NHS.
1992   The Association for Public Health, a multidisciplinary organization to promote public health policy, is created.
1992   Rio Earth Summit and Agenda 21.
1995   The Standing Nursing and Midwifery Advisory Committee (SNMAC) reports to Ministers on the contribution of nurses, midwives and health visitors to public health.
1997   Creation of a Minister of Public Health.
        White Paper: 'The New NHS – Modern, Dependable'. 3-year local health improvement programmes introduced.
1998   Green Papers: 'Our Healthier Nation' health strategy for England; 'Working together for a Healthier Scotland'; 'Better Health, Better Wales'; 'Fit for the Future' (Northern Ireland).
        Chief Medical Officer's project to strengthen the public health function.
        Health Action Zones (HAZs) – 11 pilot projects announced.
1999   Launch of the UK Public Health Association, incorporating the Public Health Alliance and the Association for Public Health.

Public health and health promotion

 The following have been identified as public health principles:

- Health for all – equality for all citizens
- A strategy for health
- Involvement of the public and patients
- Intelligence and surveillance
- Need for strong evidence base
- Importance of education, research and ethical considerations (Calman 1998).

The following have been identified as health for all principles:

- Empowerment
- Participation
- Equity
- Collaboration (WHO 1985)

Can you identify areas of overlap?

The new public health and health promotion share many principles and strategies. Indeed, the overlap is so great that one commentator has stated that: 'The principles and content of modern health promotion . . . are identical to those of the new public health' (MacDonald 1998, p. 28). Whilst there appears to be acceptance that public health is not solely reliant on medical expertise, the voice of health promotion remains marginalized. Health promoters have not been identified as particularly skilled or appropriate partners for public health.

The Chief Medical Officer is heading a project to ensure that there is a strong public health infrastructure capable of delivering the Government's new health agendas. Five main themes have been identified (DoH 1998):

- *A wider understanding of health* and of how people and organizations can contribute to health
- *Better coordination of,* and communication between, the different partners involved in promoting public health, including practitioners, academics, managers and politicians
- *An increase in capacity and capabilities* which will involve the development of public health specialists from a variety of professional backgrounds
- *Sustained development* so that public health gains are protected and built on
- *Effective joint working* between different organizations and professions.

Does it matter whether it is called public health or health promotion, as long as it is promoting the public health?

It could be argued that terminology is irrelevant so long as the job gets done. However, there is a danger in ignoring hard-won expertise and wasting resources by duplicating what is already known on the ground. This applies to the overlap of health promotion departments and public health departments, and also to local government who have strengthened their public health role.

The public health role of health workers

Many health workers have a public health role. In particular, community nurses, health promotion specialists and environmental health officers have a role in protecting and promoting the health of populations. For example, many health visitors compile community profiles which assess the health status and health needs of their local 'patch' or area. Caseload analyses provide another means of examining up-to-date information in order to ascertain trends and patterns, enabling community nurses to identify newly emerging health issues. This information can then be used to produce local health targets and to inform community nursing contracts with local commissioners of health services. For more information on health needs assessment, see Chapter 17.

A recent report by the Standing Nursing and Midwifery Advisory Committee highlighted the potential for nurses to contribute to public health work:

> Public health in nursing, midwifery and health visiting practice is about commissioning health services and providing professional care through organised collaboration in the NHS and society, to protect and promote health and well-being, prolong life and prevent ill-health in local communities, groups and populations.
>
> (SNMAC 1995, p. 5)

The examples in the box on the next page show how public health work can be undertaken even if the practitioner does not have a strategic planning role. For those whose job does include strategic planning, the opportunities for public health work are greater and more varied. For example, a locality forum could be established, bringing together health and local authorities and their communities, to share information and develop policies.

Public health principles

Three core principles which underpin public health and the WHO 'Health for All' programme are participation, equity and collaboration.

Participation

It is now accepted that the public have the right to be consulted and to have a say in the policy-making process (NHS Executive 1992).

Public health work and nurses

1. A nurse employed in a health authority public health department works at a strategic level to identify health needs, appraise health services and develop outcome indicators for strategic health objectives in commissioning. One area of work is managing the strategic purchasing programme for elderly people and for people with physical disabilities.
2. A health visitor in an NHS trust is responsible for assessing and meeting health needs at a community level. She has compiled a community health profile which identifies health needs and is used to agree local public health targets with the health authority's public health department. She works closely with local people to increase local resources for health. Projects she is involved with include accident prevention, women's health, smoking and solvent abuse, and services for children.
3. A health visitor is employed as a specialist worker for health and homelessness in a very deprived inner city area. Her role includes managing the homeless families' notification system and linking families with health visitors, ensuring local primary care services are accessible, appropriate and effective for homeless families, and having an input into commissioning strategies to ensure homeless families receive high-quality services.
4. A staff nurse in an intensive care unit explored how to promote accident prevention messages to children. This led to her linking up with local schools to provide educational sessions for 10- to 12-year-olds. Evaluation showed an increase in knowledge and behaviour change, such as wearing bicycle helmets and crossing roads more carefully.

Source: SNMAC (1995)

However, the means of public consultation range from formal to informal; one-off events to ongoing contact; reactive to proactive. Any activities undertaken to increase public participation and involvement could be said to be public health work.

 Identify ways in which you might promote public participation and accountability in your work.

Did you include the following:

■ Supporting patient participation groups in general practice including lay views in community health profiles
■ Seeking feedback from the community on service provision and using this to change practice
■ Supporting self-help groups in the community
■ Working with community groups on health issues
■ Liaising with schools and youth groups on health issues.

Equity

There is now a wealth of evidence to show that social and economic inequalities are reflected in health inequalities (Benzeval et al 1995, Drever & Whitehead 1997). The Acheson Report on health inequalities (Acheson 1998) came 18 years after the Black Report (Townsend & Davidson 1982) which first highlighted the link between poverty and ill health. Since then the UK has become an even more unequal society and the disparities in health have become more marked. More deprived and disadvantaged groups suffer higher levels of ill health and premature death than affluent and advantaged groups. There is also evidence that all people living in societies with greater inequality experience poorer health compared to more egalitarian societies (Wilkinson 1996). This provides a strong argument for advocating greater social and economic equity as a means of promoting health. Equity refers to both material resources and power (the ability to achieve desired goals). Equity, or being fair and just, is not the same as equality, which is the state of being equal. Whilst equality may be impossible to achieve, providing equal services for people with equal needs and working to reduce known inequalities in health are realistic goals.

What can you do in your health promotion role to promote equity?

Most practitioners see the promotion of equity as a political task beyond their role or competence. However, even small steps contribute to greater equity. For example, ensuring clients know their benefit entitlement and claim it, helping clients to fill out the necessary forms, or supporting the case for a welfare benefits advisory service to receive health authority funding are all aspects of working for equity. Identifying inequities in local services, such as people not registered with general practices, and supporting such groups to gain access to services, is also working for equity. Targeting areas of deprivation for more intensive interventions is another example.

Collaboration

Collaboration or partnership working is the third public health principle. Collaboration means working together with others on shared projects. Collaboration is necessary because of the many different factors affecting the public health, which means that any one agency or organization can have only a limited impact on health. By working together, more fundamental changes can be put into place, with a greater potential to promote health. Government publications have stressed the need for local authorities to consult widely with their local communities (NHS Executive 1992) and to work alongside the NHS to promote health (DoH 1998, 1999).

Coterminous boundaries, joint appointments and better resourcing have all been identified as important factors (DoH 1998).

Chapter 8 has highlighted some of the problems with collaborating across organizational boundaries, such as differences in priorities, organizational ethos, funding arrangements, competition for contracts and geographical boundaries. Enabling factors include committed individuals, joint funding and pooling of resources, shared education and training opportunities and existing projects which span different agencies.

Think of an intervention in your health promotion practice concerning the health promotion of young children or a young child.

Reflect on why you did what you did.
Could you have done something different?
Would other health promoters have done the same as you?
If you adopted a public health approach to your work, what aspects of this intervention would change?
How could you:

- increase participation?
- promote equity?
- increase collaboration and partnership working?

Conclusion

Public health is currently a high-profile issue. A key principle is replacing the medical model of health with a social model. International and national agencies that are responsible for providing the broad agenda for public health have produced a variety of supportive declarations, charters and legislation. For many, public health means the broad government functions of healthy public policy, and is a political agenda which is thought of as an activity removed from everyday practice. It is important to have a supportive public agenda, but the real challenge is to translate such lofty ideals into everyday practice, which requires a range of activities at many different levels. Central to this task are activities aimed at promoting participation, equity and collaboration.

Water fluoridation is advised by public health doctors and dentists in order to promote oral health. A powerful public lobby campaigns against water fluoridation on the grounds that it infringes personal liberty, and also questions the epidemiological evidence.

How could you make the public health case for water fluoridation in your local area?

Questions for further discussion

- What aspects of public health can you identify in your work?
- How could you build on and develop these aspects?
- Who and what could be your ally in this process?
- Do you need additional training, support or resources to develop these aspects?

Summary

This chapter has defined what public health work is and has shown how the new public health has built on the 19th century's legacy of public health reforms. The new public health draws on many partners such as environmental movements, political parties and international agencies such as the World Health Organization and the United Nations. The translation of public health work into health workers' everyday practice has been illustrated with examples. Public health work includes many different activities at different levels and this chapter has shown the diversity of what this means in practice.

Further reading

Jones L 1997 Health promotion and public policy, *and* Making and changing public policy. In: Jones L, Sidell M (eds) The challenge of promoting health: exploration and action. Open University/Macmillan, Basingstoke, chs 6, 7. *These chapters introduce and discuss key concepts in public policy for health and give examples from current practice. The contested nature of public policy is examined.*

Naidoo J, Wills J 1998 Practising health promotion: dilemmas and challenges. Baillière Tindall, London. *Chapter 4 looks in more detail at promoting equity, and Chapter 8 examines collaboration for health in more detail.*

Draper P (ed) 1991 Health through public policy: The greening of public health. Green Print, London. *This books adopts a broad perspective on public health. Different contributors look at how the environment can damage health, at the activities of industries which harm health and public watchdogs set up to protect the public health, and discuss future directions for public health.*

References

Acheson D 1998 Independent inquiry into inequalities in health: a report. Stationery Office, London

Alderslade R 1998 The Public Health Act of 1848. British Medical Journal 317: 549–550

Benzeval M, Judge K, Whitehead M 1995 Tackling inequalities in health: an agenda for action. King's Fund, London

Calman K 1998 The 1848 Public Health Act and its relevance to improving public health in England now. British Medical Journal 317: 596–598

Department of Environment, Transport and Regions 1998 Modern local government: in touch with the people (White Paper). Stationery Office, London

Department of Health (DoH) 1996 Variations in health: what can the Department of Health and the NHS do? DoH, London

Department of Health (DoH) 1997 The new NHS: modern, dependable. Stationery Office, London

Department of Health (DoH) 1998 Chief Medical Officer's project to strengthen the public health function in England: a report of emerging findings. DoH, London

Department of Health (DoH) 1999 saving lives: our healthier nation (White Paper). Stationery Office, London

Drever F, Whitehead M 1997 Health inequalities. Stationery Office, London

Longfield J 1998 The White Paper on the Food Standards Agency: how does it measure up?' Public Health Forum 2(1): 4

MacDonald T H 1998 Rethinking health promotion: a global approach. Routledge, London

McKeown T 1979 The role of medicine: dream, mirage or nemesis? Oxford University Press, Oxford

Milio N 1986 Promoting health through public policy. Canadian Public Health Association, Ottawa

Naidoo J, Wills J 1998 Practising health promotion: dilemmas and challenges. Baillière Tindall, London

NHS Executive 1992 Local voices: the views of local people in purchasing for health. Green Print, London

Standing Nursing and Midwifery Advisory Committee (SNMAC) 1995 Making it happen: public health – the contribution, role and development of nurses, midwives and health visitors. DoH, London

Taylor P, Peckham S, Turton P 1998 A public health model of primary care – from concept to reality. Public Health Alliance, Birmingham

Townsend P 1997 Think globally, act locally. In: Sidell M, Jones L, Katz J, Peberdy (eds) Debates and dilemmas in promoting health: a reader. Open University Press/Macmillan, Basingstoke

Townsend P, Davidson N 1982 Inequalities in health: the Black Report. Penguin, Harmondsworth

Townsend P, Davidson N, Whitehead M 1988 Inequalities in health: the Black Report and The Health Divide. Penguin, Harmondsworth

United Nations 1992 Rio Declaration on Environment and Development. UN, New York

Wilkinson R G 1996 Unhealthy societies: the afflictions of inequality. Routledge, London

World Commission on Environment and Development 1987 Our common future. Oxford University Press, Oxford

World Health Organization 1985 Health for all in Europe by the year 2000. Regional targets. WHO, Copenhagen

World Health Organization 1986 The Ottawa Charter for health promotion. WHO, Geneva

World Health Organization 1988 Adelaide recommendations on healthy public policy. WHO, Adelaide

World Health Organization 1992 Third international conference on health promotion (9–15 June 1991): Sundsvall, Sweden. WHO, Geneva

World Health Organization 1997 New players for a new era: leading health promotion into the 21st century. 4th International Conference on Health Promotion, Jakarta, Indonesia 21–25 July 1997. Conference Report World Health Organization, Geneva/Ministry of Health, Indonesia

10 *Working with communities and community development*

Key points

- Defining community development
- Community development in health promotion
- Working with a community development approach
- Community development activities
- Dilemmas for practice

OVERVIEW

We have seen in previous chapters how there are many different ways of working for health. This chapter focuses on community development – a strategy which aims to empower people to gain control over the factors influencing their health. Working with communities to increase their participation in decisions affecting health is an essential aspect of health promotion. This chapter begins by defining what is meant by a community and goes on to explore different ways in which health promoters can work with communities. Some of the dilemmas that confront the health promoter who wants to work in this way are discussed and illustrated using examples of community development projects.

What is the community?

The concept of community is frequently used in discussions about health and health care. In general, the context of the community is taken to be desirable; thus we have care in the community, community policing, and community education, all of which are seen as preferable to alternative (non-community) practice. In contrast to the State or the bureaucratic organization, services provided by and in the community are viewed as being more appropriate and sensitive. But what is the community which is referred to in these ways?

There are different ways of defining a community, but the most commonly cited factors are geography, culture and social stratification. These factors are viewed as being linked to the subjective feeling of belonging or identity which characterizes the concept of 'community'. Other characteristics of communities are social networks or systems of contact, and the existence of potential resources such as people's skills or knowledge.

Geography

A community may be defined on a geographical or neighbourhood basis. A well-known example is the East End of London, but this use

- Which communities do you belong to?
- Are these the same communities which your parents belonged to?
- What are the key characteristics of these communities?

of community is not restricted to working class or urban areas. It is this notion of community which gives rise to 'patch'-based work, where people such as social workers, police officers or health visitors are assigned a geographically bounded area. The assumption is that people living in the same area have the same concerns, owing to their geographical proximity.

Culture

Community may be defined in cultural terms, as in 'the Chinese community' or 'the Jewish community'. Here the assumption is that common cultural traditions may transcend geographical or other barriers, and unite otherwise scattered and disparate groups of people. There is an expectation that members of a cultural community will assist each other and share resources. The most commonly cited elements of a common cultural heritage are ethnic origin, language, religion and customs.

Social stratification

A community may be based on interests held to be common, which are usually the product of social stratification. Thus we have 'the working class community' and 'the gay community'. This definition implies that members of a community share networks of support, knowledge and resources which may transcend other boundaries, even national ones.

 Which definitions of community are being used in the following quotations?

- 'A number of individuals with something in common who may or may not acknowledge that connection' (HEA 1987)
- 'A locality which comprises networks of formal and informal relationships, which have a capacity to mobilise individual and collective responses to common adversity' (Barclay Report 1982)
- 'People with a basis of common interest and network of personal interaction, grouped either on the basis of locality or on a specific shared concern or both' (Smithies & Adams 1990, p. 9).

Most definitions of community tend to suggest that it is a homogeneous entity. However, it is obvious that any geographical community will include people whose primary identity is based on different factors, e.g. class, race, gender or sexual orientation. People who feel united by a shared interest, e.g. pensioners, or the unemployed, will also be members of other communities, geographical and otherwise. People may belong to several different communities, some of which may have more salience for the individual than others. In practice, people may find their allegiance to different communities shifting at different points in their life span.

The meaning and significance of community varies enormously. How one defines community is important because it influences how community representatives may be identified and communicated with.

Definition of terms

Community development

Community development has been defined as:

> a process by which a community identifies its needs or objectives, orders (or ranks) these needs or objectives, develops the confidence and will to work at these needs or objectives, finds the resources (internal and/or external) to deal with these needs or objectives, takes action in respect to them, and in so doing extends and develops co-operative and collaborative attitudes and practices in the community.
>
> (Ross 1955)

Community participation

The involvement of people in the community in the formal processes of policy making and implementation. Participation can vary from high to low levels of involvement.

Outreach

Outreach is the extension of a professional service into the community in order to make it more accessible. The location may be in the community, but there is no challenge to professional norms or claim to expertise. Outreach work is determined by professional priorities and the focus is on obtaining certain outcomes defined by professionals. An example of outreach is a mobile bus offering cervical cancer screening to women at their place of work. This may increase uptake of services by making them more accessible, but the type of service provision is predetermined and is not open for negotiation.

Community health projects

Projects organized to meet people's health needs in the community. Projects may be independent, for example self-help or voluntary projects, or located within the statutory services.

Key features of community development

Community development for health is: 'a process by which a community defines its own health needs, considers how those needs can be met and decides collectively on priorities for action' (CHIRU/LCHR 1987).

Community development is both a philosophy and a method. As a philosophy its key features are:

- a commitment to equality and the breaking down of hierarchies and power relationships
- an emphasis on participation and enabling all communities to be heard
- an emphasis on lay knowledge and the valuing of people's own experience
- the collectivizing of experience and seeing problems as shared
- the empowerment of individuals and communities through education, skills development and sharing and joint action.

The community development approach has been influenced by the work of Paulo Freire, a Brazilian educationalist who worked on literacy programmes with poor peasants in Peru and Brazil during the 1970s. Freire saw education as a way to liberate people from cycles of oppression. He aimed to engage the people in critical consciousness raising or 'conscientization', helping people to understand their circumstances and why they have been oppressed. The process of 'conscientization' begins with problem-posing groups which seek to break down barriers and establish a dialogue between individuals and between individuals and the facilitator. Eventually a state of 'praxis' is reached in which there is a common understanding and development of action and practice, whereby people collectively can transform their circumstances. The process is summarized as:

- reflection on aspects of reality
- search and collective identification of the root causes of that reality
- an examination of their implications
- development of a plan of action to change reality (Freire 1972).

Community development is a recognized way of working which has given rise to a specific profession – community development workers, who are generally employed by local authorities to support, facilitate and empower communities. Community development workers have their own training courses, qualifications and professional associations.

Community development and health promotion

Community development is a recurring theme in health promotion. In the 1960s the Women's Movement emphasized the need to reclaim knowledge about our bodies and control over our lives. Shared personal experience led to a new understanding of health issues as well as providing positive effects and social cohesion for participants. Black and ethnic minority groups also addressed health issues, particularly the effect of racism within the health services (Jones 1991).

In the 1970s and early 1980s numerous community development projects were set up, mostly funded and located outside the NHS. Inner city decline prompted youth work, neighbourhood centres and planning groups which drew attention to the relationship between poverty, health and inequalities in service provision (Rosenthal 1983). Within the health services, community development approaches remained marginalized.

In the latter part of the 1980s there was widespread lip service to the notion of community development, stimulated in part by the World Health Organization.

'The people have a right and a duty to participate individually and collectively in the planning and implementation of their health care' (WHO 1978).

'Health for all will be achieved by people themselves. A well-informed, well-motivated and actively *participating community* is a key element for the attainment of the common goal' (WHO 1985, p. 5, original emphasis).

'Health promotion works through concrete and effective community action in setting priorities, making decisions, planning strategies and implementing them to achieve better health. At the heart of this process is the empowerment of communities, their ownership and control of their own endeavours and destinies' (WHO 1986).

'Community action is central to the fostering of health public policy' (WHO Adelaide 1988).

'Health promotion is carried out by and with people, not on or to people. It improves the ability of individuals to take action, and the capacity of groups, organisations or communities to influence the determinants of health. Improving the capacity of communities for health promotion requires practical education, leadership training and access to resources.' (WHO 1997).

Community development has been seen as the central defining strategy for health promotion (Green & Raeburn 1990). By the mid-1980s the Community Health Initiatives Resource Unit estimated that there were 10 000 local projects in existence. By the 1990s the lead health promotion agencies for developing strategies were under pressure as community development was seen as too radical. Its focus on structural causes of inequality such as class, race and gender, was not acceptable to New Right political ideology (see Ch. 7 for more discussion of this). The Community and Professional Development Division of the Health Education Authority (HEA) was disbanded. The National Community Health Resource (NCHR) lost its funding from the HEA and Community Health UK (CHUK) lost its funding from the Department of Health.

Yet the 1990s also saw an emphasis on the concept of 'community'. Strategies for service delivery were linked to the notion of community, and care in the community, community policing and community education emerged as key policies.

What do you think contributed to this emphasis on working with 'the community'?

The focus on the community needs to be seen in relation to the developing crisis in the role of welfare state provision and broader debates around accountability. Chapter 7 has shown how the New Right concern to retreat from welfare was linked to a focus on individuals as consumers of services. Locality or 'patch' planning, a focus on primary care and an emphasis on participation and 'consumer involvement' were all strategies designed to achieve these aims.

The New Labour Government elected in 1997 has also emphasized the importance of working with the community, albeit from a different set of political values (see Ch. 7 for more details of the different political philosophies). Chapter 15 looks at how neighbourhoods are being used as settings for health promotion. Community development is on the ascendency again, and now there is a greater acceptance of the link between vibrant communities and good health.

 Crosshands Healthy Communities Project

The Crosshands Healthy Communities Project is based at the Crosshands Health Centre in the Gwendraeth Valley in Wales. It aims to promote healthy, dynamic local communities and to develop effective strategies to address community health needs. The project is funded by Health Promotion Wales, the Llanelli/Dinefwr NHS Trust, Menter Cwm Gwendraeth and the Crosshands GP Practice. The project was launched in 1997 with the appointment of a healthy community coordinator who acts as a facilitator encouraging partnerships between local agencies and the community. Key tasks include:

- Profiling to identify existing community facilities, services and resources
- Networking and linking between service providers and community groups and local organizations
- Developing structures, e.g. the Healthy Community Alliance
- Collaborative projects, e.g. needs assessment studies on drugs and alcohol, sexual health and mental health of young people.

Such approaches are supported by evidence of the health-enhancing effects of social support and community involvement. A research project investigating four wards of varying health and socio-economic status in Luton indicates that the healthier wards had higher levels of 'social capital' characterized by trust in others and in organizations, and participation in formal and informal social networks (HEA 1998).

Community development may therefore be applauded as a radical health promotion strategy which challenges inequalities and aims to increase participation. However, community development is not necessarily radical. In the 19th century, community development was used as a means of controlling the UK's colonies in the face of demands for self-government. The emphasis on people deciding their own needs and helping themselves can be used as a means of reducing state expenditure on services and to mislead people about the extent of their control.

Working with a community development approach

The ways in which community development is carried out vary enormously. Yet there are three elements which are common to all community development work:

User led

In contrast to professionally determined priorities, community development starts with priorities identified by and common to communities. This means starting out with people's concepts of health which are typically more broadly based than those of health workers. Coulter (1987) found that working-class people identified social, economic and environmental factors, such as unemployment, pollution, housing and income, as the most important influences on their health. (This is discussed in greater detail in Ch. 1.) Problems and concerns are seen as interlinked and not solely to do with 'health' or 'housing'.

The key task of a community development worker is to build a picture of the community, identifying key individuals, groups and resources, and get to know the community formally and informally. Building networks and identifying 'communities' takes time.

> The role of the community worker is to build on initial research and contact with people living and working in the community, so that the needs identified can be expanded upon and solutions developed. The worker's overall role would be to support and facilitate that process, particularly in terms of existing organisational structures and the creation of new ones.
>
> (Thornley 1997, p. 64)

An important aspect of community development work is legitimizing people's knowledge about health and illness and giving this a voice. Not only does this pose a challenge to medical dominance; it is also very different from the systematic research into needs which we describe in Chapter 17. Establishing the needs of the community also means a shift towards more participatory and locality-based involvement. Later in this chapter we look at how communities can be enabled to participate in health decisions.

Focus on process

The process of enabling communities to promote health is viewed as a positive activity in its own right. Community development entails greater participation and this process will itself enhance self-confidence, self-esteem and feelings of being in control, which are themselves health-promoting factors. Whether this activity is directed towards a specific health issue such as coronary heart disease, or more general issues, such as transport or housing, is not crucial, for the skills which are gained are transferable to different contexts.

The role of the community development worker may be:

■ to encourage personal development, e.g. through a self-help group
■ to develop skills, e.g. lobbying or working with committees
■ to provide practical support, e.g. child care facilities, a meeting place, training or transport.

Those involved in community development work recognize the knowledge and experience in that community and aim to build up its capabilities. This will mean giving people time to develop these skills. Consequently, there may be no immediate or tangible outcomes of community development work.

Focus on the needs of disadvantaged and vulnerable groups

The third characteristic is that community development acknowledges health inequalities and prioritizes activity with disadvantaged and vulnerable groups. Instead of focusing on individual lifestyles, community development focuses on the social determinants of ill health. Its aim is to empower people to act together to influence the social, economic, political and environmental issues which affect them. This may mean:

■ working to promote the health of disadvantaged groups
■ increasing the accessibility of services
■ influencing the commissioning of services

■ **How important do you think community development is as a health promotion strategy?**
■ **How does it compare with other approaches such as the medical preventive, individual empowerment, educational, behaviour change or social change approaches?**

Table 10.1
Advantages and disadvantages of the community development approach

Advantages	Disadvantages
Starts with people's concerns, so it is more likely to gain support	Time consuming
Focuses on root causes of ill health, not symptoms	Results are often not tangible or quantifiable
Creates awareness of the social causes of ill health	Evaluation is difficult
The process of involvement is enabling and leads to greater confidence	Without evaluation, gaining funding is difficult
The process includes acquiring skills which are transferable, for example communication skills, lobbying skills	Health promoters may find their role contradictory. To whom are they ultimately accountable – employer or community?
If health promoter and people meet as equals, it extends principle of democratic accountability	Work is usually with small groups of people
	Draws attention away from macro issues and may focus on local neighbourhoods

- acting as an advocate and representing the interests of disadvantaged groups
- building a social profile of the community, highlighting the relationship to health status.

The community development approach is challenging. It offers the prospect of change for health but there are many practical difficulties to overcome (Table 10.1).

Types of activities involved in community development

A large number of different activities may be included in the term community development. Smithies & Adams (1990) propose five different categories of community action for health. These are:

- formal participation in decision-making mechanisms
- community action
- facilitating processes which enable the community
- professional and community interface
- strategic support.

Formal participation

The emphasis in community development on increasing people's power and control means increasing their participation in decision-making. Participation may be thought of as a ladder which includes many different activities (Fig. 10.1). At the low or weak end, it may mean consultation to 'rubber stamp' plans already drawn up by official agencies. At the high or strong end of the spectrum, it may mean control over the setting of priorities and implementation of programmes.

Figure 10.1
Arnstein's ladder of participation. Adapted from Arnstein (1969).

8	Citizen control		Citizens are involved in planning and decision-making through joint committees, delegated representatives or complete control
7	Delegated power	} Degrees of citizen power	
6	Partnership		
5	Placation		
4	Consultation	} Degrees of tokenism	Citizens have a voice but may not be heeded
3	Informing		
2	Therapy	} Non-participation	Those with power educate or cure Citizens are recipients
1	Manipulation		

Consider the following examples of participation. Where would you place them on Arnstein's ladder?

How could they be moved up the ladder?

- A public forum to discuss the provision of mental health services
- The attendance of a mother at a court hearing about the care of her child
- The use of care plans for elderly people living in residential homes
- An inner city locality project funded by local and health authorities: a health visitor is given a 0.5 secondment to lead the project; the focus is on providing appropriate preventive services.

Community action

Community action is any activity undertaken by a community in order to effect change. This includes lobbying authorities to provide services, and the provision of voluntary or self-help services to address needs.

Trojan et al (1991) conducted a survey of about 1700 community organizations in Hamburg. The findings of the survey were that between 75% and 85% of all health-related community organizations were actively engaged in providing social support, undertaking social action for better health, supporting networks within communities, and seeking to empower people. These activities are all important to health promotion. They conclude that 'To a great extent, therefore, promoting health means strengthening community organisations' (Trojan et al 1991, p. 456).

There is a growing body of research linking civic involvement and health (Wilkinson 1996). Networks and support established through community action promote the sense of coherence which Antonovsky (1993) has suggested is protective of health.

Facilitating processes

Facilitating processes are those activities which are designed to increase and enhance people's skills in working for change. This may include providing appropriate training, and developing and supporting viable networks within communities.

> **The Loftus Good Grub Club**
>
> The Loftus Good Grub Club was started in 1996 with funding from Tees Health Authority. The aim was to improve the diets of women on a low income and to reduce social isolation. The project was publicized on local radio and via schools and community groups. The Loftus Good Grub Club focuses on cheap, easy family meals and getting fit. The project negotiated discounted rates with the local leisure centre to promote exercise and has produced cook books and made a profit through catering for buffets. Some of the women involved have gained certificates in food handling. The project is now self-sufficient.

Many community nurses compile community profiles. How could these be used to open up the professional/community interface?

Professional and community interface

The professional and community interface needs to be open and flexible if community development is to achieve real change. This can be achieved by a reorientation of professionals and official agencies so that community concerns are seen as legitimate. Organizational culture tends to be inward-looking, and this needs to be changed so that community views are actively sought and valued as part of the planning and provision of services.

Strategic support

Strategic support refers to organizational policies and initiatives which endorse community development and enable it to take place. Strategic support may function at different levels, neighbourhood, city, region or nationwide.

> **Tower Hamlets Health Strategy Group**
>
> Tower Hamlets Health Strategy Group is a voluntary sector organization in East London which was set up over 10 years ago. It is funded by grants from health authorities, the local authority, single regeneration budget money and charitable trusts. A major part of its work is to undertake research to develop and evaluate innovative health service provision which addresses the needs of groups not currently well served.
>
> Source: Curtis & Taket (1996)

- **What positive outcomes have been attributed to community development health promotion projects?**
- **Are these outcomes unique to community development?**

Dilemmas in community development practice

The question of whether the community development worker is engaged in radical practice or supporting the status quo is at the root of much of the ambiguity surrounding practice. Common dilemmas facing the community development worker relate to funding, accountability, acceptability, the role of the professional and evaluation.

Funding

Most community development projects are funded by statutory agencies, such as health and education authorities, sometimes in partnership, through joint funding. Other projects which might come under the label 'community development' belong in the voluntary sector, and are funded from a variety of sources including direct government grants and independent fund-raising. Most community development work is funded in the short term only. Lack of security and the impossibility of guaranteeing an input in the long term increases the problems of planning and evaluating such work. Insecure funding arrangements can also subvert a project's focus, leading workers to spend time fund-raising instead of working around defined issues.

Accountability

All community development workers have a dual accountability: to their employers and to their communities. Funding agencies naturally require projects to be accountable, and this can lead to problems where the priorities of the community and the agency are not the same. Organizational objectives such as service take-up may become incorporated into the community development worker's role.

Community and worker responses to issues may also differ. For example, both may identify safety as a priority, but whereas the worker may respond by advocating structural changes such as better lighting and common responsibility for shared areas, the community might respond by advocating increased vigilance or the exclusion of specific groups, families or individuals.

Community development workers may feel themselves to be trapped in the role of mediator – informing statutory services about community needs and informing the community about how services work so that people can participate.

Acceptability

Employing authorities often view community development as not quite respectable. Community development may be seen as absorbing unacceptably large amounts of time and resources for dubious results. Community development tends to focus on small numbers of people whereas employers tend to be responsible for large populations. The long-term nature and diffuse outcomes of community development are at odds with the organizational need to allocate resources on the basis of demonstrable results.

Issues which are raised through a community development approach (such as discrimination in service provision) may be unacceptable to employing authorities. By allying themselves with dissent, community development workers may be seen as betraying the organization.

Community development workers may also find that they need to establish and negotiate their role before they are accepted by a community. The role of the worker is ambiguous. Their status and employment sets them apart from the community in which they are working. Relationships of trust may need to be created before any other work can take place

Role of the professional

Community development also poses problems for workers whose primary training lies in other areas.

Problems may arise from the different kind of client–worker relationship envisaged in professional training and community development work. Professional workers are taught a particular area of expertise and tend to assume that they know what is best for their clients. They may be sensitive to individual circumstances but the secondary socialization encountered during professional training reinforces the notion of expertise.

A health visitor wishes to adopt a community development approach in her work. She has identified setting up a postnatal mothers' group as an appropriate project.

■ What arguments might she use in favour of this kind of work?
■ What arguments might her manager use against it?

The health visitor might argue that such work is important for health because it increases self-esteem, autonomy and confidence, and a sense of belonging. She could argue that such work is effective. For example, postnatal networking amongst mothers could prove effective in reducing mental illness amongst this client group (Brown & Harris 1978). The health visitor might also argue that time spent on setting up the group will reduce claims on her time in future, and is therefore a cost-effective option.

The health visitor's manager might respond that there is not enough time to carry out such work. Full caseloads and many other priority claims (such as visiting all new mothers and carrying out child development check-ups) mean there is no spare time available for other activities. The manager might also argue that such activities need to be thoroughly evaluated and of proven effectiveness before resources can be committed.

Sociologists argue that professional culture is actually an occupational strategy designed to increase the status and rewards of the professional group (Freidson 1986, Johnson 1972). By acquiring professional jargon, expertise and qualifications, professionals can justify their right to practice and defend their area of work.

By contrast, community development workers see their role as that of catalyst and facilitator rather than expert. Their task is to enable a community to express its needs, and support the community in meeting those needs themselves. This requires a different worker–client relationship, based on egalitarianism and the sharing of knowledge. For professionals, whose identity is bound up in their work role, this can be a difficult switch to make.

The skills involved in community work also tend to be different from those acquired in professional training (unless this includes community development). Key skills concern process rather than content and include:

■ organizational skills, e.g. developing appropriate management structures such as management committees or steering groups
■ communication skills, e.g. consultation and communication with a variety of groups including community groups, funding agency and co-workers
■ evaluation skills, e.g. monitoring the impact of interventions and self-evaluation.

- **Which of these skills are covered in your professional training?**
- **How much time is devoted to these areas compared to other areas in the curriculum?**
- **Do you think your professional training has equipped you to practise community development?**

Evaluation

Evaluating the impact of community development work raises many questions which are discussed in greater detail in Chapter 14. What is impressive is the positive feedback from communities and workers who have been involved in community development around health issues. This is a consistent finding from many different projects, although the local scale of such work means such findings are not easily disseminated to a broader audience. To take just one example, a report of the Hartcliffe Health and Environment Action Group, a group based in a deprived outer city housing estate in Bristol, states that:

> From the health education point of view, this project can be seen to be instrumental in promoting people's health. A significant number of those involved would, in all probability, never otherwise have had access to information about health, health services and the support and opportunity for personal growth which has evidently been presented through their participation in this group.
>
> (Roberts 1992, unpublished dissertation, p. 54)

This is typical of the enthusiasm many workers feel, which is itself a reflection of the feedback they receive from the people involved. A member of the Hartcliffe group puts it succinctly: 'I don't feel like a spectator now' (Roberts 1992, p. 37). However, these kinds of outcomes are difficult to express concisely, or to put in quantitative terms.

Empowerment as a process of developing understanding and influence over personal, social and economic forces is difficult to measure. Evaluation may focus on:

- outcomes, e.g. changes in service provision, increased social networking, achievement of educational qualifications, behavioural changes, more open decision making
- process, e.g. shifts in awareness of power, development of self-esteem, enhanced negotiating skills.

A review of more than 40 community development projects has found a range of evaluation methods, many developing new ways of involving the community in the design of the evaluation, as informants and in developing future work (Beattie 1995).

Despite these difficulties, it is important to evaluate community development. Ongoing or formative evaluation provides a means for results and outcomes to be fed back into a project, allowing it to be modified if necessary.

Conclusion

Community development does not fit tidily into most health promoters' working lives. In contrast to how most health promotion workers have been trained, community development relies upon a different set of assumptions about the nature of health and a different set of skills. This can make it a problematic activity to undertake. However, practitioners who have espoused community development are enthusiastic about its potential and outcomes. It is claimed to be the most ethical and effective form of health promotion, and one which makes a real impact on people's lives.

> What (inner city community health projects) are doing is creating a climate in which some of the most oppressed and deprived sections of our urban communities can find a voice with which to challenge the forces which both determine their health and control the quantity and quality of health services to which they have access.
>
> (Rosenthal 1983)

Community development does appear to address many of the problems inherent in more traditional forms of health promotion. It avoids victim-blaming, addresses structural causes of inequalities in health, and seeks to empower people. This goes some way to explain its popularity with health promoters.

Community development has been endorsed both at the international level, by various WHO declarations, and at the local level, by project workers. It is not such a popular option at the middle level of large-scale organizations, including the NHS. This is in part due to the practical difficulties of implementation and evaluation. However, there are also ideological conflicts if community development is to be practised within the NHS. It has been stated that community development represents a challenge to the medical model of health, and previous experience in the UK has also demonstrated that it is perceived as an overtly political strategy. The political implications of community development have been attacked from both the right and left wings of the political spectrum. Community development has been viewed as both a subversive left-wing activity, and a subtle means of policing and controlling communities.

A global review of community projects has shown that they do tackle broader influences on health and promote health behaviour change in individuals (Gillies 1997).

 Community development in Costa Rica

A comprehensive community development programme in Costa Rica involved links across government departments, health and local authorities working together, local people contributing to decision-making through local social action committees, needs assessments, educational opportunities for women and micro-enterprise developments to boost income in the poorest groups. The programme led to improved infant mortality rates, improved access to services and improved social, economic and physical environments. The key elements of success were:

- Involvement of local people in identifying needs
- Committed and open partnerships between agencies
- Involvement of local people in planning and decision-making through local action committees
- Training and support for volunteers, peer educators and local networks.

Source: Gillies (1997)

New primary care groups need to shape services by assessing local health needs and working in partnership with local agencies. Community development strategies could help PCGs to be more accountable and focus on social determinants of health (Burton & Harrison 1996, Freeman et al 1997).

Questions for further discussion

- Would you consider adopting a community development approach in your work?
- Do you think community development has advantages over other health promotion strategies?

Summary

This chapter has examined the history and theoretical underpinnings of community development as an approach to health promotion. We have seen that community development is often viewed by workers as the most ethical and effective means of promoting health. At the same time, its practice poses dilemmas for the health promoter and its evaluation is fraught with problems. However, we would argue that the reasons put forward for the privileged position of community development are sound. Practical difficulties should not obstruct the continuing development and spread of this health promotion strategy. On the contrary, what is needed is a more open outlook from statutory organizations, and a willingness to experiment with this kind of strategy.

Further reading

Jones L, Sidell M 1997 The challenge of promoting health: exploration and action. Open University and Macmillan, Basingstoke. *An accessible textbook which explores the potential for communities to be involved in promoting their own health.*

Smithies J, Adams L 1990 Community participating in health promotion. HEA, London. *A brief and clear summary of different British community health promotion projects. Includes a useful glossary of key terms.*

References

Antonovsky A 1993 The sense of coherence as a determinant of health. In: Beattie A, Gott M, Jones L, Sidell M. Health and wellbeing: a reader. Macmillan/Open university, Basingstoke, pp 202–214

Arnstein S R 1971 Eight rungs on the ladder of citizen participation. In: Cahn SE, Passelt BA. Citizen participation: effecting community change. Praeger, New York

Barclay Report on Social Work 1982 National Institute for Social Work. Social workers: their role and tasks. Bedford Square Press, London

Beattie A 1995 Evaluation in community development for health: an opportunity for dialogue. Health Education Journal 54: 465–471

Burton P, Harrison L (eds) 1996 Identifying local health needs: new community based approaches. Policy Press, Bristol

Brown G, Harris T 1978 The social origins of depression. Tavistock, London

Community Health Initiatives Resource Unit/London Community Health Resource 1987 Guide to community health projects. NCVO, London

Coulter A 1987 Lifestyles and social class: implications for primary care. Journal of the Royal College of General Practitioners 37: 533–536

Curtis S, Taket A 1996 Health and societies. Arnold, London

Freeman R, Gillam S, Shearin C, Pratt J 1997 Community development and involvement in primary care. King's Fund, London

Freidson E 1986 Professional powers: a study of the institutionalization of formal knowledge. University of Chicago Press, Chicago

Freire P 1972 Pedagogy of the oppressed. Penguin, Harmondsworth

Gillies P 1997 The effectiveness of alliances or partnerships for health promotion. Conference working paper. 4th International Conference on Health Promotion, Jakarta, Indonesia

Green L W, Raeburn J 1990 Community wide change: theory and practice. In: Bracht N (ed) Health promotion at the community level. Sage, California

Health Education Authority 1987 Leaflet on community department. HEC, London

Health Education Authority 1998 Towards healthier communities. Annual report 1997/98. HEC, London

Johnson T 1972 Professions and power. Macmillan, London

Jones J 1991 Community development and health education: concepts and philosophy. In: Open University Health Education Unit. Community development and health education. Open University Press, Milton Keynes, vol 1

Roberts SE 1992 Healthy participation: an evaluative study of the Hartcliffe Health and Environmental Action Group, a community development project in Bristol. (Unpublished MSc dissertation)

Rosenthal H 1983 Neighbourhood health projects – some new approaches to health and community work in some parts of the United Kingdom. Community Development Journal 18: 120–130

Ross M 1955 Community organisations: theories and principles. Harper and Brothers, New York

Smithies J, Adams L 1990 Community participation in health promotion. HEA, London

Thornley P 1997 Working at the local level. In: Jones L, Sidell M (eds) The challenge of promoting health: exploration and action. Open University and Macmillan, Buckingham

Trojan A, Hildebrandt H, Deneke C, Faltis M 1991 The role of community groups and voluntary organisations in health promotion. In: Badura B, Kickbusch I (eds) Health promotion research: towards a new social epidemiology. WHO Regional Publications, Copenhagen

Wilkinson R 1996 Unhealthy societies: the afflictions of inequality. Routledge, London

World Health Organization 1978 Alma Ata 1978: primary health care. WHO, Geneva

World Health Organization 1985 Targets for health for all. WHO Regional Office for Europe, Copenhagen

World Health Organization 1986 The Ottawa charter for health promotion. Health Promotion 1: iii–v

World Health Organization 1988 Adelaide recommendation on health public policy. WHO, Adelaide

World Health Organization 1997 New players for a new era: leading health promotion into the 21st century. 4th International Conference on Health Promotion, Jakarta, Indonesia 21–25 July 1997. Conference Report World Health Organization, Geneva/Ministry of Health, Indonesia

11 *Helping people to change*

OVERVIEW

People's health behaviour or lifestyles have been regarded as the cause of many modern diseases. Therefore a main focus of health promotion has been on modifying those aspects of behaviour which are known to have an impact on health.

In previous chapters we have argued that such an approach is unlikely to be effective unless it acknowledges how people's behaviour may be a response to, and maintained by, the environment in which they live. Many health promoters, however, see their role as helping people to live their lives to its best potential, which may involve some change in their health behaviour.

This chapter is concerned with those aspects of health behaviour that people can control. Understanding why people behave in certain ways and how they can be helped to maintain chosen behaviours is central to self-empowerment. This chapter explores the usefulness of social psychology which offers several theoretical models that identify the determinants of behaviour change. This can contribute to, if not the prediction, then at least an understanding of how people make decisions about their health. This can be a useful tool in planning health promotion interventions. The influence of specific factors such as individual self-esteem or people's perceptions of control over their lives needs to be taken into account by the health promoter in order to offer practical support and positive experiences in making choices.

Key points

- The role of beliefs, attitudes and values in health-related decisions
- The influence of social norms on health behaviour
- The concept of locus of control
- Health promotion strategies to change attitudes or behaviour

Several theories have attempted to explain the influence of different variables on an individual's health related behaviour:

- the Health Belief Model (Becker 1974)
- the Theory of Reasoned Action (Ajzen & Fishbein 1980)
- the Stages of Change Model (Prochaska & DiClemente 1984).

This chapter explores the application of these models of behaviour change to health, and considers various strategies used to change attitudes or behaviour.

Definitions

According to social psychology theories of behaviour change, people's behaviour is partly determined by their attitude to that behaviour. An individual's **attitude** to a specific action and the intention to adopt it are influenced by **beliefs**, **motivation** which comes from the person's **values**, **attitudes** and **drives** or **instincts**, and the influences from **social norms**.

Beliefs.   A belief is based on the information a person has about an object or action. It links the object to some attribute. For example, a person believes that potatoes (object) are fattening (an attribute). Theories of health-related behaviour change are based on the idea that an individual's behaviour will be based on their beliefs. In this example, the person will cut down on potatoes if they wish to lose weight. If this person is encouraged to believe that potatoes are not fattening but a useful bulk food, then they may include them in their diet. In other words, that information can influence beliefs which will then, in turn, influence behaviour. This simple model is sometimes referred to as the Knowledge–Attitudes–Behaviour (KAB) model. Of course, behaviour change is never quite as simple as that. Information alone is neither necessary nor sufficient for behaviour change. The health risks of smoking are well known and yet over 30% of the population continue to smoke.

Values.   These are acquired through socialization and are those emotionally charged beliefs which make up what a person thinks is important. A person's values will influence a whole range of feelings about family, friendships, career and so on. For example, values relating to sex and gender give rise to a number of attitudes towards motherhood, employment of women, body image, breast feeding and sexuality.

Attitudes.   These are more specific than values and describe relatively stable feelings towards particular issues. There is no clear association between people's attitudes and their behaviour. Sometimes changing attitudes may stimulate a change in behaviour and sometimes behaviour change may influence attitudes. For example, many people continue to smoke despite a negative attitude to smoking. Yet once the behaviour is stopped, they may develop vehement anti-smoking views.

People's attitudes are made up of two components:

- cognitive – the knowledge and information they possess
- affective – their feelings and emotions and evaluation of what is important.

Attitudes are very hard to change. They may be changed by providing more or different information, or by increasing a person's skills. For example, a person's attitude towards the benefits of exercise might be influenced by providing information about different types of physical activity and their effects on the body. It might also be influenced by improved performance which motivates the person and encourages him or her to think of exercise as enjoyable.

Festinger (1957) used the term 'cognitive dissonance' to describe a person's mental state when new information is given which is counter to that already held. This prompts the person either to reject the new information (as unreliable or inappropriate) or to adopt attitudes and behaviour which would fit with it.

 How do people respond to information about the risks to their health from particular behaviours?

Some people may become concerned and change when presented with information about health risks. Others may make some change such as switching to a lower-risk substitute (e.g. low-fat spread). Others may deny their risk, perhaps by underestimating the frequency or amount of their current behaviour.

Drives.   The term 'drive' is used in the Health Action Model (Tones 1994) to describe strong motivating factors such as hunger, thirst, sex and pain. It is also used to describe motivations which can become drives, such as addiction. Some studies suggest that addiction is the consequence of frequently repeated acts which become a habit and its base is a psychological fear of withdrawal (Davies 1992). Social learning theory (Bandura 1977) uses the term 'instinct' to describe behaviours which are not learned but are present at birth. Instincts can override attitudes and beliefs. Hunger, for example, can easily override a person's favourable attitude and intention to diet.

The practitioner needs to understand what contributes to people's decision-making about health and what makes some people more amenable to change than others. The social cognition models which we shall now consider highlight the following as important:

- people's views about the cause and prevention of ill health
- the extent to which people feel they can control their life and make changes
- whether they believe change is necessary
- whether change is perceived to be beneficial in the long term, outweighing any difficulties and problems which may be involved.

These theoretical models try to unpack the relative importance of these factors, recognizing that what people say is not necessarily a guide to what they will do, and that there are numerous antecedent and situational variables.

The Health Belief Model

The Health Belief Model is probably the best-known theoretical model highlighting the function of beliefs in decision-making (see Fig. 11.1). This model, originally proposed by Rosenstock (1966) and modified by Becker (1974), has been used to predict protective health behaviour, such as screening or vaccination uptake and compliance with medical advice (e.g. Gillam 1991). The model suggests that whether or not people change their behaviour will be influenced by an evaluation of its feasibility and its benefits weighed against its costs. In other words, people considering changing their behaviour engage in a cost–benefit or utility analysis. This may include their beliefs concerning the likelihood of the illness or injury happening to them (their susceptibility); the severity of the illness or

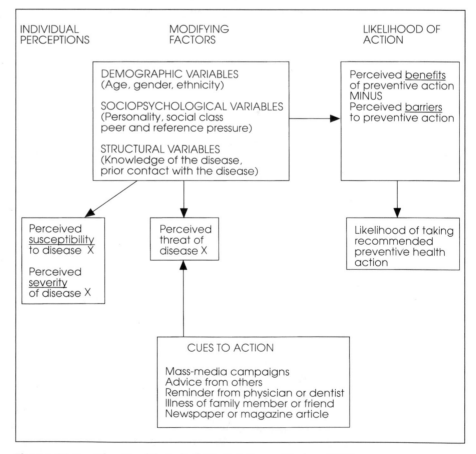

Figure 11.1 *The Health Belief Model. From Becker 1974.*

injury; and the efficacy of the action and whether it will have some personal benefit, or how likely it is to protect the person from the illness or injury.

For a behaviour change to take place, individuals:

- must have an incentive to change
- feel threatened by their current behaviour
- feel a change would be beneficial in some way and have few adverse consequences
- must feel competent to carry out the change.

 Consider the following situation and then try to apply the Health Belief Model to see if you can predict how the woman might respond.

A mother of three children under five receives a card from her GP informing her that her youngest child should receive an Hib injection to protect him from meningitis. The woman works at a local factory as an hourly paid packer. Her mother cares for the children whilst she is at work, but has no transport.

If we are to use the Health Belief Model as a model for predicting health behaviour, we would see the mother as a rational problem-solver who would not only be aware of the causes of Hib meningitis but also the risks of contracting it (the child's susceptibility and severity). We would assume that the mother would have been made aware of the efficacy of the vaccine and be aware of its protection against one type of meningitis only (*Haemophilus influenzae* B). She would also be aware of any possible side-effects or contraindications. If the mother has had previous children vaccinated with no adverse effects or had this child or other children immunized against other diseases, she is more likely to view this vaccination favourably and have confidence in its effectiveness. In using this model as a predictor of behaviour, we need to take into account the perceived barriers and costs to taking this action. The mother would need to ask her own mother to take the child to the doctor. The child's grandmother may be unwilling or unable to take three children on public transport. Or the mother would have to take time off work with consequent loss of earnings.

Most learning theories are based on the premise that people's behaviour is guided by consequences. If these are positive or deemed to be positive, then the person is more likely to engage in that behaviour. These explanations which see behaviour as a simple response to positive or negative rewards do not seem to account for the persistence of health behaviours which have apparently negative consequences, such as smoking or drinking and driving. Obviously short-term gratification is a greater incentive than possible long-term harm.

Becker suggests that individuals are influenced by how vulnerable they perceive themselves to be to an illness, injury or danger (their **susceptibility**) and how serious they consider it to be (**severity**). People's perception and assessment of risk is central to the application of this model. Most people make a rough assessment about whether they are at risk. This seems to be influenced by three factors: personal experience; ability to control the situation; and a kind of general feeling that 'the illness or danger is thoroughly nasty and able to kill easily' (British Medical Association 1987). However, in many situations people have an unrealistic optimism that 'it won't happen to me' (Weinstein 1984).

Consideration of these variables in relation to AIDS shows the difficulties faced by AIDS educators. Many heterosexual people have an 'illusion of invulnerability' (Phillips 1993), and do not make a realistic assessment of personal risk because the social representation of AIDS is of a disease associated with gay men and injecting drug users. In a study of young people, Clift and colleagues (Clift et al 1989) found that students estimated their own risk of HIV infection to be less than that of their peers. In the absence of perceived risk, the perceived costs of using a condom – loss of pleasure, expense, interruption of lovemaking – may be seen as greater than any benefits.

Since beliefs may be affected by experience, direct contact with those who have a condition can powerfully affect attitudes exposing stereotypes and prejudice. For example, contact with a person who is HIV positive or who is living with AIDS can change beliefs about the fatality of the disease, and about whom is affected and how.

Those who work with young people find perceptions of risk are very different. Risk-taking is an important task of adolescence and part of separation from family. It is hard for young people to appreciate the long-term effects of, for example, smoking when 25 can seem old.

Many health education campaigns have attempted to motivate people to change their behaviour through fear or guilt. Drink–drive

Questioner: **'How do you think you'll be in say ten years' time, in terms of health?'**

K (age 16) **'Dead!'**

T (age 15) **'I don't want to think about tomorrow, let alone ten bloody years.'**

Source: HEA (1993)

campaigns at Christmas show the devastating effects on families of road accident fatalities; smoking prevention posters urge parents not to 'teach your children how to smoke'. Although fear can encourage a negative attitude and even an intention to change, such feelings tend to disappear over time and when faced with a real decision-making situation.

Being very frightened can also lead to denial and an avoidance of the message (Montazeri et al 1998). Protection Motivation Theory (Rogers 1975) suggests that fear only works if the threat is perceived as serious and likely to occur if the person does not follow the recommended advice.

The Health Belief Model suggests that people need to have some kind of cue to take action to change a behaviour or make a health-related decision. The issue needs to become salient or relevant. The cue could be noticing a change in one's internal state or appearance. For example, a pregnant woman stops smoking when she feels the baby move. It could be an external trigger, such as a change in circumstance like change in job or income, or the death or illness of someone close. It could be a comment from a 'significant other' or a newspaper article. Health care workers can be significant others. For example, GPs' advice is taken seriously. The GP has expertise, is trustworthy and has authority, leading the patient to desire to comply. The effects of persuasive communications on attitudes are discussed more fully in Chapter 12 on mass media.

> **Considerable changes in sexual behaviour have taken place among gay and bisexual men in response to AIDS. However, there is a high incidence of homosexually active men engaging in what is known to be a potentially risky sexual activity, unprotected receptive anal sex.**
>
> ■ Consider how the Health Belief Model could be used to explain this health behaviour.
> ■ What reasons could you offer for individuals not carrying out their intentions to act in ways that are perceived as beneficial?

The Health Belief Model has been widely criticized. Some of these criticisms relate to its lack of weighting for different factors – all cues to preventive action, for example, are seen as equally salient. Stainton Rogers offers a strong critique of psychological models which attempt to explain complex behaviour by assuming that 'the whole is no more than the (albeit complex) "sum of the parts"; that actions are informed and chosen via analysis of a set of conceptual components isolated from one another. They have no place for the kinds of interwoven, articulated arguments and stories which form the fabric of conversation and of media messages'

(Stainton Rogers 1993, p. 55). The model may not be particularly helpful in predicting behaviour or identifying those elements that are important in influencing people to change, but it does highlight the range and complexity of factors involved.

Theory of Reasoned Action and Theory of Planned Behaviour

According to the Theory of Reasoned Action (Ajzen & Fishbein 1980) behaviour is dependent on two variables:

■ attitudes – beliefs about the consequences of the behaviour and an appraisal of the positive and negative aspects of making a change
■ subjective norms –what 'significant others' do and expect and the degree to which the person wants to conform and be like others.

These two influences combine to form an intention.

Ajzen & Fishbein (1980) acknowledge that people do not necessarily behave consistently with their intentions. The ability to predict behaviour will be influenced by the stability of a person's belief. Stability is determined by strength of belief, how long it has been held, whether it is reinforced by other groups to which the individual belongs, whether it is related to and integrated with other attitudes and beliefs, and how clear or structured it is.

The Theory of Reasoned Action differs from the Health Belief Model in that it places importance on social norms as a major influence on behaviour. Figure 11.2 shows the significance of this factor in the Theory of Reasoned Action. Social pressure may be

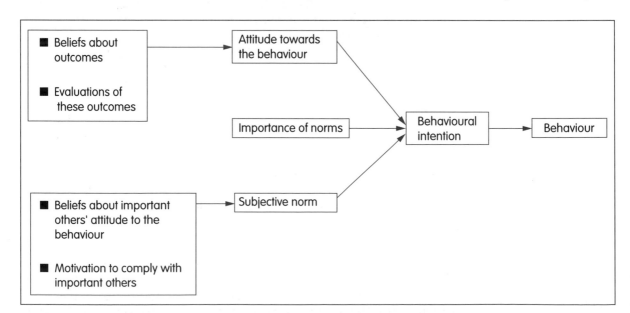

Figure 11.2   *The Theory of Reasoned Action. From Ajzen & Fishbein 1980.*

exerted through societal norms (such as those relating to weight and body image), community norms, the peer group and the beliefs of 'significant others' (such as parents or partners).

The motivation to comply with perceived social pressure from 'significant others' could cause individuals to behave in a way that they believe these other people or groups would think is right. The influence of so-called peer group pressure (even if it does not amount to pressure) can be very powerful within a small group if the individual values membership of that group or wants to belong to it. Young people who associate with older and mixed-sex peer groups and those whose best friends smoke are more likely to smoke themselves (HEA 1996).

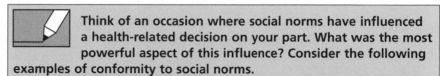

Think of an occasion where social norms have influenced a health-related decision on your part. What was the most powerful aspect of this influence? Consider the following examples of conformity to social norms.

- An example of public acceptance and private autonomy: 'Ann goes on holiday with a group of friends. On the first evening it becomes apparent that no-one smokes. Rather than ask if anyone minds if she does, Ann retires early to bed and has a solitary cigarette.'
- An example of temporary acceptance of group mores: 'Bill works in a predominantly male office. At the end of the day, five or six people adjourn to a local bar. The men are eager to establish themselves by buying a round of drinks. Bill waits until everyone has finished before offering to buy a round by which time someone else has got to the bar. Bill usually only drinks one pint of beer but he stays until everyone has bought a round – six pints.

The role of modelling has been particularly important in health promotion. Concern has been expressed that indirect modelling of behaviour may come from the media. For example, people on television are able to drink heavily without any apparent ill effects (Hansen 1986). A study of tobacco use in films has shown that this is far higher than its prevalence in society. Between 1991 and 1996, 80% of male leads in films smoked (Stockwell & Glantz 1997). Direct modelling is sometimes assumed to be less influential, but models who have status and credibility, such as musicians and people in sport have been used to present health promotion messages. If

Should health promoters 'practise what they preach'?

Think of some examples where practitioners' behaviour may be at odds with the health improvement they wish to promote.

people are influenced by role models, then health promoters may themselves be taken as exemplars.

Some health promotion programmes use the influence of the peer group to promote positive health, e.g. smokebusters clubs in schools. In the USA, gay men identified as popular opinion leaders (or 'gay heroes') were trained to give positive messages about safer sex to their peers (Kelly et al 1992). The rationale is that 'significant others' have credibility, are able to communicate in appropriate ways and are models to follow, although doubts may be expressed about the skills and information that peer educators possess (Wilton et al 1995).

Social norms include peer group or family beliefs, but also what are perceived to be 'general' norms as conveyed by, for example, the mass media. What is important is what the individual believes other people do, not the actual extent of the activity. The Joint Breastfeeding Initiative has, for example, complained that the low number of young mothers who choose to breast feed is partly due to their perception that other women bottle feed. The World Health Organization have identified the importance of formal and informal social networks to support individuals and give people assistance in the pursuit of health (WHO 1986). Group techniques, such as those used by Alcoholics Anonymous, appear to have some success by getting clients to identify with the group through personal testimony and a public commitment, which encourages the group to then provide support for each other.

Bandura's (1977) social learning theory suggests that the health choices people make are related to:

A study of family eating patterns (Charles & Kerr 1986) highlighted women's views about what constitutes a proper meal – 'it means separate little piles on a plate'. What do you think are current social norms about child nutrition?

■ outcome expectancies (whether an action will lead to a particular outcome)
■ self-efficacy (whether people believe they can change).

Perceptions of self-efficacy are based on people's assessment of themselves – whether they have the knowledge and skills to make changes in their behaviour and whether external factors such as time and money will allow that change. Personal judgement of worth expressed in the attitudes people hold towards themselves is also part of a sense of self-efficacy. We talk of high or low self-esteem in the sense of feeling more or less worthwhile and valued. Self-concept is a global term which refers to all those beliefs which people have about themselves – about their abilities and their attributes. It includes ideas about appearance, intelligence and physical skills. It is built and modified through our perceptions of the way other people behave towards us, how we are accepted and affirmed, or rejected and criticized. It will thus also derive from having a network of social support.

The development of self-concept and self-esteem has been at the centre of work in health education and promotion. It is assumed that

How might a person's self-concept influence her eating behaviour?

people with high self-esteem are likely to feel confident about themselves and have social and life skills which will enhance their feelings of personal efficacy. Because of these feelings of personal effectiveness, the person's self-esteem is enhanced.

Many health education programmes, particularly those targeted at young people, have been based on the premise that there is a relationship between self-esteem and health behaviour. Those who engage in health-damaging behaviour such as drug-taking are thought to have low self-esteem reinforced by poor social relationships (Tones & Tilford 1994, p. 30). However, there is an argument that the majority of young people who use drugs casually are more confident and more risk-taking and may, according to all attitude measures, have higher self-esteem (Chapman 1992).

Drug education and sex education programmes have focused on boosting self-esteem by equipping young people with efficacy skills like resisting peer group pressure and self-awareness. However, what takes place in a classroom may bear little relation to the social context in which the behaviour takes place.

Intention and behaviour in sexual decision-making

Thompson & Holland (1995) found that 77% of a sample of young women had the knowledge and the intention to use a condom but only 23% had ever done so. The Theory of Reasoned Action helps to highlight two factors which might explain why using condoms might be difficult for young women:

■ Social norms do not support condom use. They are perceived as associated with casual sex. Contraceptive culture for young women focuses on the Pill.
■ Self-efficacy – young women lack the power and control to negotiate safer sex.

Ajzen further developed the Theory of Reasoned Action and recast it as the Theory of Planned Behaviour (Ajzen 1991) (Fig. 11.3). This model incorporated another variable – that people's behaviour is a consequence of their perceived control. People differ in the extent to which they think they can make changes in their lives. Social learning theory suggests that the ways in which people explain the things that happen to them is a product of their childhood experiences. Those who are rewarded for their successes, and punished consistently and fairly will come to believe that they are in control of their lives. Those who have inconsistent rewards or punishments irrespective of their behaviour are more likely to see events as a consequence of chance and their own role as irrelevant (Rotter 1954).

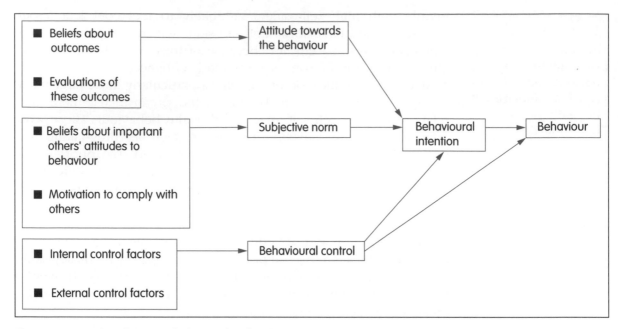

Figure 11.3   *The Theory of Planned Behaviour. From Ajzen 1991.*

Control in the context of health can be understood in terms of:

■ internal locus of control (the extent to which individuals believe that they are responsible for their own health)
■ external locus of control (people who believe that their actions are influenced by powerful others, chance, fate or luck).

Research has focused on categorizing attitudes to health by using a locus of control measure such as a multiple choice inventory. It has been assumed that those who have a strong internal locus of control will see themselves as more coping, and more able to act decisively and capably and will be those people who undertake preventive health actions or change to more healthy behaviours. So far it has generally been found that there is only a weak relationship between feelings of control and specific behaviours, although associations have been found with smoking cessation and weight loss and the propensity to use preventive medical services (Wallston et al 1978). Indeed, a lifestyle survey of 9000 adults found that 'unhealthy' kinds of behaviour are more likely to be associated with an internal locus of control (Blaxter 1990). At the same time, those who recorded positive or responsible attitudes to health were also more likely to have a high locus of control. This confirms the argument earlier in this chapter that specific behaviour cannot necessarily be predicted from attitudes.

Stainton Rogers has written a highly critical account of the work on locus of control suggesting that most research has only established self-evident differences between groups of people

What strategies can practitioners use to help build their clients' confidence so that they feel more able to make changes in their health behaviour?

which had little to do with their health beliefs. People who register as 'externals' on the multi-dimensional health locus of control scale are those with lower levels of education, and of lower socio-economic class – in other words, people who have every reason to believe that they do not have much control over their lives or health status (Stainton Rogers 1993).

The Stages of Change Model

Increasingly, primary care workers have taken on the role of assessment and advice in brief interventions (Rollnick et al 1992). Chapter 16 discusses the evidence of effectiveness of such advice in general practice and the ways in which screening and opportunistic health promotion have become routine in primary care.

Practitioners have guidelines on who might be regarded as at risk according to various normative measures, e.g. body mass index or blood cholesterol levels. They then try to encourage clients to change those aspects of their behaviour which may be putting them at risk. As we have seen, behaviour change may be a lengthy and complex process and not simply the result of a quick decision.

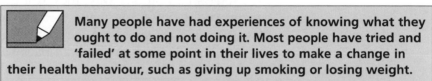

Many people have had experiences of knowing what they ought to do and not doing it. Most people have tried and 'failed' at some point in their lives to make a change in their health behaviour, such as giving up smoking or losing weight.

Think about one of your experiences of failing to make a change. Why do you think the change did not last:

- Lack of motivation?
- Lack of support?
- Lack of knowledge?
- Lack of time or other resource?

Now think about a change you have managed to make. Why do you think you were able to stick to this decision?

The work of Prochaska & DiClemente (1984, 1986) in developing a stage model of behaviour acquisition is important in showing that any change we make is not final but part of an ongoing cycle of change. Their work has focused on encouraging change in addictive behaviours, although the model can be used to show that most people go through a number of stages when trying to change or acquire behaviours. Figure 11.4 illustrates this process and identifies the following stages:

Precontemplation. Those in the precontemplation stage have not considered changing their lifestyle or become aware of any potential risks in their health behaviour. When they becomes aware of a problem, they may progress to the next stage.

Contemplation.   Although individuals are aware of the benefits of change, they are not yet ready and may be seeking information or help to make that decision. This stage may last a short while or several years. Some people never progress beyond this stage.

Preparing to change.   When the perceived benefits seem to outweigh the costs and when the change seems possible as well as worthwhile, the individual may be ready to change, perhaps seeking some extra support.

Making the change.   The early days of change require positive decisions by the individual to do things differently. A clear goal, a realistic plan, support and rewards are features of this stage.

Maintenance.   The new behaviour is sustained and the person moves into a healthier lifestyle. For some people maintaining the new behaviour is difficult and the person may revert or 'relapse' back to any of the previous stages.

Prochaska et al (1992) argue that whilst few people go through each stage in an orderly way, they will go through each stage. This has proved helpful for many health care workers who find it reassuring that a 'relapse' on the part of their clients is not a failure, but that the individual can go both backwards and forwards through

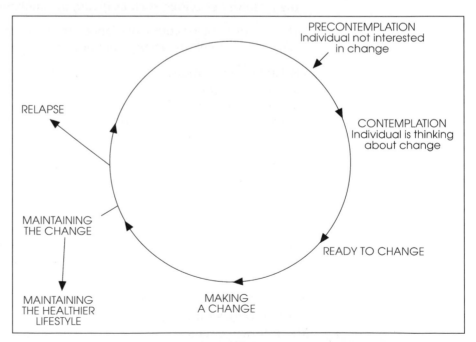

Figure 11.4   *The Stages of Change Model. After Prochaska & DiClemente 1984.*

a series of cycles of change – like a revolving door. Thus a smoker may stop smoking many times before finally giving up completely. Nevertheless the client is still aware of the benefits of giving up smoking and health care workers may be able to focus on such small changes, which can provide themselves and their clients with a sense of achievement and identifiable progress.

Whilst individuals may not have an awareness of contemplating, actioning and maintaining change, the intention will be based on individuals deciding that it is in their best interests to change. The key to successful interventions then is for a client to be motivated. Health promoters must bear in mind that their clients may not share their perceptions about the worth of a particular behaviour. However, evidence from a study of nurses helping people to stop smoking, showed that where clients are strongly involved in the planning process they are more likely to be motivated (MacLeod Clark & Dines 1993).

 How might you help someone to decide to make a change in her health behaviour?

■ What questions might you use to help the client explore her situation?
■ How would you identify her readiness to change?
■ How would you help someone to weigh up the pros and cons of making a change?
■ What support would you offer to help someone to stick to the change she makes?
■ How would you help her to cope with difficult situations or setbacks?

 Consider the following list of factors identified in the Allied Dunbar National Fitness Survey (Sports Council/HEA 1992) which motivated people to take exercise:

■ To feel in good shape physically
■ To feel a sense of achievement
■ To improve or maintain health
■ To get out of doors.

Now consider the factors identified as barriers to participation:

■ Not being the sporty type
■ Do not enjoy it
■ Need to rest and relax in spare time
■ Have not got time.

Suggest how you would support someone in his decision to take up regular exercise.

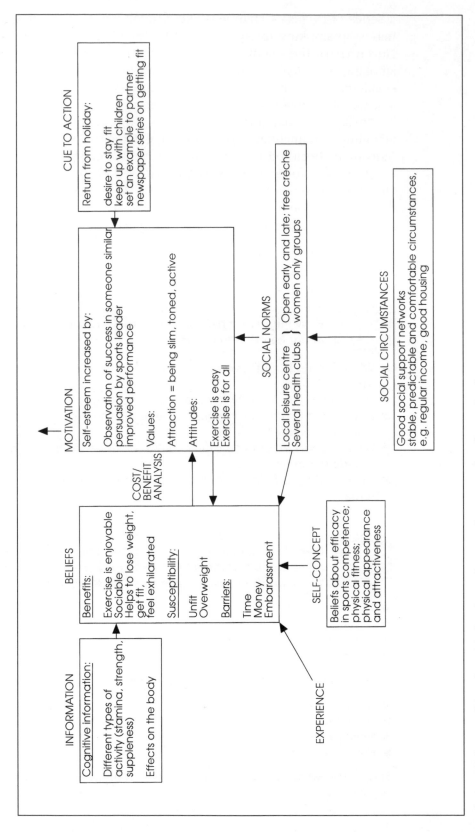

Figure 11.5   *Health-related behaviour change: the example of exercise in women.*

Identifying a precontemplative stage is important because it reminds health care workers to be aware that a client may not be ready to change and therefore their work should focus on other issues, perhaps ensuring a 'safer' lifestyle. For example, an injecting drug user who chooses to continue to use drugs may be advised to use a needle exchange scheme.

The Stages of Change Model differs from the other models of behaviour change described in this chapter because it is principally about how people change and not why people do not change.

Figure 11.5 is a diagrammatic representation of some of the influences on a person's decision to take up an exercise programme. It shows how confidence to participate in physical activity could be built through positive attributions such as fitness and weight loss and through successful performance. Social support networks will also be crucial in maintaining commitment.

All these models of behaviour change suggest that people are involved in a rational processing of information when they make a decision. People are not usually so consciously rational as this study of the health beliefs of working class mothers in South Wales illustrates:

> In the subjects we studied there was little evidence of a rational approach to the personal decision-making process i.e. a weighing up of the advantages and disadvantages of a particular change followed by a decision to act. Instead any change was a consequence not just of thought but also a mix of emotion, habit, impulse, social influences and bolshie lack of forethought, which is so typically human.
>
> (Pill & Stott 1990)

The prerequisites of change

Pill & Stott's study of self-initiated change shows the importance of precipitating life events and the minor part played by health concerns. For example, women who gave up smoking did so to save money and those who took up exercise did so to join in with their children.

The importance of considering the social context and everyday life is brought out clearly by this study which showed that eventually most women reverted to their original behaviours because of the influence of partners or children, or because it was too difficult to juggle personal and family priorities.

The evidence from people who have changed their health behaviour suggests that there are certain minimum conditions required for that change to take place (RUHBC 1989).

1. The change must be self-initiated
Some people react adversely or wish to contain any attempt to look at their 'unhealthy behaviour'. To some people, their behaviour may

not seem 'unhealthy' at all but may constitute a clear source of well-being, its benefits far outweighing its risks. There is a clear message here for those health promoters who work with individual clients and who are sometimes accused of 'telling people what to do' – people will only change if they want to.

2. The behaviour must become salient

Most health-related behaviours including smoking, alcohol use, eating and exercise (or lack of it) are habitual, and built into the flow of everyday life such that the individual does not give them much thought. For a change to occur, that behaviour or habit must be called into question by some other activity or event so that the behaviour becomes 'salient'. For example, a smoker going to live with a non-smoker causes the smoking behaviour to be reappraised. The death of a relative from breast cancer may similarly prompt a woman to go for screening.

3. The salience of the behaviour must appear over a period of time

The habitual behaviour needs to become difficult to maintain. The new behaviour must, in turn, become part of everyday life. For example, one reason why people on diets often resume their previous eating pattern is because they are made constantly aware of the diet and it is never allowed to become a habit. Similarly, exercise is often not maintained because it requires effort, hence the advice to reluctant 'couch potatoes' to build physical activity into their daily life by walking to work or running up stairs rather than going out to exercise at a pool or gym.

4. The behaviour is not part of the individual's coping strategies

People have various sources of comfort and solace, and will resist change to these behaviours. It is sometimes possible to enable clients to identify alternative coping strategies. For example, a person who eats chocolate when depressed may be encouraged to become physiologically aroused by taking up jogging.

5. The individual's life should not be problematic or uncertain

There is a limit to a person's capacity to adapt and change. For example, those living on low incomes will be stretched by coping with poverty and its uncertainties. Having to make changes in their health behaviour may be too much to expect for people whose lives are already problematic.

6. Social support is available

The presence and interest of other people provides reinforcement and keeps the behaviour salient. Changing one's behaviour can be stressful and individuals need support. The influence of peer group pressure and support is not given sufficient weight in the various psychological theories of change. The World Health Organization recognized the important role for the health promoter in stimulating and maintaining social support for individuals and groups (WHO 1986).

Think about an attempt you have made to enhance your health, e.g. giving up smoking, losing weight.

- Were you successful in the change?
- What influenced you to make the change?
- Can you identify any specific triggers that prompted you to make the change?
- How do your family and friends regard the behaviour?
- What were the costs and benefits of making the change?

Look at the list of minimum conditions above, do any of these factors help to explain your success or failure in making the health-related behaviour change?

Conclusion

The application of social psychology to health promotion has attracted criticism because it is believed that behaviour is not the most important determinant of health, and working to change attitudes and behaviour minimizes the structural inequalities which limit people's potential for health. Nevertheless, behaviour change remains a feature of many approaches to health promotion and we have argued in this book that this must be accompanied by programmes which attempt to provide the environmental conditions that make the healthy choice the easier choice. The role of health education and promotion is neatly summarized by Whitehead & Tones:

> One level involves primarily influencing beliefs (assuming that attempts to directly 'plug into' motivation by creating fear or otherwise generate emotional responses are of dubious value both ethically and in terms of effectiveness). The other level is concerned with providing the understanding and skills needed to translate intention into practice. Health education is also concerned to foster healthy public policy in order to encourage

the development of a health-promoting environment that both will facilitate intentions to make healthy choices and will signal the unacceptability of unhealthy practices.

(Whitehead & Tones 1991, p. 13)

What is clear from this outline of psychological theories of behaviour change is that none provides a full explanation. However, the variables identified by these models do appear in people's accounts of their health behaviour:

■ perceptions of risk and vulnerability
■ perceptions of the severity of the disease
■ perceived effectiveness of the behaviour in contributing to better health
■ perception of own ability to make a change
■ perception of how significant others evaluate the behaviour.

Whilst these models may not help to predict who will adopt preventive health practices, they can help to plan programmes of education by making clear those factors which influence decisions.

Although the efficacy of breast self-examination has been questioned, 90% of breast cancers are detected by women themselves (CMO 1991). There is value then in promoting early detection methods including breast awareness and mammography for those eligible. Using a model of behaviour change may help in planning programmes on breast cancer and its detection:

■ Women are not well informed about the risk factors for breast cancer
■ They cannot make a realistic assessment of their own susceptibility
■ Personal risks tend to be over-estimated which can result in fear and denial
■ Women believe that most people with cancer will not be cured
■ Women are not confident in their ability to detect a breast lump
■ Women regard screening as an inconvenience.

Source: Pitts (1993)

Key elements in a successful campaign might be:

1. The provision of accurate information to all women
2. Information to enable individuals to identify their personal risk
3. A campaign to emphasize that the quality of living with cancer is improved with treatment even when the disease is not curable
4. Breast awareness to be taught by all health care workers
5. Improvements in the call/recall system
6. Publicizing the campaign through women's networks to engender social support.

Questions for further discussion

- Do social psychology theories help you to understand the reasons why people may or may not change their health behaviour?
- What factors should health promoters take into account when helping clients to change their health behaviour?

Summary

This chapter has reviewed the role of psychosocial factors in health behaviour and discussed three theoretical models. These models have been used to explain and predict health-related decisions, such as screening or compliance to a medical regimen. All the models identify some common variables which influence the likelihood of a person adopting 'healthy' behaviours: beliefs about the efficacy of the new behaviour; motivation and whether they value their health enough to change; normative pressures and the influence of significant people around them. The limitations of the role of social psychology in health promotion are outlined but it is concluded that an understanding of those factors influencing individual behaviour can help in planning appropriate health promotion interventions.

Further reading

Bennett P, Murphy S 1997 Psychology and health promotion. Open University, Buckingham. *A very useful textbook which examines how behaviour and the social environment contribute to health status.*

Downie RS, Tannahill A, Tannahill C 1996 Health promotion: models and values, 2nd edn. Oxford Medical Publications, Oxford. *Chapters 7, 8 and 9 include useful attempts to describe and define the role of health and beliefs, attitudes and values.*

Ogden J 1996 Health psychology: a textbook. Open University, Buckingham. *An accessible textbook on psychological theory integrating case studies and examples of research studies.*

Payne S, Walker J 1996 Psychology for nurses and the caring professions. Open University, Buckingham. *A clear and comprehensive introduction to social psychology.*

Research Unit in Health and Behavioural Change 1989 Changing the public health. Wiley, Chichester. *Chapter 5 is a packed account of research findings relating to behaviour change. The chapter outlines the limitations of social psychology models and suggests its own theory of behaviour change.*

Tones K, Tilford S 1994 Health education: effectiveness, efficiency and equity. Chapman & Hall, London. *Chapter 3 provides a short but clear account of the theoretical models which seek to explain the relationship between knowledge, beliefs, attitudes, social pressures and environmental constraints. It concentrates on the Health Action Model.*

References

Ajzen I 1991 The theory of planned behaviour. Organisational Behaviour and Human Decision Processes 50: 179–211

Ajzen I, Fishbein M 1980 Understanding attitudes and predicting social behaviour. Prentice Hall, Englewood Cliffs

Bandura A 1977 Social learning theory. Prentice Hall, Englewood Cliffs

Becker M H (ed) 1974 The Health Belief Model and personal health behaviour. Slack, Thorofare, New Jersey

Blaxter M 1990 Health and lifestyles. Tavistock/Routledge, London

British Medical Association 1987 Living with risk. Wiley, Chichester

Chapman C 1992 Drugs issues for schools. Institute for the Study of Drug Dependence, London

Charles N, Kerr M 1986 Issues of responsibility and control in the feeding of families. In: Rodmell S, Watt A (eds) The politics of health education: raising the issues. Routledge and Kegan Paul, London, pp 57–76

Chief Medical Officer 1991 Statement on women's health and breast awareness. Department of Health, London

Clift S M, Stears D, Legg S, Memon A, Ryan L 1989 The HIV/AIDS education and young people project: report on phase one. AVERT, Horsham

Davies J B 1992 The myth of addiction. Harwood, Reading

Festinger L 1957 A theory of cognitive dissonance. University Press, Stanford

Gillam S 1991 Understanding the uptake of cervical cancer screening: the contribution of Health Belief Model. British Journal of General Practice 41: 510–513

Hansen A 1986 The portrayal of alcohol on television. Health Education Journal 45: 3

Health Education Authority 1993 The health action pack. HEA, London

Health Education Authority 1996 Smoking update. HEA, London

Kelly J A, St Lawrence J S, Stevenson L Y 1992 Community AIDS/HIV risk reduction: the effects of endorsements by popular people in three cities. American Journal of Public Health 82: 1483–1489

MacLeod Clark J, Dines A 1993 Nurses working with people who wish to stop smoking. In: Dines A, Cribb A (eds) Health promotion: concepts and practice. Blackwell, Oxford, pp 67–84

Montazeri A, McGhee S, McEwan J 1998 Fear inducing and positive image strategies in health education campaigns. Journal of the Institute of Health Promotion and Education 36(3): 68–75

Phillips K 1993 Primary prevention of AIDS. In: Pitts M, Phillips K (eds) The psychology of health. Routledge and Kegan Paul, London

Pill R M, Stott N C H 1990 Making changes: a study of working class mothers and the changes made in their health related behaviour over five years. University of Wales College of Medicine, Cardiff

Pitts M, Phillips K (eds) 1993 The psychology of health. Routledge, London

Prochaska J O, DiClemente C 1984 The transtheoretical approach: crossing traditional foundations of change. Don Jones/Irwin, Harnewood, IL

Prochaska J O, DiClemente C C 1986 Towards a comprehensive model of change. In: Miller W R, Heather N (eds) Treating addictive behaviours: processes of change. New York, Plenum

Prochaska J O, DiClemente C, Norcross J C 1992 In search of how people change. American Psychologist 47: 1102–1114

Research Unit in Health and Behavioural Change 1989 Changing the public health. Wiley, Chichester

Rogers R W 1975 A protection motivation theory of fear appeals and attitude change. Journal of Psychology 91: 93–114

Rollnick S, Heather N, Bell A 1992 Negotiating behaviour change in medical settings: the development of brief motivational interviewing. Journal of Mental Health 1: 25–37

Rosenstock I 1966 Why people use health services. Millbank Memorial Fund Quarterly 44: 94–121

Rotter J B 1954 Social learning and clinical psychology. Prentice Hall, Englewood Cliffs

Sports Council/HEA 1992 Allied Dunbar national fitness survey. Sports Council/Health Education Authority, London

Stainton Rogers W 1993 Explaining health and illness: an exploration of diversity. Harvester, Hemel Hempstead

Stockwell T F, Glantz S A 1997 Tobacco use in popular films. Tobacco Control 6: 282–284

Thompson R, Holland J 1994 Young women and safer (hetero) sex: context, constraints and strategies. In: Wilkinson S, Kitzinger C (eds) Women and health: feminist perspectives. Taylor Francis, Basingstoke

Tones K, Tilford S 1994 Health education; effectiveness, efficiency and equity. Chapman & Hall, London

Wallston K A, Wallston B S, DeVellis R F 1978 Locus of control and health: a review of the literature. Health Education Monographs 6: 107–117

Weinstein N 1984 Why it won't happen to me; perceptions of risk factors and susceptibility. Health Psychology 3: 431–457

Whitehead M, Tones K 1991 Avoiding the pitfalls. HEA, London

Wilton T, Keeble S, Doyal L, Walsh A 1995 The effectiveness of peer education in health promotion: theory and practice. HEA, London

World Health Organization 1986 Lifestyles and health. Social Science Medicine 22: 117–124

12 *Using the mass media in health promotion*

OVERVIEW

Mass media are powerful agents of communication, reaching large numbers of people. Over 80% of the population cite the media as their most important source of health information (Office of Health Economics 1994). It is also the means by which we are persuaded to buy a vast array of products and lifestyles which create ill health, such as tobacco, alcohol and fast cars. Its use in health promotion has a long history.

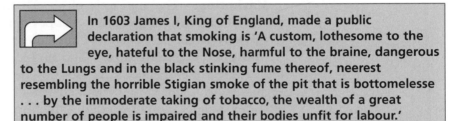

In 1603 James I, King of England, made a public declaration that smoking is 'A custom, lothesome to the eye, hateful to the Nose, harmful to the braine, dangerous to the Lungs and in the black stinking fume thereof, neerest resembling the horrible Stigian smoke of the pit that is bottomelesse . . . by the immoderate taking of tobacco, the wealth of a great number of people is impaired and their bodies unfit for labour.'

The powerful effects of propaganda during the Second World War were influential in persuading health promoters to adopt a similar strategy. In 1953 John Burton, the editor of the *Health Education Journal,* stated that:

> The first 10 years of our existence could well be called the era of propaganda. Health education has been realised mainly in terms of mass publicity on all fronts. Ad hoc exhortations have been directed at the public following closely the patterns of commercial advertising. In addition much energy and ingenuity has been expended on exhibitions and displays of all kinds, and even on carnivals.

(Burton, cited in Tones 1993, p. 128)

However, by this time there had already developed a concern that such a strategy was not working and that the role of the mass media in health promotion needed to be redefined:

Many (have come) to feel that mass publicity methods were expensive and relatively ineffective in changing people's health habits and beliefs, and that health education would have to be planned on a more personal basis.

(Burton, cited in Tones 1993, p. 128)

This chapter looks at the potential and limitations of using the mass media to promote health. Their high profile makes using them a popular choice of strategy and planned advertising campaigns are an important element in many national health strategies.

Definitions

Mass communication. Any form of communication with the public that does not depend on person-to-person contact.

Mass media. Any printed or audio-visual material designed to reach a mass audience. This includes newspapers, magazines, radio, television, billboards, exhibition displays, posters and leaflets.

Message. A cultural communication encoded in signs and symbols.

Marketing. The sum total of all activities (the marketing mix) designed to persuade people to adopt certain behaviours.

Advertising. One component of the marketing mix.

Audience segmentation. The division of a mixed population into more homogeneous groups or market segments. Market segments are defined by certain shared characteristics which affect attitudes, beliefs and knowledge. Targeting specific market segments allows for more specific messages which will have a greater effect.

The nature of media effects

Views on the effects of the mass media have shifted from an early belief that the mass media could produce dramatic changes in attitudes and behaviour to the opposite view that the media have negligible effects. A review by Gatherer et al (1979) of 49 evaluated studies of mass media campaigns stated that 'the effect is not very great, especially on the individual'. Today there is a more tempered view, which regards the media as influential in certain circumstances and in specific ways. Tones & Tilford (1994) concluded that 'Mass media (campaigns) can serve a very useful purpose in health education when their inherent limitations are recognised'. Four main models of how the media affects audiences have been suggested.

Direct effects

This model likens the effects of the mass media to a hypodermic syringe that has an immediate and direct effect on its audience. It assumes a passive audience who can be swayed by manipulative mass media. This view prompted the development of political broadcasts intended to shift voting intentions.

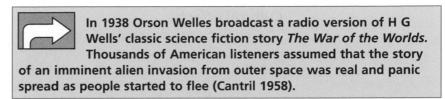

In 1938 Orson Welles broadcast a radio version of H G Wells' classic science fiction story *The War of the Worlds*. Thousands of American listeners assumed that the story of an imminent alien invasion from outer space was real and panic spread as people started to flee (Cantril 1958).

This view has since been replaced by an aerosol spray analogy: 'Rather than being a hypodermic needle, we now begin to look at mass communication as a sort of aerosol spray. As you spray it on the surface, some of it hits the target: most of it drifts away; and very little of it penetrates' (Mendelsohn 1968).

This view underlines the Labour party strategy to abandon party political broadcasts except at election time in favour of more interpersonal techniques of persuasion, such as telephone cold calling. Nevertheless, the belief that the media are inherently persuasive and influential remains popular and accounts for their widespread use as a strategy to promote health.

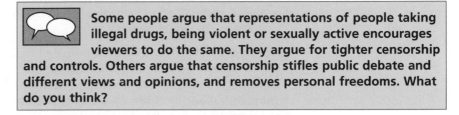

Some people argue that representations of people taking illegal drugs, being violent or sexually active encourages viewers to do the same. They argue for tighter censorship and controls. Others argue that censorship stifles public debate and different views and opinions, and removes personal freedoms. What do you think?

Two-step model

This model suggests that mass communication influences key opinion leaders who are active members of the mass media audience. These opinion leaders then spread ideas to other people through interpersonal means of communication (Katz & Lazarsfeld 1955).

The process of diffusing innovation or new ideas through a population suggests that there is a slow initial uptake followed by rapid acceptance, as opinion leaders communicate the benefits, and then a final slowing as a minority resist acceptance or change. This suggests that the mass media may be important in raising awareness and communicating basic information, but interpersonal sources, such as friends and known 'experts', are most influential in persuading people to make changes.

Uses and gratifications

This model tends to see the audience as more active in selecting and interpreting communications. It suggests that people use the media to meet their own needs – reinforcing existing beliefs or rejecting or reinterpreting communications that do not fit their existing values or beliefs.

Cultural effects

This model sees the media as having a key role in creating beliefs and values about health, medicine, disease and illness. The ways in which these are presented, from the kindly doctor in soap operas, to news bulletins on miracle cures and high-tech interventions, all contribute to people's understanding of health (see, for example, Lupton 1994).

 Monitor media coverage on television, in magazines, on radio, in broadsheet and tabloid newspapers for items about health over a 1-week period.

Karpf (1988) identifies four frameworks for health coverage:

■ Medical dominance, e.g. about medical breakthroughs, high-technology interventions
■ Consumerism, e.g. self-help stories about how to choose and access health services
■ 'Look after Yourself', e.g. healthier lifestyle items
■ Social, political and environmental, e.g. policy changes and how these might affect health.

Does the media coverage you monitored fit into these categories? Which categories were least/most common?
How much of the coverage was in entertainment programmes?
Think about and find some examples of how the following are represented in popular media culture:

■ Doctors
■ Hospitals and health care services
■ Sickness and injury
■ Health.

Communication is concerned with the transmission of messages from a sender to a receiver. The media are cultural communications which are indirect, leaving scope for different interpretations or readings of the same content.

Messages are coded into signs and symbols which have meaning within specific codes. The message is encoded by the sender, and decoded by the receiver (see Fig. 12.1). The intention is that messages should be decoded and understood according to the intentions of the sender; but there is ample opportunity for messages to be decoded in different ways, as the following example illustrates.

Figure 12.1 *Media messages.*

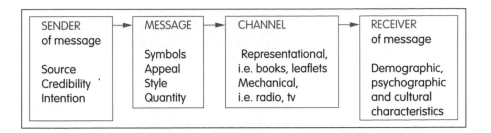

SENDER of message	MESSAGE	CHANNEL	RECEIVER of message
Source Credibility Intention	Symbols Appeal Style Quantity	Representational, i.e. books, leaflets Mechanical, i.e. radio, tv	Demographic, psychographic and cultural characteristics

In 1986 and 1987 the Government launched a major media campaign on AIDS, including a leaflet delivery to all households. One advertisement featured a picture of an iceberg with the slogan 'Don't die of ignorance'.

■ How many possible interpretations of this advertising illustration and slogan are there?
■ What do you think was the intended message?
■ Do you think that this message was successfully communicated?

The intention was that people should recognize that HIV infection is preventable, be motivated to acquire correct information on prevention and practise safer sex. However, many people connected the ominous picture of icebergs and the word 'die' with HIV/AIDS. This reinforced their belief that sex, death and HIV are related but also raised anxiety levels. Knowledge increased, but so too did people's perception of their own behaviour as low risk (perhaps as a means of dealing with their anxiety), making it unlikely that they would change their behaviour (Wober 1988). It is in the nature of mass media that there is no immediate feedback, so messages which are decoded in ways not intended may survive and become reinforced through repetition or repeated exposure.

The role of mass media

Mass communication has been used in health promotion to:

■ raise public awareness through:
  ❑ providing information
  ❑ reminding the population of the effects of their health-damaging behaviour and the benefits of adopting healthy behaviours and lifestyles
■ create a climate of opinion conducive to policy change through maintaining the salience of an issue and making sure it is thought about.
■ shift attitudes and prompt behaviour change through stressing the ill-effects of health-damaging behaviour and the benefits of preventive behaviour.

Find an example of a planned health promotion campaign with each of the above aims.

The campaign to reduce drink-driving has, at different times, reflected all of these aims:

■ Using shock tactics with re-enactments of accidents and depictions of injuries to raise awareness of drink-driving as a health issue, and to motivate drivers to stop drinking
■ Creating a climate of disapproval by suggesting that drink-drivers will be social outcasts and can get a criminal record
■ Maintaining the salience of the issue by showing the consequences of drink-driving and linking victims with perpetrators.

There are two main ways in which mass media are used:

1. Planned campaigns and advertising. This has the advantage of reaching large numbers of people from all social classes and population groups quickly. Messages can be developed and targeted to meet specific objectives.
2. Unpaid publicity and media advocacy. This has the advantage of low cost and a greater credibility, as messages are not seen as being directly promoted by health organizations.

Planned campaigns

Mass media campaigns have been widely used by national health promotion agencies in the UK to promote various health messages. Different media including billboards, press advertisements and radio announcements have been used, but television is the principal medium because, although it is expensive, it reaches much larger audiences and recall has been shown to be better.

The value of such campaigns in contributing to behaviour change is much disputed. Evaluation of the extensive HIV/AIDS campaign in the 1980s found no evidence of a reduction in sexual partners or increased use of condoms among heterosexuals (DHSS 1987a). The drug prevention campaign 'Heroin Screws You Up' which took place over the same period similarly showed no evidence of influencing those young people who might contemplate heroin use (DHSS 1987b). The Stanford Three Communities Study in America investigated the effect of the mass media and interpersonal communication in reducing people's coronary heart disease risk score through their adoption of healthy behaviours. The group exposed to both forms of communication achieved a reduction in CHD risk 20% greater than that achieved by the group exposed to mass media only (Davis 1987).

No Smoking Day

'No Smoking Day' is a major annual health promotion event which has been running since 1984. Its aims are:

- To encourage and assist smokers to give up for the day
- To bring the day to the attention of as many people as possible
- To involve as many people as possible in activities related to smoking education
- In the long-term, to assist those wishing to give up smoking to do so for good.

Its strategy is twofold: a public relations campaign and supporting local organizers. 10% of the budget is allocated to research and evaluation. The event is evaluated by quantitative survey data and qualitative research into local activities. Evaluation of the 1989 'Day' found:

- High prompted awareness of the campaign (86%)
- 19% of smokers claimed to have tried to participate in the 'Day', of which 41% claimed to have quit for the whole day
- 3 months later, 0.5% smokers had quit and were still not smoking.

Source: McGuire (1992)

Although the behaviour changes attributable to the National No Smoking Day media campaign are small, the effects are still considerable. Reid (1996) calculates that 1% of 8 million smokers is giving up equivalent to 80 000 individuals or the output of 10 000 smoking cessation groups with 32 smokers each and a quit rate of 25%.

Smoking campaigns are somewhat different from other initiatives and are more likely to be successful because:

- Public opinion is already against smoking and in support of the campaign's goals.
- 70% of smokers are already motivated to change and want to give up and so the message is credible for them.

The 'Sunsmart' campaign in Victoria, Australia, is an example of a successful campaign which led to significant attitudinal shifts, increased hat-wearing, sunscreen use and reduced sunburn prevalence. 48% of those surveyed took additional precautions and most attributed this directly to the campaign (Hill 1993). There are several factors that contributed to the success of the Australian campaign compared to the UK campaign 'Sun Know How':

- Public opinion was already favourably disposed to sun protection.
- Behaviours could be easily adopted without need of further professional advice or support.

> Look at the examples in Figure 12.2 of a Health Education
> Authority campaign targeted at young adults. The
> campaign aims to shock young people into stopping
> smoking. What is your response to this strategy?
>
> The evidence on whether fear is an effective strategy is not
> consistent. Early studies showed that people may attend, comprehend
> and retain information when shocked, but may also become resistant
> or deny the relevance of the message (Montazeri et al 1998).

Figure 12.2 *The national smoking education campaign: resources for young adults.*

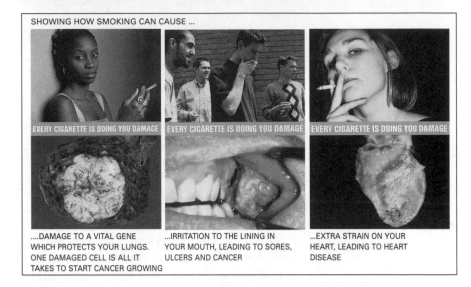

In a review of the most effective interventions to reduce smoking
prevalence, Reid et al (1992) concluded:

- The campaign was very well resourced with a budget of half a
  million pounds each year for a campaign directed at 4.3 million
  people.

Extensive reviews of media campaigns now conclude that they may
be successful if their goals are reasonable and there is no expectation
of immediate results. Tones & Tilford (1994) refer to the hierarchy of
communication effects which suggests that simple awareness or
market penetration is relatively easy to achieve; to inform or reinforce
attitudes is more difficult, and to have any effect on behaviour is even
more difficult. They identify certain preconditions for success:

- favourable public opinion which is most likely when there has
  been extensive market research at the design stage
- time available for the presentation of complex information
- support through interpersonal communication.

In a review of the most effective interventions to reduce smoking
prevalence, Reid et al (1992) concluded:

Paid advertising has formed the most conspicuous part of mass
media campaigns which coincided with major declines in

prevalence both in the United States and Australia. . . . Paid advertising is therefore a leading intervention, with a probable direct effect on smokers and the capacity to enhance the value of community based interventions.

(Reid et al 1992, p. 191)

 Unpaid media coverage

The Royal National Institute for the Blind organized a campaign in 1997 to promote regular eye tests, especially for those at risk of eye disease. There was national advertising and two leaflets, 'Half an Hour Could Save Your Sight' and 'Open Your Eyes'. The RNIB achieved:

12 mentions on national television
5 regional television pieces
20 radio and 60 regional radio mentions
4 national press features and 200 in the local press.

Unpaid media coverage

The term 'unplanned' is used to describe media coverage that is not specifically paid for as part of a campaign. Health promotion has become increasingly concerned to generate news stories. Campaigns can extend their reach enormously through unpaid coverage.

The mass media have no responsibility to promote health and so if they address such issues it is because the issues are inherently newsworthy, or have been packaged by health promoters to become newsworthy. The tendency to sensationalize means that it is the emotional, the dramatic or the tragic that gets space. Stories tend to relate to individuals, and issues which concern population groups such as older people or the determinants of health thus get ignored. The emphasis on behavioural journalism means that personalities or real-life case studies are also prominent. Newsworthiness depends less on the importance of an issue than on its immediate impact, which is often heightened by being linked to celebrities in emotive ways.

 Newsworthiness of health issues

Media coverage of AIDS in the USA was relatively unaffected by the increasing number of people with AIDS or scientific discoveries. However, as soon as important media celebrities (Rock Hudson, Magic Johnson) were diagnosed as having AIDS, media coverage soared.

Source: Wallack et al (1993)

Giving a local spin to general stories will also ensure coverage in regional media, as shown above in the amount of local coverage achieved by the RNIB in its mass campaign.

Whilst such tactics may increase coverage of the work of health promoters and put across health messages, the ability of the media to distort and sensationalize should always be remembered. An editorial in *The Observer* newspaper in 1994 commented: 'There is nothing quite so irresponsible as the media in hot pursuit of a health scare and nothing quite so gullible as the public presented with one'. The editorial had been prompted by a concern about necrotizing fasciitis (a tissue-destroying disease caused by a strain of bacteria) which was neither new nor on the increase, but which had prompted headlines such as 'Killer bug eats my body' or 'Flesh-eater on the move'.

Reid observes that media interest can be generated by the commissioning of surveys or research reports (Reid 1996). However, such reports frequently result in health scares because of misunderstanding of statistics and the concept of risk. A recent research study which linked MMR vaccine to the development of autism and Crohn's disease in young children, led to a drop in MMR uptake immediately following the press reports.

Take a current issue which has received a lot of media coverage, e.g. food safety, young people's drug use, institutional racism.

■ What is helpful and useful about such coverage?
■ What is unhelpful and not useful?
■ On balance, would you try to get more or less media coverage?

Whilst the generation of unpaid publicity can be effective and at minimal cost, it is difficult to sustain a high level of coverage for more than a few days. Health promoters need persistence and creativity to keep issues prominent in the media. There is also a need for media training for health promoters in skills such as writing press releases, networking and design in order to access and use the media to their full potential.

Media advocacy

Public policy is rarely a consequence of direct approaches to policy makers and increasingly there is a recognition that public opinion can influence decisions. Media advocacy is a particular strategy of using the media to try to generate public concern about the ways in which the legislative, economic or environmental context affects public health.

Media advocacy is a strategy to advance public health objectives such as the passing of new laws or policies. Media advocacy objectives are:

- to get an issue discussed
- to get an issue discussed differently
- to discredit opponents
- to bring in new voices
- to introduce new facts or perspectives
- to shift risk perceptions.

Chapman & Lupton (1994) emphasize the importance of the media in achieving policy change: 'There are few instances in the recent history of public health where advocacy staged through the news media has not played a pivotal role in effecting the changes sought by public health workers.' They cite examples of successful media advocacy in Australia in achieving tighter gun control and the fencing in of garden pools to prevent accidental drownings. One of the most successful media advocacy campaigns was the Billboardists Utilising Graffiti Against Unhealthy Promotions (BUGA-UP), which targeted tobacco advertising (Fig. 12.3). In the UK, to avoid the illegality of billboard defacing, the Group Against Smoking in Public (GASP) used the media to draw attention to the effects of smoking by entering the painting shown in Figure 12.4 for a portrait award.

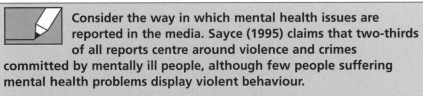

Consider the way in which mental health issues are reported in the media. Sayce (1995) claims that two-thirds of all reports centre around violence and crimes committed by mentally ill people, although few people suffering mental health problems display violent behaviour.

How could the media be actively used to get mental health issues discussed differently?

Figure 12.3 *Defaced billboard. Courtesy of Cecilia Farren.*

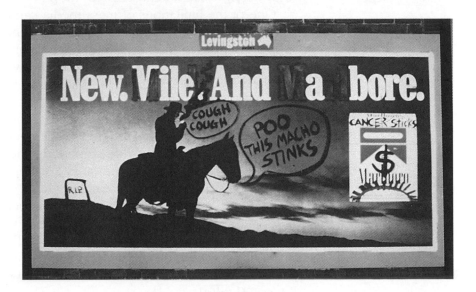

Figure 12.4 *The early death of Jackie Filbert. Courtesy of Cecilia Farren.*

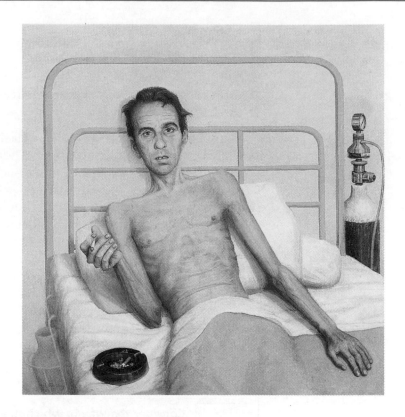

Social marketing

Just as commercial companies are able to get the public to buy products (even those they may not really need), so health promoters should be able to get people to choose healthy behaviours. Some of the techniques of marketing are now being widely used in health promotion to influence the acceptability of healthy lifestyles so that they seem desirable and easy to adopt.

One of the limitations of mass media campaigns is that they are a one-way communication process and tend to adopt a uniform population message. Increasingly, health promoters are making use of social marketing techniques that allow specific groups to be targeted (Naidoo & Wills 1998). Marketing segments the population into different subgroups based on attitudes and behaviour as well as more crude socio-economic and demographic variables.

Commercial marketing is based on the idea of 'exchange' – that the marketer tries to provide something the consumer wants at an acceptable price. Health promoters are beginning to recognize the importance of formative research, which carefully identifies what people see as the benefits of particular health behaviours so that these can be incorporated into the campaign message. In a sense this is merely an application of the Health Belief Model (see Ch. 11) which suggests that for people to make a change in their health behaviour they need to see the benefits outweighing costs such as time and effort.

'Be All You Can Be'

Using positive images which seek to establish an association between a health behaviour and a desired lifestyle is still a relatively untapped approach.

The Scottish Health Education Group (now the Health Education Board for Scotland) tried this approach in the 1980s with a campaign to promote physical activity and mental well-being called 'Be All You Can Be'. The report concluded that the campaign 'conceptually has moved health education into a new dimension, introducing for the first time a style of corporate branding with its own images that subsume the problem specific perspective' (Leathar 1988).

Marketing a commercial product is very different from trying to sell health. Advertising typically mobilizes existing predispositions, whereas health promotion typically tries to counter them. For example, advertising associates the product (beer, crisps) with something people desire, such as fun. All too often, health promotion messages are about not indulging, and therefore by implication, not having fun (don't drink and drive, eat less fat). Advertising is selling things in the here and now, to be immediately consumed and enjoyed. By contrast, health promotion messages are often about foregoing present enjoyment for future benefits.

As we have seen, selling a product is a complex and carefully researched process. The needs of the market have to be identified, messages developed which will appeal to the market segment that is being targeted, and a comparison made of different media

The marketing mix: the four Ps:

■ Product – the product or behaviour and its key characteristics which can contribute to the product image
■ Price – the value of the product and how important it is to the audience
■ Place – where the product is available
■ Promotion – the means by which the product is promoted (advertising, publicity, personal communication).

Choose an issue which you think could be promoted through an advertising campaign, e.g. sun safety, sensible drinking, safer sex, cancer awareness.

Decide on the market or target audience for the campaign.

■ How would you present the issue? Identify a key slogan and illustration for the campaign.

channels and their relative effectiveness in reaching a general and the targeted population. Together these aspects make up the marketing mix.

What the mass media can and cannot do

Research and evaluation of the use of the mass media in health promotion has led to a reassessment of their potential and limitations (see particularly Tones & Tilford 1994). It is now accepted that the mass media can:

■ raise consciousness about health issues, e.g. drink-driving
■ help place health on the public agenda, e.g. recycling
■ convey simple information and single messages, e.g. put babies to sleep on their backs
■ change behaviour if other enabling factors are present, e.g. encourage smokers already committed to giving up.

Factors which enable behaviour change include existing motivation, supportive circumstances and advocating simple one-off behaviour change (e.g. carry a donor card, install a smoke alarm).
Using the media is more effective if:

■ they are part of an integrated campaign including other elements such as one-to-one advice
■ the information is new and presented in an emotional context
■ the information is seen as being relevant for 'people like me'.

The mass media cannot:

■ convey complex information, e.g. the relative risks of different kinds of fat in the diet
■ teach skills, e.g. how to negotiate safer sex
■ shift people's attitudes or beliefs; if messages are presented which challenge basic beliefs, it is more likely that the message will be ignored, dismissed, or interpreted to mean something else
■ change behaviour in the absence of other enabling factors.

Communication tools

Many health promoters use print media in their work. Leaflets and pamphlets have been used to educate the public since the beginning of the century. When the Central Council for Health Education was established in 1927 it listed the provision of better and cheaper leaflets as its main aim. The greatest use of written material is to support one-to-one interactions with clients and patients. As only 50% of information can be recalled by patients 5 minutes after a consultation, this seems an effective use of leaflets. However, in a recent survey of GPs less than 50% use written material and 30% expressed reservations that it might disrupt the doctor–patient

How could written material be more effectively used in one-to-one interactions?

relationship (Tapper Jones et al 1998). In a review of strategies for changing eating behaviour, information-giving through the use of standard leaflets has not been shown to be effective (Hunt 1995) and many leaflets are used inappropriately and are thus of limited value (Murphy & Smith 1993). Leaflets intended for mass use may not be targeted or distributed to particular groups and so frequently become unread waste paper. Wicke (1994) found, for example, that less than 10% of people read or took a leaflet from displays in health service waiting areas.

There are numerous leaflets available on a wide range of topics. Some are produced by health promotion agencies and successfully combine good design with information. There is clear guidance on design and production for health promoters who wish to develop their own materials (see, for example, Ewles & Simnett 1999). Many commercial organizations also produce materials free of charge. These may not directly advertise products but the independence and quality of their information needs to be carefully scrutinized.

In contrast to the print media that have been widely used in health promotion for some time, multimedia tools and other new technologies are beginning to offer opportunities for the dissemination of information. Digital television will allow the delivery of information directly to people's homes. The worldwide web offers the possibility of interactive dialogue and for the public to select the information they require. The Health Education Authority has developed several websites, including ones to encourage people to be more active and to help people give up smoking. They have also produced an innovative CD-ROM to educate young people about drugs, which offers an interactive route. Telemedicine, including the new helpline, NHS Direct, offers a two-way dialogue allowing people who are unable to access primary care to ask questions and get feedback about their symptoms.

These new technologies offer a completely different starting point for communication than simply providing information. It is possible that existing human interaction – conversations, the cafe, support groups – can all be harnessed to link health information with the important element of sociability.

Many claims have been made for the Internet as a medium for health promotion:

- that it is interactive
- that it enables the individual to maintain privacy and control (especially important in sexual health promotion)
- that it is value free.

Do you agree with these assertions?

See Anderson (1988) and Anthony (1996) for more information.

Conclusion

The mass media are significant partners for health, but ones that need to be understood and used according to their own priorities. To expect a mass media campaign to produce large shifts in behaviour and contribute directly to reduced morbidity and mortality is unrealistic. But the media can work for health by supporting individual and social change.

On an individual level, the mass media can supplement, but not substitute for, one-to-one education and advice. Even with sophisticated marketing and audience research, the mass media remain a fairly blunt instrument with little opportunity for feedback or clarification. However, the media can raise awareness, provide information and motivate people to change if their environment is supportive. The media can also be used to advocate for the public health by shifting public opinion and encouraging the formation of healthy public policies. Whilst this is a relatively new strategy in the UK, experience from other countries is encouraging (Chapman & Lupton 1994, Wallack et al 1993).

Questions for further discussion

■ How could you use the media to raise public awareness of a health issue and get the issue discussed in a way which is health promoting?
■ What criteria would you use to decide whether or not to use a printed leaflet or pamphlet?

Summary

This chapter has looked at the ways in which mass media are used to promote health. It has discussed different strategies including advertising as part of a planned campaign and the marketing of health messages. There is now greater awareness of how to use the mass media more effectively and this chapter looked at how media coverage can be generated and used to influence public opinion. It has contrasted print media with new multimedia technologies to show how effective communication combines information with the key element of interaction.

Further reading

Egger G, Donovan R, Spark R 1993 Health and the media: principles and practice for health promotion. McGraw Hill, Sydney. *A comprehensive and accessible guide to using different media for health promotion. Combines practical advice, examples and theoretical underpinning.*

Tones K, Tilford S 1994 Health education: effectiveness efficiency. Chapman & Hall, London. *Includes detailed accounts of evaluated mass-media campaigns.*

References

Anderson W 1998 Sexual health in cyberspace. Health Education Authority, London

Anthony D 1996 Health on the Internet. Blackwell, Oxford

Cantril H 1958 The invasion from Mars. In: Maccoby E E, Newcombe T M, Hartley E L (eds) Readings in social psychology. Henry Holt, New York

Chapman S, Lupton D 1994 The fight for public health: principles and practice of media advocacy. BMJ Publishing, London

Davis A M 1987 Heart health campaigns. Health Education Journal 46: 3–10

Department of Health and Social Security (DHSS) 1987a AIDS: monitoring response to the public education campaign February 1986–February 1987. HMSO, London

Department of Health and Social Security (DHSS) 1987b Anti-heroin campaign: stage five research evaluation. HMSO, London

Ewles L, Simnett I 1999 Promoting health: a practical guide, 4th edn. Baillière Tindall, Edinburgh

Gatherer A, Parfit J, Porter E, Vessey M 1979 Is health education effective? Health Education Council, London

Hill D 1993 Changes in sun related attitude and behaviours, and reduced sunburn prevalence in a population at high risk of melanoma. European Journal of Cancer Prevention 2: 447–456

Hunt P 1995 Development and evaluation of the 'Changing What You Eat' resources for primary care. Health Education Journal 54: 405–414

Karpf A 1988 Doctoring the media. Routledge and Kegan Paul, London,

Katz E, Lazarsfeld P 1955 Personal influence: the part played by people in the flow of mass communication. Free Press, Glencoe, Illinois

Leathar D S 1988 The development and assessment of mass media campaigns: Be All You Can Be, case history, part 2. Journal of Institute of Health Education 26: 85–93

Lupton D 1994 Medicine as culture. Sage, London

McGuire C 1992 Pausing for breath. A review of no smoking day research 1984–1991. HEA, London

Mendelsohn H 1968 Which shall it be: mass education or mass persuasion for health?' American Journal of Public Health 58: 131–137

Montazeri A, McGhee S, McEwan J 1998 Fear inducing and positive image strategies in health education campaigns. International Journal of Health Promotion and Education 36(3): 68–75

Murphy S, Smith C 1993 Crutches, confetti: or useful tools? Professionals' views on and use of health education leaflets. Health Education Research 8(2): 205–215

Naidoo J, Wills J 1998 Practising health promotion: dilemmas and challenges. Baillière Tindall, London

Office of Health Economics 1994 Health and the Consumer 30, May 1994. OHE, London

Reid D 1996 Health education via mass communications – how effective? Health Education Journal 55(3): 332–344

Reid D, Killoran A, McNeill A, Chambers J 1992 Choosing the most effective health promotion options for reducing a nation's smoking prevalence. Tobacco Control 1: 185–197

Sayce L 1995 An ill wind in a climate of fear. Guardian, 18 January

Tapper Jones L, Smail S, Pill R, Havard Davies R 1998 General practitioners' use of written materials during consultations. British Medical Journal 269: 908–909

Tones K 1993 Changing theory and practice: trends in methods, strategies and settings in health education. Health Education Journal 52: 126–139

Tones K, Tilford S 1994 Health education: effectiveness efficiency and equity. Chapman & Hall, London

Wallack L, Dorfman L, Jernigan D, Themba M 1993 Media advocacy and public health: power for prevention. Sage, California

Wicke D M 1994 Effectiveness of waiting room noticeboard as a vehicle for health education. Family Practice 11(3): 292–295

Wober J M 1988 Informing the British public about AIDS. Health Education Research 3: 19–24

SECTION 3

Settings for Health Promotion

This section is concerned with the settings which can promote health. It is in settings that we live our lives – at school, at work, in neighbourhoods and in our contact with health services. How can these settings be made more conducive to health?

Introduction to settings for health promotion

Health promotion has been carried out in particular settings for many years. Workplaces and schools, for example, have provided established channels to reach defined populations. The concept of a settings approach to health promotion, however, first emerged in the 1980s. The Ottawa Charter (WHO 1986) stated that 'health is created and lived by people within the settings of their everyday life: where they learn, work, play and love'. As we have seen in this book the focus of health promotion activity is moving away from identifying the diseases and conditions contributing to ill health and the groups at risk, to identifying the complex interplay of factors which create health. It is in settings – at school, at work, in our neighbourhood and in our contact with health services – that we live our lives and it is these contexts or settings which need to be made more conducive to health:

'By the year 2000, all settings of social life and activity, such as the city, school, workplace, neighbourhood and home, should provide greater opportunities for promoting health ...' (WHO 1991, p. 64).

The first and best-known example of settings-based health promotion is the 'Healthy Cities' project. Originally this was a small project initiated by the World Health Organization in 1986 to put the Ottawa Charter and 'Health for All principles' (WHO 1985, 1986) into practice. It has subsequently expanded to become a world wide movement incorporating over 600 cities. Parallel initiatives have been developed and are coordinated by European Networks in schools, hospitals, workplaces, prisons and universities. The UK health strategies have all referred to the importance of settings. *The Health of the Nation* published in 1992 stated that settings 'offer between them the potential to involve most people in the country' (DoH 1992). *Our Healthier Nation* (DoH 1998) identifies schools, workplaces and neighbourhoods as providing 'opportunities to focus the drive against inequalities and improve health overall'.

The World Health Organization has actively pursued a settings-based approach and a few writers (Baric 1993, Baric 1994, Grossman & Scala 1993, Kickbusch 1995) have drawn on organization and management theory to develop practice in this area. Grossman & Scala (1993) have argued that whereas health services provide a system for addressing illness, no system exists to address health. Therefore 'health' must enter each system and find a place in organizations and institutions which were created and structured for other purposes. The culture of a school, for example, is geared to educational objectives and whilst pupil well-being may be an avowed aim it will be less evident than educational attainment. The settings approach builds a concern for health into the fabric of the system and makes sure that the routine activities of the system are committed to and take account of health.

The settings approach is a long-term one. In most cases it is being implemented through defined projects which are designed to:

■ introduce specific interventions to create healthy working and living environments
■ develop health policies
■ integrate health into quality, audit and evaluation procedures to build evidence of how health can make the system perform better.

This section looks at health promotion in four key settings:

■ workplace
■ schools
■ neighbourhoods
■ primary health care and hospitals.

Each setting is addressed in a separate chapter but it is important to remember that the settings are not discrete but coexist as part of a wider independent system. Schools, workplaces, primary health care and hospitals are all in neighbourhoods and there is a constant flow of people within and between the settings. Tones & Tilford (1994) have argued that the approach is unlikely to have any long-term impact on population health until 'different settings have congruent aims and opearate synergistically'.

Each of the following chapters examines why the setting is appropriate for health promotion, identifying the factors of the settings which affect health and outlining some health-promoting initiatives which have been developed in that setting.

References

Baric L 1993 The settings approach: implications for policy and strategy. Journal of the Institute of Health Education 30(1): 17–24

Baric L 1994 Health promotion and health education in practice: the organisational model. Barns Publications, Altrincham

Department of Health (DoH) 1998 Our healthier nation. Stationery Office, London

Department of Health (DoH) 1992 The health of the nation. HMSO, London

Grossman R, Scala K 1993 Health promotion and organisational development: developing strategies for health. WHO, Copenhagen

Kickbusch I 1995 An overview to the settings based approach to health promotion. In: Theaker T, Thompson J The settings based approach to health promotion: report of an international working conference 17–29 November 1993. Hertfordshire Health Promotion, Welwyn Garden City

Tones K, Tilford S 1994 Health education: effectiveness, efficiency and equity. Chapman & Hall, London

WHO 1991 HFA European region targets. WHO, Copenhagen

World Health Organization 1985 targets for health for all. WHO Regional Office for Europe, Copenhagen

World Health Organization 1986 Ottawa charter for health promotion. WHO, Geneva

13 *Health promotion in the workplace*

Key points

- The workplace setting
- Relationship between work and health
- Responsibility for workplace health
- Health promotion in the workplace

OVERVIEW

There is a potential workforce in the UK of 25.5 million people. Because adults spend 60% of their waking hours at work, the workplace is significant both in affecting people's health and as a context in which to promote health.

This chapter looks at the workplace as a social system and ways in which it can contribute to ill health. It goes on to look at ways in which health promotion has been implemented in the workplace which have tended to be around the major lifestyle risk factors and employers' legal responsibilities to provide a safe working environment. Examples of effective workplace health promotion are included with a summary of those factors identified as key to successful interventions.

Why is the workplace a key setting for health promotion?

There are two main reasons for prioritizing the workplace. It gives access to a target group, healthy adults, who are often difficult to reach in other ways. Employees in the workplace are a captive audience for health promotion. It is easy to follow up interventions and encourage participation in health programmes because there are established modes of communication. Adult men are least likely to come into contact with health services, so the workplace provides a useful route to reach the 85% of men under 64 who are economically active (Central Statistical Office 1995). The cohesion of the working community also provides peer pressure and support. The other reason for promoting health in the workplace is to ensure that people are protected from the harm to their health that certain jobs may cause.

The relationship between work and health

The relationship between work and health is complex. In general, attention has focused on the effects of work on health, although it

Work-related ill health

- 18% of deaths each year are work-related.
- 6% adults (2.2 million) suffer ill health associated with work.
- 12 million working days are lost annually through work-related illness, 23 million through workplace injuries, 80 million through stress-related illness.
- The costs of ill health at work are equivalent to 2–3% of the Gross National Product.

Source: Health Education Authority (1997)

is also acknowledged that poor health will have negative effects on the capacity for paid employment. There is evidence that paid work is good for your health and unemployment can be linked to ill health. Work is beneficial for health because it provides an income, a sense of self-worth, and social networks of colleagues and friends. However, work may also harm health, and most research has concentrated on this aspect of the relationship.

Think of a recent work experience.

- In what ways do you think work contributed to your health?
- In what ways do you think work had a negative impact on your health?
- Overall, would you say that work was a positive or a negative influence on your health?

The workplace can affect health in many different ways. Table 13.1 provides a means of classifying these different kinds of relationship.

Table 13.1 *The relationship between work and health*

	Direct relationship	Indirect relationship
Hazards	Handling chemicals and toxic materials as part of the job	Job provides access to dangerous drugs
Risky behaviour	Lifting loads and people as part of the job	Excessive drinking associated with work culture
General work environment	Stress generated by work conditions	Lifestyle risk behaviours, e.g. smoking as coping strategy

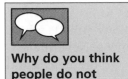

Why do you think people do not always report injuries at work?

Hazards tend to be what people think of first when health in the workplace is mentioned. Most legislation is directed towards the containment of hazards, and safety legislation has been enshrined in numerous Factory Acts since the mid-19th century. Work that involves handling hazardous or toxic materials may have a direct negative effect on health (e.g. cancers caused by asbestos or occupational asthma). Work which provides easy access to hazardous substances is also linked to associated ill health. For example, doctors and pharmacists have high rates of suicide associated with drug overdose.

Table 13.2 shows that the workplace is implicated in a number of fatal and serious injuries. The number appears to be declining, owing partly to the shift away from employment in manufacturing and extraction industries to service industries where the risks are lower. It is likely, however, that the true extent of work-related injuries is under-reported, partly because of the way in which data are collected and partly because many employees do not take time off. Surveys of back pain among nurses, for example, have found that despite 'no manual lifting' policies, many nurses continue lifting and experience pain, but do not report it and continue to work (Hignett 1996). The 1989 General Household Survey found that 22% of people treated in hospital accident and emergency departments had suffered their accidents at work (OPCS 1991).

The workplace is characterized by fragmented information which is collected by different bodies (including the Health and Safety Executive [HSE] and occupational health services). This poses obvious difficulties when trying to plan and implement a health promotion intervention. In an attempt to get a wider and more complete picture of workplace accidents, the Health and Safety Executive now include questions about occupational accidents addressed to employees in addition to the accident data which employers must compile.

Table 13.2 *Fatal and major injury rates per 100 000 employees: 1986/87–1993/94*

	1986/87	1987/88	1988/89	1989/90	1990/91	1991/92	1992/93	1993/94
Agriculture	145	169	158	150	169	157	174	183
Energy	336	289	308	260	246	231	203	180
Manufacturing	147	144	146	147	138	130	126	127
Construction	293	287	296	308	291	281	247	216
Services	58	56	53	54	56	50	53	53
All industries	**101**	**96**	**94**	**93**	**91**	**83**	**82**	**81**

Source: Health and Safety Commission Annual Report 1994/5

Health is often affected through risky behaviour or changed routines. Risky behaviour is the preferred explanation for most official accounts of accidents and injuries sustained in the workplace (Watterson 1986). There are extensive regulations to cover manual handling (Manual Handling Operations Regulations 1992) which require employers to provide training and equipment. Nevertheless, the employee is expected to 'take reasonable care for the health and safety of themselves and any others who may be affected by their acts and omissions'. This approach extends to the workplace the victim-blaming ideology of some brands of health promotion. Behaviour which carries health risks may be an integral part of the job or part of the work culture. For example, bartenders have high rates of alcohol-related ill health because drinking heavily is associated with work.

The general work environment and its effects on health is the most neglected aspect of the work–health relationship. This is due in part to ideological or political reasons, and in part to the fact that such a generalized relationship is hard to research or prove. Because the relationship between work and health is to a large extent indirect, it is often difficult to trace ill health to what happens in the workplace. This in turn leads to the true impact on health from work being underestimated. Focusing on the work environment instead of individual workers' behaviour shifts responsibility on to the employer and has resource implications.

Although the relationship is difficult to quantify, strong evidence implicating the importance to health of the general work environment is becoming available (Sanders 1993, Theorell 1991). There is a body of research demonstrating that certain factors associated with some types of work, such as repetitive tasks, lack of autonomy and pressures to meet deadlines, have harmful effects on health. The Whitehall II study (Marmot 1996) has shown that work conditions are responsible for the mortality and morbidity differences between different grades in the civil service. In particular, low control by workers over what they do and how they do it contributes to stress. Long-term exposure to stress results in poor health and may also lead to less healthy lifestyle choices, such as smoking.

The impact of work on psychological health has been the subject of recent litigation. Recently in the UK, John Walker, a social services officer successfully sued Northumberland County Council for work-related stress, establishing 'that employers have a duty to care not only for the physical but also the mental well-being of their employees' (Cooper & Earnshaw 1998, p. 16). In another case, North Essex Mental Health Trust admitted that an employee's suicide was due to work-related stress. The family's QC stated that 'the death was undoubtedly caused by stress, which together with an unpleasant management regime had pushed him over the edge' (Payne 1998, p. 15).

Look at the following factors which might contribute to stress at work. Have you ever experienced any of these stressors? How did they impact on your health?

■ Stressors intrinsic to the job, e.g. physical conditions (noise, lack of space), information technology (equipment breakdown, lack of training), too much work (overload), too little work and lack of stimulation (underload).

■ Role of the individual in the organization, e.g. role conflict (between work and home), role ambiguity (uncertainty about extent of responsibilities or degree of authority), role responsibility (anxiety about motivating or disciplining others).

■ Career development, e.g. lack of job security, thwarted ambition, lack of progression.

■ Relationships with others, e.g. interpersonal conflicts, conflicts with managers.

■ Organizational culture, e.g. degree of control, performance appraisal, ability to participate in decision-making.

Source: Cooper & Williams (1994)

There are two main ways in which workplace stress is being addressed. The traditional approach has been to see the individual as unable to cope with the demands and pressures and therefore in need of support. Many large workplaces offer stress management courses, counselling services and employee assistance programmes to help people adjust to new skills.

Organizational approaches to stress are still rare despite a growing literature linking stress with organizational factors, such as lack of control or lack of consultation over changes. These approaches start from the view that illness and stressed behaviour are responses to factors in the workplace of which individuals may not even be aware.

'Accept that work stress is a problem for the organisation, not the individual. Forget about blaming individuals. It's everyone's problem. Although individual responses may vary, stress at work is a collective problem. Both the sources of stress and the remedies are often beyond the control of individuals. It is not enough to say that individuals must learn to cope better by practising relaxation or counselling. Changes may be needed in the workplace itself to reduce or eliminate the sources of stress' (Jee & Reason 1989, p. 17).

What could your organization do to reduce stress at work?

An international survey of stress intervention programmes (ILO 1992) concluded that task and work reorganization is the most successful form of intervention. It describes various system solutions to improve communication, the creation of autonomous work groups and whole organization interventions to restructure relations between management and unions. These interventions do not obviate the need for individual support, but follow an earlier stage of raising staff awareness of stress and its causes (increasingly this is being done through stress audits, such as the Health Education Authority's 'Positive Stress at Work' training pack).

Responsibility for workplace health

The relationship between work and health may appear substantial but it is viewed in different ways by different groups of people. One of the defining characteristics of the workplace setting is that it brings together a variety of groups who have different agendas with regard to work and health. The key parties are workers or employees and their trade unions or staff associations, employers and managers, occupational health staff, health and safety officers, environmental health officers and specialist health promoters.

Workers

It has always been a priority for workers' organizations to ensure that employees are working in safe and healthy conditions. With 700 workplace deaths and 170 000 major injuries each year, safety and hazards are obviously of key importance.

Membership of trade unions has, however, declined since the mid-1970s when membership was just under two-fifths (Rose 1993). Changing patterns of employment also mean that part-time (mainly female) workers make up a quarter of the working population. So although consultation with unions is an important means of reaching workers, it does not reach everyone. As the key target group, workers need to be fully involved at all stages of the development and implementation of health promotion programmes. The setting up of liaison committees and employee advisory boards has been shown to be useful (Sorensen et al 1990) and research has also shown that effective health promotion programmes are associated with full staff participation (HEA 1998).

British Rail introduced an alcohol policy in 1993 to comply with the Transport and Works Act. Employees face dismissal if they are found to have a blood alcohol level over the legal limit.

■ What are the interests of British Rail?
■ Why might the workforce object to such a policy?
■ Is such a policy health-promoting?

Employers and managers

Employers and managers have as their first priority the viability of the organization. Health is relevant in so far as it can be shown to be linked to organizational goals. Examples of 'hard' benefits are improvements in productivity due to lower rates of sickness, absenteeism and staff turnover, and improved recruitment and retention of trained staff. 'Soft' benefits, such as enhanced corporate image, are also influential.

Employers are responsible for the health, safety and welfare of all their employees under the Health and Safety at Work Act (1974). Awareness of this responsibility varies. Bunt (1993) notes that 97% of private sector employers consider that measures to protect employees' health at work are adequate. This is in strong contrast to the views of their employees, of whom only 8% agree. Other aspects of workplace health promotion are often seen as a benefit rather than integral to the working environment (Mills 1996).

 Employer responsibilities might be:

■ making healthy choices easy for staff
■ creating flexible working arrangements that are compatible with employees' home lives
■ ensuring a smoke-free environment.

Consider your current or a recent place of work. Can you identify ways in which each of these recommendations was carried out?

Occupational health staff

In many European countries occupational health is a statutory part of health care. In the UK there is no requirement for employers to provide an occupational health service, other than first aid, and only about 50% of workers have access to a health professional at work (Health Education Authority 1997). The main functions of an occupational health service are:

■ surveillance of the work environment, e.g. the effects of new technologies
■ initiatives and advice on the control of hazards
■ surveillance of the health of employees, e.g. assessment of fitness to work, analysis of sickness-absence
■ organization of first aid and emergency response
■ adaptation of work and the environment to the worker.

The workplace has experienced considerable change and uncertainty in the last 20 years. There has been a rapid growth in the service sector, a fragmentation of large organizations and a huge increase in information technology. The provision for health in companies thus needs to be seen alongside policies on employment, the work environment and overall company policy. Lisle (1996) questions whether occupational health services are sufficiently proactive and dynamic to help to create healthy organizations.

Think of a workplace you are familiar with.

■ In what ways were people expected to adapt to the job?
■ In what ways was the job adapted to meet the health needs of people?
■ Which approach is preferable, and why?

Health and safety officers

Health and safety officers are responsible for ensuring that workplaces conform to safety legislation. They have powers to force workplaces to comply with health and safety regulations, and to impose penalties in the case of non-compliance. Responsibility for workplaces is divided between the Health and Safety Executive and environmental health officers employed by local authorities. Health and safety officers have experienced a reduction in funding together with an increased workload owing to the increased numbers of small businesses and recent European Community (EC) legislation.

In addition, trade unions may appoint safety representatives to represent their employees and under EU law all employees, whether in a trade union or not, have the right to health and safety representation. There are more than 90 000 lay safety representatives in the UK and more than 70% of workers have access to one of these officials (Trades Union Congress 1992, cited in Beishon & Veale 1996).

Health promotion specialists

Health promotion specialists may be involved in health promotion activities in the workplace. They provide a specialist resource for coordinating and motivating others to adopt such activities. This service may be provided by NHS departments, voluntary organizations or private companies.

Health promotion in the workplace

Health promotion in the workplace falls into the following categories:

■ first aid and medical treatment
■ pre-employment screening
■ protection from accidents

You are a health promoter trying to get workplaces to adopt a CHD prevention programme.

What kinds of reasons or evidence would persuade each of the following groups to participate?

■ Workers
■ Managers
■ Occupational health staff
■ Health and safety officers.

Workers will need to be convinced that the programme concerns their health and is not a covert means of introducing new work practices or conditions, or of using health surveillance to screen employees. Managers will want reassurance that the programme has benefits, preferably economic, for the organization. Occupational health staff will want their professional role to be acknowledged and maintained, and not undermined, by the programme. Health and safety officers will need a clear link to be established between the programme and their role if they are to participate. For example, passive smoking or exposure to environmental tobacco smoke (ETS) may constitute a health hazard and thus be a suitable topic to address. Above all, the different groups will need to meet to share perspectives and build trusting relationships if such a programme is to be successful.

■ control of hazards and infections
■ education and advice about healthy lifestyles and practices
■ policies and regulations to provide a healthier environment
■ provision of services, e.g. exercise facilities, screening, counselling.

There is widespread acceptance of the requirement to provide safe working conditions. Table 13.3 shows some of the key examples of health and safety legislation. Compared to other developed countries, however, the UK has far less workplace health promotion (Philo et al 1992). There is no legal requirement for occupational health services, and health promotion programmes are developed on an ad hoc basis with little evaluation (HEA 1998, Oakley et al 1994).

Health promotion programmes in the workplace are still not widespread. A survey by the Health Education Authority in 1993 found that 40% of all workplaces were involved in health promotion during the previous year but that this was more likely in large workplaces (HEA 1993). Programmes included smoking cessation, alcohol counselling, exercise and fitness interventions, general health screening and stress management courses.

Workplace health promotion tends to focus on individual lifestyle interventions. Oakley et al (1994) in their review of workplace interventions cite the following types of programmes:

- programmes to increase awareness of risk factors for disease
- single-session events to motivate employees to change an aspect of their lifestyle
- team or departmental competitions to promote behaviour change
- buddy or peer support systems
- feedback to maintain participation.

 Smoking at work

Smoking is the area where there is most widespread health promotion activity. 39% of women and 23% of men are exposed to environmental tobacco smoke (ETS) at work and it has been estimated that it may contribute to 300 excess lung cancer deaths in non-smokers. Smoking interventions at work are concerned either to protect non-smokers through the introduction of smoking policies or to help individuals to stop smoking, such as individual advice, nicotine replacement or cash incentives.

31% of workplaces have a total ban on smoking and 47% allow smoking in restricted areas. There is evidence that a workplace ban or limitation on smoking can lead to an overall reduction in tobacco consumption. In 1992 an employee successfully sued Stockport Borough Council for health damage from ETS.

- Do you think smoking should be banned completely in offices, workplaces and colleges?
- Does the place where you work or study have a smoking policy?
- Is this a total or limited ban?
- How widely is the policy observed (are there places for example that smokers go)?
- What do you think might make the policy more widely implemented?

See Bostock 1994, HEA 1997 for further information.

There is evidence that health promotion in the workplace is effective. Most of this evidence comes from the USA where initiatives are well-established and there is an incentive to reduce employer-borne health insurance costs. Bovell (1992) argues that although it may be difficult to show clear financial benefits, there are benefits in other areas, such as reduced absenteeism, increased productivity, improved staff morale and considerably reduced staff turnover. However, there is little evidence that health promotion in the workplace affects individual behaviour. The Multiple Risk Factor Intervention Trial (MRFIT) in the USA in the 1970s included multiple interventions but produced only minimal changes in smoking and eating behaviour even though it focused on men at the highest risk of coronary heart disease and there was intensive intervention over

Table 13.3 *Key dates in health and safety legislation*	1833	Factory Act	Established Factory inspectorate with powers to prosecute employers providing unsafe working conditions
	1875	Factories and Workshop Act	Centralized Inspectorate; Chief Inspector appointed
	1897	Workmen's Compensation Act	Introduced the concept of employer's liability and benefits regardless of who was to blame for accidents
	1956	Agriculture Act	Extended legislation to agricultural sector
	1972	EMAS	Employment Medical Advisory Service created to give advice and medical monitoring
	1974	Health and Safety at Work Act	Placed a legal duty on employers to train, inform, instruct and supervise employees to protect their health and safety Established the Health and Safety Commission (HSC) and the Health and Safety Executive (HSE) which incorporated EMAS
	1990	Control of Substances Hazardous to Health (COSHH)	Placed duties on employers to protect employees from the substances they have to work with. Included six key steps: (i) Assessment of risk (ii) Prevention or control of exposure (iii) Use of control measures (iv) Maintenance, examination and testing of control measures (v) Health surveillance (vi) Information, instruction and training
	1992	Management of Health and Safety at Work Regulations	Implemented six EEC directives on health and safety at work. Regulations cover: (i) Health and safety management (ii) Work equipment safety (iii) Manual handling of loads (iv) Workplace conditions (v) Personal protective equipment (vi) Display screen equipment

a 6-year period (MRFIT 1982). Although the rationale for workplace health promotion is that there is a potentially high level of participation and low level of attrition, owing to a stable and 'captive' population, most evaluations have shown that participation in workplace programmes is low (20–40% for on-site programmes) and participants tend to be the most motivated and least at-risk employees (Lovato & Green 1990).

 CHD prevention in the workplace

Programmes to reduce coronary heart disease in older men are difficult to design and sustain. Dorset Health Promotion Agency in England conducted a detailed needs assessment with men aged 40–55 and found that in order to appeal to this group, interventions should:

■ incorporate peer support
■ use an approach incorporating competitive teamwork
■ recognize motivating factors, e.g. desire for improved 'performance, personal vanity'.

Nine workplaces each represented by teams of eight men were organized into a competition to reduce weight and increase fitness. Each month a league table was circulated to all participants, and at the end of the 6-month 'season' prizes were awarded to the winning team and individual. Workplaces varied in the additional support offered to their teams – some allowed staff to exercise in work time or paid for education sessions in work time.

Evaluation showed a very low drop-out rate with all the participants completing the whole 6 months. Over 70% showed a reduction in their body mass index (BMI) and 58% increased their physical fitness. Over 80% of those who were followed up 8 months after the end of the intervention had maintained or improved their weight loss and had made some other changes towards a healthier lifestyle.

Source: Dorset Health Promotion Agency (1998)

A recent effectiveness review carried out by the Health Education Authority (1998) identified the following features for successful interventions:

■ support from senior management
■ involvement and participation of staff at all levels in the planning and implementation
■ focus on definable and modifiable risk factors which are a priority for a specified group of workers (e.g. stress or work-related cancer)
■ programmes tailored to individual organizations
■ good resourcing.

The review draws attention to the ways in which most programmes focus on health-related knowledge, values and behaviour of individuals and do not look at other aspects of the social and material context in which employees live. It recommends integrated programmes which include population-based policy initiatives and individual and group interventions.

Health at work in the NHS

In 1992 the Health at Work in the NHS initiative was introduced to encourage the NHS to become an exemplar health-promoting organization. In 1995 the Health at Work award scheme introduced standards which workplaces need to meet to become healthy workplaces:

- Raising awareness of the importance of health
- Developing and implementing policies on smoking, alcohol and HIV/AIDS
- Promoting and facilitating healthy eating, physical activity and positive mental and physical health
- Exploring how the workplace can contribute to sustainable development
- Reviewing health and safety legislation and implementing training policies to reinforce health-promoting behaviour
- Supporting positive approaches to improving staff attendance and reducing staff turnover.

Workplaces are encouraged to move from a healthy lifestyle approach of information-giving to a more strategic approach where workplace organization is modified to promote health.

Over 100 organizations have achieved awards including several local authorities, the Home Office and large commercial organizations including IBM, Hewlett Packard and Nissan Motors.

In 1999 the Healthy Workplace initiative was launched to develop examples of good practice.

Identify initiatives from your workplace which might meet these standards.

Conclusion

A body of evidence is becoming available which demonstrates the tangible benefits to be derived from workplace health promotion programmes. Research is also beginning to identify what factors are associated with effective and successful programmes. The challenge now is to increase the coverage of health promotion in the workplace schemes, in terms of both the number of organizations and the scope of the programmes. Another challenge is to reach the increasing number of part-time and home workers whose relationship with a workplace and employer is less defined.

Most programmes focus on individual lifestyle advice, monitoring and education. Unless the organizational context is also considered and modified, such programmes are likely to have a limited effect.

Health promotion in the workplace would receive a great impetus if legislation provided incentives to participate. Health promoters can support interventions by facilitating the process of liaison and dialogue amongst all staff. They can also assist by providing specialist input on organizing, planning, implementing and evaluating activities. Tangible benefits need to be demonstrated in order to win managerial support.

Questions for further discussion

■ What are the potential and limitations of health promotion in workplace settings?
■ How should health promotion address the changes in work patterns in the 21st century (e.g. increased part-time working and short-term contracts, teleworking and home-working and increased information technology)?

Summary

This chapter has looked at the reasons for prioritizing the workplace as a setting for health promotion. It has outlined the different ways in which workplaces attempt to protect employees' health and may seek to enhance health by enabling employees to gain control over their personal health, the working environment and their work organization. It has shown that many groups may be involved in workplace health and these may have different agendas. Making health a priority for workplaces is a difficult task. The effectiveness of different approaches to health promotion including policy development and lifestyle interventions has been examined.

Further reading

Daykin N, Doyal L (eds) 1999 Health at work: critical perspectives. Macmillan, London. *A critical account of the relationship between health and work.*

Health Education Authority 1997 Health update: workplace health. HEA, London. *This is a comprehensive summary of workplace health promotion including the costs of ill health in the workplace, examples of specific programmes and a review of the evidence of effectiveness.*

Health Education Authority 1998 Effectiveness of health promotion interventions in the workplace. HEA, London. *A review of interventions, most of which are based in the USA. The review includes studies based on participatory methods. Most of the programmes identified are targeted at individuals.*

Sanders D 1993 Workplace health promotion: a review of the literature. Oxford Regional Health Authority, Oxford. *A detailed review of interventions in the UK with some examples from USA and Canada. The report identifies effective smoking- and stress-reduction programmes.*

Scriven A, Orme J 1996 Health promotion: professional perspectives. Macmillan, Basingstoke. *Section six provides an accessible summary of health promotion in the workplace, examines the contributions of trade unions and the occupational health services and offers a detailed case study of how different partners need to collaborate to promote health at work.*

References

Beishon M, Veale S 1996 Trade unions and health promotion. In: Scriven A, Orme J (eds) Health promotion: professional perspectives. Macmillan, Basingstoke

Bostock Y 1994 Working smoking policy. HEA, London

Bovell V 1992 The economic benefits of health promotion in the workplace. In: Action on Health at Work seminar. HEA, London

Bunt K 1993 Occupational health provision at work. Health and Safety Executive Research Report 57. HSE, London

Central Statistical Office 1995 Employment Gazette 103(6). HMSO, London

Cooper C L, Earnshaw J 1998 The price of stress. Nursing Standard 12–16

Cooper C L, Williams S 1994 Creating healthy work organisations. Wiley, Chichester

Department of Health (DoH) 1998 Our healthier nation. Stationery Office, London

Dorset Health Promotion Agency 1998 'Keeping it up': promoting weight loss in men aged 40–55. Working Together for Better Health: conference abstracts. International Conference. Health Promotion Wales, Cardiff

Health Education Authority 1993 Health promotion in the workplace: a summary. HEA, London

Health Education Authority 1997 Health update: workplace health. HEA, London

Health Education Authority 1998 Effectiveness of health promotion interventions in the workplace. HEA, London

Health and Safety Commission 1995 Fatal and major injury rates 1986–1994. In: annual report 1994/5. HSC, London

Hignett S 1996 Work related back pain in nurses. Journal of Advanced Nursing 23(6): 1238–1246

International Labour Organization 1992 Conditions of work digest 11(2): preventing stress at work. ILO, Geneva

Jee M, Reason L 1989 Action on stress at work. HEA, London

Lisle J 1996 The role of occupational health services in promoting health. In: Scriven A, Orme J (eds)

Health promotion: professional perspectives. Macmillan, Basingstoke

Lovato C Y, Green L W 1990 Maintaining employee participation in workplace health promotion programs. Health Education Quarterly 17(1): 73–88

Marmot M 1996 The social pattern of health and disease. In: Blane D, Brunner E, Wilkinson R (eds) Health and social organisation. Routledge, London

Mills M 1996 Body and soul. People Management (Sept): 36–38

Multiple Risk Factor Intervention Trial Research Group 1982 The Multiple Risk Factor Intervention Trial –risk factor changes and mortality results. Journal of the American Medical Association 248: 1465–1476

Oakley A, France-Dawson M, Holland J, Fullerton D, Kelly P, Arnold S 1994 Review of effectiveness of workplace health promotion interventions: a summary document for the Health Education Authority. Social Science Research Unit, Institute of Education, London

Office of Population Censuses and Surveys 1991 General household survey 1989. HMSO, London

Payne D 1998 Stressed to death. Nursing Times 98

Philo J, Russell J, Pettersson G 1992 Health at work: a needs assessment in South West Thames Regional Health Authority. SWTRHA, London

Rose P (ed) 1993 Social trends 23. Central Statistical Office, HMSO, London

Sanders D 1993 Workplace health promotion: a review of the literature. Oxford Regional Health Authority, Oxford

Sorensen G, Hunt M K, Morris D H et al 1990 Promoting healthy eating patterns in the worksite: the Treatwell intervention model. Health Education Research 5(4): 505–515

Theorell T 1991 Health promotion in the workplace. In: Badura B, Kickbusch I (eds) health promotion research: towards a new social epidemiology. WHO, Copenhagen

Watterson A 1986 Occupational health and illness: the politics of hazard education. In: Rodmell S, Watt A (eds) The politics of health education: raising the issues. Routledge and Kegan Paul, London

14 *Health promotion in schools*

OVERVIEW

The view that schools can promote the health and welfare of young people has a long history. The development of a school health service, the requirement for school boards to provide meals and the provision of physical education are examples of how the school was seen as a key setting in which a captive audience could be encouraged to adopt lifestyles conducive to good health.

The concept of a health-promoting school is a relatively new one. 'The health promoting school aims at achieving healthy lifestyles for the total school population by developing supportive environments conducive to the promotion of health. It offers opportunities for, and requires commitments to, the provision of a safe and health-enhancing social and physical environment' (World Health Organization 1993). The school is seen as a total environment in which many aspects affect the health of its pupils and staff including its organization, ethos and culture and its layout, in addition to any teaching about health issues and the provision of medical and nursing services. This chapter looks at the physical, mental and social well-being of young people and how schools can be powerful agents in the promotion of good health through the curriculum and everyday practices.

The World Health Organization has described health as a resource for living. Educational achievement is also part of all children's entitlement. This chapter argues that a healthy school is a positive learning environment which can contribute to improving educational attainment.

Why the school is a key setting for health promotion

School is seen as an important context for health promotion, principally because it reaches a large proportion of the population for many years. The emphasis on schools is also a recognition that the learning of health-related knowledge, attitudes and behaviour begins at an early age. The Health Education Authority Primary

Schools Project (Williams et al 1989) showed that teachers often underestimate the wealth of information young children bring to their learning about health.

Reflect on your own experience of health promotion when you were at school. Do you regard your experience as adequate and appropriate?

Consider each of the following statements about the aims for health promotion for young people and indicate how important you would rate each.

	Very important	Important	Not very important	Not important at all

Health promotion should:

1. Provide information about how the body works
2. Foster positive personal and social relationships
3. Teach young people to keep fit and feel good
4. Equip young people with the skills to make informed and responsible decisions
5. Inform young people about local services and how to get help
6. Teach young people about the dangers of certain behaviours, such as taking drugs
7. Help young people to express their feelings and emotions
8. Teach young people how to say 'no'
9. Show young people the wonders of the human body so they do not damage it
10. Put young people off unhealthy behaviour by emphasizing the risks to their health
11. Prepare young people for parenthood
12. Provide information about human sexuality, puberty and contraception
13. Teach young people how to reduce their risk from drug-taking or sexual activity (safer sex and safer drug-taking)
14. Prepare young people to be active citizens
15. Show young people how to cope with stress
16. Equip young people with the skills to negotiate and be assertive in relationships
17. Help to build young people's self-esteem.

Relationship between schools, education and health

Adolescence is a time of great change, when young people often acquire lifetime habits and attitudes. Part of growing up is risk-taking, but problems arise when young people are unaware of the scale of risk involved. Whilst adolescence is characterized by powerful peer group attachments, the school setting provides an opportunity to communicate with young people and provides learning opportunities and a safe environment to practise new skills.

There is little evidence that young people who engage in health-damaging behaviours necessarily adopt this as a lifestyle. 'Young people follow health careers, engaging with, and disengaging from, multiple risk at different points in their lives' (Aggleton 1996, p. 88). There are, however, economic, societal and individual factors which affect the decisions young people take, the response they have to health issues and the values and norms of their particular culture. Economic disadvantage, lack of community and neighbourhood support and low school achievement have been identified as factors predisposing young people to health risks.

The effects of smoking, excessive alcohol consumption, drug use and low levels of exercise may not be evident until later life. There is some evidence, however, that health risks for young people do cluster together. Among 9- to 15-year-olds, for example, regular smokers drink more than twice as much per week as non-smokers and are over 50% more likely to use illegal drugs (HEA 1991b). Sexual risk-taking and accident proneness may be consequences of these behaviours.

There is a relationship between health and education and the ability to learn. Young people's experiences in school influence the development of their self-esteem, self-perception and their health behaviours. Pupils who dislike school and who rate their own achievement as low, tend to start smoking and drinking earlier and are more likely to be regular users of tobacco and alcohol (European Network of Health Promoting Schools 1997). It also seems that learning is quicker, more comprehensive and more enjoyable if children are healthy (WHO 1995).

What factors would you identify as important in promoting a health-enhancing lifestyle for young people?

How schools can influence well-being

- The school system and its objective of developing and evaluating academic performance puts a strain on many young people.
- Young people may feel isolated or excluded from activities in breaks and have few opportunities to develop support from teachers or fellow students, and so feel unsafe and stressed.
- Disturbances in class and teachers' attempts to calm students down can inhibit learning.
- Codes of behaviour and rules may be inconsistently applied or perceived as unfair.
- Young people may feel unsafe as a consequence of bullying.

Source: WHO Cross National Study of Health Behaviour in School-Aged Children (King et al 1996)

The context for health promotion in schools

The development of health education and promotion in schools has reflected many approaches to health promotion. Health education before the Second World War tended to reflect the medical view of health. Although it was part of teachers' training, it was a fringe subject and almost exclusively concerned with hygiene and fitness. Education in the 1960s saw a swing to being child-centred and educational methods sought to develop autonomy and responsibility through discovery learning. Health education emerged as a complex theme of well-being and fulfilment of maximum potential.

The Schools Council Health Education Project 13–18 (1982) saw health education as concerned with making informed decisions and the development of self-esteem. Health themes ranged from the physiological to environmental and community health – a multidimensional view which reflected the holistic concept of the World Health Organization. Subsequent projects have sought to develop social and life-skills, such as being assertive, making relationships, managing conflict, working in groups and influencing people (Gray & Hill 1992, HEA 1989, 1991a, Hopson & Scally 1980, 1982, 1985, 1987). Health promotion in schools is now closely linked to personal and social development and the pastoral curriculum. The aim is for young people to be in charge of their own lives and the role of the school is to develop self-esteem and self-awareness. Emphasis is placed on the *process* of education, and finding teaching and learning strategies which encourage reflection and personal awareness. The direction and organization of the health promotion programme also aim to reflect the needs of the children and young people.

Alongside the attempts to promote autonomy and decision-making skills are more traditional information-giving approaches. Behind such an approach is the simple assumption that people are rational decision-makers whose behaviour will change once they have information about how to live more healthily. Much health promotion in schools therefore entails the provision of information about the health-damaging effects of certain behaviours, such as smoking and taking drugs.

The provision of sex education in schools reflects these distinct views of health promotion. On the one hand there are national calls to reduce teenage pregnancies, reduce the spread of HIV infection and warn young people of sexual health risks. On the other hand there are calls to promote family values which it is claimed will act as a check on sexual activity, and in the USA there is a strong move towards abstinence education. Sex education is regularly surrounded by moral panic, health scares and political argument.

Although most schools have some general sex education, surveys consistently show that young people perceive this as 'too little, too

The 1993 Education act requires schools to:

- Make provision for sex education
- Make a policy statement available to parents
- Allow parents to request the exclusion of their child from all or part of sex education other than those elements which form part of the statutory National Curriculum
- Publish in a prospectus a summary of the content and organization of the sex education programme.

Do these arrangements mark a commitment to sex education?

late'. Few schools consult pupils about their needs and there seems a gap between what schools think it is important to provide, and what young people want to know. The focus in schools is on physiology and biology, rather than emotional and sexual feelings (Radat & Speed 1994).

Sex education and drug education are both subjects which have generated considerable concern and controversy. Specific sums of money have been earmarked since 1986 for curriculum development and training in these areas, reflecting the belief that schools provide important settings in which young people can be alerted to health risks. There has also been a long-standing debate about the likely effects of education on behaviour with a widespread belief that it may encourage early experimentation. The evidence from the Netherlands and Sweden, and from an analysis of data from the UK National Survey of Sexual Attitudes and Lifestyles, seems to be that, if anything, comprehensive and early sex education programmes, combined with accessible health care services, are likely to postpone sexual initiation (Wellings et al 1995).

Aggleton (1996) summarizes the findings from numerous studies and identifies the following as likely to promote the sexual and reproductive health of young people:

- provision of relevant information
- exercises and activities to encourage personal appraisal of risk and self-awareness
- skills training in negotiation and communication
- awareness of, and access to, appropriate health services and condoms.

Barriers to promoting health in schools

Section 1 of the 1988 Education Reform Act places a statutory responsibility on schools to provide a broad and balanced curriculum that:

- promotes the spiritual, moral, cultural, mental and physical development of pupils
- prepares pupils for the opportunities, responsibilities and experience of adult life.

Yet health education and promotion is not well established in schools. The number of primary schools with a policy on health education and promotion rose from 17% in 1978 to 80% in 1993, and in secondary schools the increase was from 68% in 1981 to 89% in 1993 (Lewis 1993). Yet few schools have a planned programme with specialist teachers. Most health promotion is taught by teachers from another subject specialism (usually science) who may not be familiar with participative teaching methods, and are likely to favour the physiological at the expense of the personal and social.

The introduction of a National Curriculum in 1990 and regular pupil assessment has squeezed curriculum time. Health education was identified as a cross-curricular theme lacking the status of core and foundation subjects. Despite attempts to slim down the national curriculum following the enquiry by Ron Dearing, chair of the School Curriculum and Assessment Authority in 1995, and a further review in 1998, there remains little time for personal, social and health education (PSHE). The introduction of league tables of schools based on academic results has also placed pressure on schools to devote the curriculum to academic subjects. In secondary schools, brief timetabled sessions are the most popular means of giving time to those areas which do not command subject status. In primary schools the emphasis on literacy and numeracy leaves little time for topic work. PSHE is also marginalized in relation to staffing, in-service training and advisory services (Jamison 1993).

 What topics or themes would you expect to find taught in health education and promotion in schools?

The National Curriculum for schools is under review but currently includes nine core and foundation subjects. There are also five cross-curricular themes of which health education is one. Although part of the National Curriculum, there is no legal requirement to teach health education. The National Curriculum guidance offers nine components or topic areas for health education:

- Substance use and misuse
- Sex education
- Family life education
- Safety
- Health-related exercise
- Food and nutrition
- Personal hygiene
- Environmental aspects
- Psychological aspects.

The future development and delivery of health promotion will also depend on initial teacher education. As Scriven (1996) points out, moves to more school-based training for teachers disadvantage health promotion as it is already marginalized in the curriculum, and students may be unable to observe it being taught. Primary and secondary training courses only receive funding for courses in core and foundation subjects and students are unable to choose health studies as a major part of their degree programme.

The health-promoting school

Health promotion is not just something which takes place in the curriculum. Many aspects of school can be health promoting or health inhibiting. Educationalists have long talked of a 'hidden curriculum' and the way in which messages can be transmitted through children and young people's daily experience of their surroundings and relationships at school. For example, the state of many school toilets might suggest that hygiene is not valued or that the pupils do not require (or deserve) cleanliness or care. Many aspects of a school institution can promote health: especially the physical environment; the nature of relationships between all those in the school; the reciprocal relationship with the community; the quality of the learning experience; the systems of discipline, care and support; and the general ethos of the school.

If education for the health of young people is to focus on more than individual behaviour and be health *promotion*, it needs to acknowledge the influence of the school itself as a health-promoting environment and as part of a wider community.

The European Network of Health Promoting Schools was launched in 1992 as an initiative of the World Health Organization, involving 40 countries, each of which supports a network of pilot schools. The aim is to develop good practice in how schools can contribute to the health of pupils, teachers and the wider community. Each country has developed the project in different ways and many are now incorporating the principles into mainstream provision. Each is guided by the 12 WHO criteria for a health-promoting school (WHO 1993) (see box on page 288).

In the UK, healthy school award schemes have been popular. As with other award schemes for hospitals and workplaces, the scheme encourages institutions to work towards specific targets. A basic level is to ensure that systems are in place to ensure that specific aspects of health are able to be incorporated into a school. The whole school approach means focusing on:

Policies and practices. The policies that a school develops represent its values. Schools may have policies on equal opportunities, discipline and rewards, health and safety, drugs and

The 12 WHO criteria for a health-promoting school

1. Active promotion of the self-esteem of all pupils by demonstrating that everyone can make a contribution to the life of the school.
2. Development of good relations between staff and pupils and among pupils in the daily life of the school.
3. Clarification for staff and pupils of the social aims of the school.
4. Provision of stimulating challenges for all pupils through a wide range of activities.
5. Use of every opportunity to improve the physical environment of the school.
6. Development of good links between school, home and community.
7. Development of good links among associated primary and secondary schools to plan a coherent health education curriculum.
8. Active promotion of the health and well-being of school and staff.
9. Consideration of the role of staff as exemplars in health-related issues.
10. Consideration of the complementary role of school meals (if provided) to the health education curriculum.
11. Realization of the potential of specialist services in the community for advice and support in health education.
12. Development of the education potential of school health services beyond routine screening and towards active support for the curriculum.

the management of drug-related incidents and various curriculum issues including sex education. Policies may be merely 'paper exercises' unless they have been influenced by wide consultation within the school and community, have been clearly written and disseminated and are consistently applied. The practices of a school can be evidenced in its daily life and the ways in which decisions are taken. Democratic participation by pupils is a key element in a health-promoting school.

The Ottawa Charter describes health promotion as a process of 'enabling people to take more control over and improve their health' (WHO 1986). How can pupils in schools be enabled to make decisions about their education and their health?

Ethos.   The quality of social interactions among pupils, between staff and pupils and between the staff contribute to the ethos or climate in a school. Increasingly, schools are recognizing that healthy schools which value positive relationships, prioritize learning and build self-esteem also drive up educational standards. In primary schools, children and teachers may participate in 'circle time' in which they discuss feelings about issues that arise in class or at home, such as bullying, feelings of failure or achievement, separation and loss.

Curriculum.   The characteristics of an effective curriculum have been widely debated. It is generally agreed that it should offer learning experiences appropriate to the social and cognitive development of pupils and that an ongoing and progressive programme or spiral curriculum, in which the same topics are revisited, is most effective. In the UK as noted earlier, there is no statutory provision for health promotion and its integration in the curriculum is patchy. Health promotion lends itself to teaching and learning methods which are learner-centred and participatory, but the drive to push up standards has meant many teachers reverting to traditional didactic (commonly known as 'chalk and talk') methods.

 Health promotion for pre-school children

A comprehensive programme for 4- to 6-year-olds has been developed in Luxembourg. It focuses not only on imparting knowledge but also on developing emotional awareness. A multidisciplinary approach allows for the use of stories, games, painting, singing, drama and role play. The topics are seen as being relevant to the child's experience, provide a base for the continuation of health promotion in later school experience, and encourage links to be made to family life. They include short sequences of 20–30 minutes to:

- Acquaint the child with its body and develop positive feelings about it
- Introduce the child to body and dental care and the need for this to be a personal responsibility
- Raise awareness of nutrition and healthy snacks in a joint meeting with parents and carers
- Develop critical attitudes to television
- Introduce children to active ways of spending leisure time including drama, painting and dance
- Introduce children to relaxation methods

Source: European Network of Health Promoting Schools (1997)

Environment.   The physical environment and layout of a school may be stimulating or depressing. Schools should provide a clean and safe environment with no litter or graffiti, clean toilets and a welcoming but secure entrance. There should be areas for play, for social interaction and for quiet study or reading.

Think back to your primary school and try to picture the playground area. Was it a health-promoting environment?

Links with the community.   Partnerships with parents may vary from information about school events and fund-raising requests, consultation about uniform or meals provision to the active involvement of all parents in decision-making about the curriculum, pastoral care and resource issues. Parents may also become involved in school life through reading schemes, practical parenting classes and breakfast clubs. A survey of parents' views on health education and promotion found that many parents did not know what schools were doing and had not been consulted about health promotion despite the fact that they saw school as a major influence on young people's health awareness (National Foundation for Educational Research 1997).

'Society School'

A school in Belgium identified the need to socially integrate its diverse ethnic groups. One way to do this was to involve parents in school activities. The school took the approach of celebrating its multiculturalism by asking parents to prepare a snack food from their traditional foods for all the children in the school. Many parents participated, also providing decorations and music. All parents were invited to the school for a free meal. Parents reported that this project broke down their initial hesitation about coming into the school and enabled them to build relationships with other parents.

Source: European Network of Health Promoting Schools (1997)

Schools are also part of a wider community and should be open to that community. Many agencies and services can provide support to schools. For example, the police and emergency services often provide educational sessions concerning accident prevention.

Choose one of the following aims and make a list of indicators in the broad areas of policy, curriculum, ethos, environment and community links that would demonstrate that the school was health-promoting.

■ Establishment of a safe and secure environment.
■ School ethos based on the promotion of mutual respect and understanding.
■ Promotion of physical activity.
■ An approach to food and nutrition which promotes the importance of healthy eating.
■ An informed and coherent approach to substance use.
■ An approach to sex and relationships that supports and informs pupils.

Effective interventions

Health promotion interventions in schools differ substantially in their nature, ranging from programmes providing physiological information to life skills to abstinence-oriented programmes, in addition to the comprehensive whole-school approaches outlined above. Many curriculum programmes aim to have outcomes relevant to risk reduction, such as increased knowledge or changes in behaviour. Programmes may thus be specific to a particular health issue (e.g. smoking education) or more generic life skills programmes aiming to develop self-esteem and social and communication skills.

Schools are dynamic communities and there are many varied influences on young people both within and outside the school setting, so demonstrating the particular effect of health promotion is extremely difficult. The majority of interventions aim to develop health-enhancing behaviours. These health outcomes will not be apparent until later in life. For example, the Australian 'no hat – no play' policy will not demonstrate an effect on skin cancer rates until well into adulthood.

In general, school-based curriculum initiatives seem to have a limited effect. Smoking education has a long history and there is some evidence that programmes focusing on social norms and the development of refusal skills may contribute to short-term behaviour change (Reid et al 1995), but the effectiveness of such approaches is greater when the education takes place in the context of a whole-school policy of non-smoking. Reviews of drug education also conclude that programmes focusing on identifying and resisting peer pressure and the exploration of social norms concerning drug use may result in appreciable delays in the onset of taking drugs (Dorn & Murji 1992, HEA 1997). Peersman et al (1996) in their review of sexual health interventions concluded that few evaluated interventions in schools have shown any impact on sexual activity or contraceptive behaviour, although in the short term sex education may delay the onset of first intercourse and reduce the number of partners.

 Evaluating the health-promoting school

The holistic nature of the health-promoting school concept means that it is particularly difficult to evaluate and demands a range of research methodologies. An evaluation of the Wessex Healthy Schools Award in 10 intervention and 5 control schools showed positive changes in school management, raised awareness of the school's health-promoting role and some effect on pupil behaviour. Pupils in the intervention schools were less likely to start smoking or use drugs.

Source: Moon et al (1998)

Conclusion

Schools are widely seen as having a key role in health promotion. This is particularly so when there is public and media concern over health issues. Then the young are seen as a key target population for the provision of information and encouragement of 'responsible' attitudes. For example, concern over the spread of HIV infection led the Government in 1991 to include HIV/AIDS education in the statutory National Curriculum for Science. At that time, the provision of sex education was at the discretion of school governing bodies. After intense lobbying by religious groups, HIV education (except its biological aspects) was withdrawn from the National Curriculum in 1994.

Concern over youth crime has led some to call for more emphasis on personal, social and health education, others to call for more religious and moral education, and still others to call for a return to 'basics', formal discipline and school uniform, so that would-be truants could be easily identified. Great are society's expectations of schools and teachers. Yet we must be realistic and recognize that school-based health promotion is only one influence on young people's behaviour. Health promotion in schools is most likely to be effective where:

- it addresses the needs of young people and starts from where they are in terms of knowledge and experience
- it is supported by an institution which is itself health promoting
- it is supported by broader health promotion in the community
- it is delivered by committed and informed teachers with curriculum time and resources that reflect its importance.

Recent educational changes concerned with school improvement and educational standards are being linked with the process of developing healthy schools in line with government policy to produce a coherent and integrated strategy for health across all departments. The school setting is seen as crucial in terms of the access it provides to young people and its potential to provide a positive learning environment. Problem-solving, communication and analytical skills developed through personal social and health education programmes contribute to learning and the ability of young people to take control over their health.

Questions for further discussion

■ How can the core health promotion principles of collaboration, participation, empowerment and equity be incorporated into the school structure and management?

■ What are the barriers to developing health-promoting schools?

Summary

This chapter has examined the reasons why schools are a key setting for health promotion. The ways in which schools can increase young people's understanding about health issues and help them to make informed choices about their health behaviour, help them to feel good about themselves and others and foster the development of communication and decision-making skills have been identified. This chapter has shown how the whole school needs to be health promoting so that what is taught is reinforced by all aspects of school life. Evidence about the effectiveness of health promotion in schools has been considered. Recent national policy developments have supported the concept of the healthy school but there remain significant barriers to the development of health promotion in schools.

Further reading

Aggleton P 1996 Health promotion and young people. HEA, London. *A concise summary of young people's health in relation to key issues, their risk-taking and protective behaviours and the effectiveness of different interventions.*

European Network of Health Promoting Schools publish a newsletter and is coordinated in England by the Health Education Authority, Trevelyan House, 30 Great Peter Street, London SW1P 2HW.

Perkins E R, Simnett I, Wright L 1999 Evidence based health promotion. Wiley, Chichester. *Chapter 8 provides a rationale for working in school settings and evidence of effective interventions in sex and relationships education and drug and alcohol education.*

Ryder J, Campbell L 1988 Balancing acts in personal, social and health education. Routledge, London. *Useful for providing an insight into curriculum organization and active learning methods.*

Scriven A, Orme J 1996 Health promotion: professional perspectives. Macmillan, Basingstoke. *Section 4 looks at the potential for health promotion in education settings including schools, youth clubs, further education and the school health service.*

Tones K, Tilford S 1994 Health education: effectiveness, efficiency and equity. Chapman & Hall, London. *Chapter 4 provides an overview of school health education and evidence of its effectiveness.*

References

Aggleton P 1996 Health promotion and young people. HEA, London

Dorn N, Murji K 1992 Drug prevention: a review of the English language literature, Institute for the Study of Drug Dependence. Research Monograph 5. ISDD, London

European Network of Health Promoting Schools 1997 The health promotion school – an investment in education, health and democracy: conference case study book, Thessaloniki-Halkidiki 1–5 May. WHO, Copenhagen

Gray G, Hill F 1992 Health action pack: health education for 16–19. HEA/National Extension College, London

Health Education Authority 1989 Health for life 1 and 2. HEA/Nelson, London

Health Education Authority 1991a Health and self. HEA/Forbes, London

Health Education Authority 1991b Tomorrow's young adults. HEA, London

Health Education Authority 1997 Health promotion with young people for the prevention of substance misuse. HEA, London

Hopson B, Scally M 1980, 1982, 1985, 1987 Life skills teaching programmes 1, 2, 3, 4. Lifeskills Associates, Leeds

Jamison J 1993 Health Education in schools: a survey of policy and implementation. Health Education Journal 52:2.

King A, Wold B, Tudor-Smith C, Harel Y 1996 The health of youth: a cross national survey. WHO, Copenhagen

Lewis D 1993 Oh for those halcyon days: a review of school health education over 50 years. Health Education Journal 52(3): 161–171

Moon A, Mullee M, Thompson R, Speller V, Roderick P 1998 Do healthy school award schemes make a difference? Working together for better health: International Conference 23–25 September, Cardiff

National Foundation for Educational Research 1997. Parents' views of health education: summary of key findings from the ENHPS survey of parents. NFER, London

Peersman G, Oakley A, Oliver S, Thomas J 1996 Review of effectiveness of sexual health promotion interventions for young people. London Social Science Research Unit, Institute of Education, London University, London

Radat K, Speed M 1994 Sex education, sexual behaviour and attitudes of young people. In: Glanz A, McVey D, Glass R (eds) Talking about it: young people, sexual behaviour and HIV. HEA, London

Reid D, McNeill A, Glynn T 1995 Reducing the prevalence of smoking in youth: an international review. Tobacco Control 4: 266–277

Schools Council/HEC Project 1982 Health education 13–18. Forbes, London

Scriven A 1996 The impact of recent government policy on the provision of health education in schools. In: Scriven A, Orme J (eds) Health promotion: professional perspectives. Macmillan, Basingstoke

Wellings K, Wadsworth J, Johnson A M, Field J, Whitaker L, Field B 1995 Provision of sex education and early sexual experience: the relation examined. British Medical Journal 311: 417–421

Williams T, Wetton N, Moon A 1989 A Picture of health. HEA, London

World Health Organization 1986 Ottawa charter for health promotion. WHO, Geneva

World Health Organization 1993 The European network of health promoting schools. WHO, Copenhagen

World Health Organization 1995 WHO expert committee on comprehensive school health education and promotion. WHO, Geneva

15 *Health promotion in neighbourhoods*

OVERVIEW

Neighbourhoods have been identified as important settings for health promotion in a number of policy documents (White Paper 1997, DoH 1999).

> People relate closely to their neighbourhoods, and are likely to be healthier when they live in neighbourhoods where there is a sense of pride and belonging. Evidence . . . shows how social cohesion and strong social networks benefit health.
>
> (DoH 1999, p. 52)

This chapter examines the concept of 'neighbourhood' and why it has grown in popularity in recent years. The linked concept of social capital to describe neighbourly relationships and networks is explored. The usefulness of the neighbourhood as a setting for health promotion is discussed. Neighbourhoods include different levels or structures such as the neighbourhood environment, services and people, which may all be used as a springboard for health promotion. Examples of various initiatives which focus on the neighbourhood setting are given as examples of good practice.

Defining neighbourhoods

The terms 'neighbourhood' and 'community' are frequently used. Are they the same thing?

Neighbourhoods are defined as small localities with a distinct identity forged by a community of people who know each other and the provision of essential services such as post offices, shops and health centres. Lay networks and support systems are an important element. Neighbourhoods will often be bounded by geographical features such as major roads, railways or green areas and may be urban or rural. The key factor is that residents define their local neighbourhood themselves and feel they have an investment in its future, the services provided and its appearance. In the modern world where transactions are increasingly fragmented and anonymous, and where the overarching symbols of community, such as religion and nationhood, are less cohesive and meaningful, the role of the neighbourhood in promoting identity and self-esteem is more important. Neighbourhoods provide the immediate environment where people live, work and play, and for many more vulnerable groups, such as older people and those on low income, most of their lives are lived in one neighbourhood.

- **How would you define your neighbourhood?**
- **In what ways does your neighbourhood support health?**
- **In what ways does it compromise health?**

Why neighbourhoods are a key setting for health promotion

The Government's White Paper on public health for England has identified neighbourhoods as an important setting for health promotion. This reflects two popular views:

The White Paper on health promotion and public health 'Saving lives: our Healthier Nation' suggests that neighbourhoods are a particularly important setting for health'.

Why might this be?

- that deep-seated health problems can only be tackled by people themselves and therefore there is a need to harness local energies and commitment
- that neighbourhoods can in themselves promote health.

Neighbourhoods are a key setting for health promotion because they provide the infrastructure for health. Neighbourhoods are where the physical and social environments interact with service provision to provide an overall environment which has enormous potential to support people's health. Neighbourhoods include:

- *The physical environment*, e.g. the degree of air and noise pollution, quality of housing, amount of traffic and the availability of green space.
- *The social environment* refers to the amount of social interaction between residents, the number of community or voluntary groups or organizations operating in the area and the extent of mutual self-help activities. The concept of social capital, which refers to relationships of trust and regard between people, and organizations they have contact with, is relevant to both the social environment and services provided.
- *Services* provided in neighbourhoods include places such as shops, post offices, health services, places of worship, sports facilities, community halls, transport systems or outreach workers from statutory agencies, e.g. housing and welfare officers' weekly sessions held in the community hall.

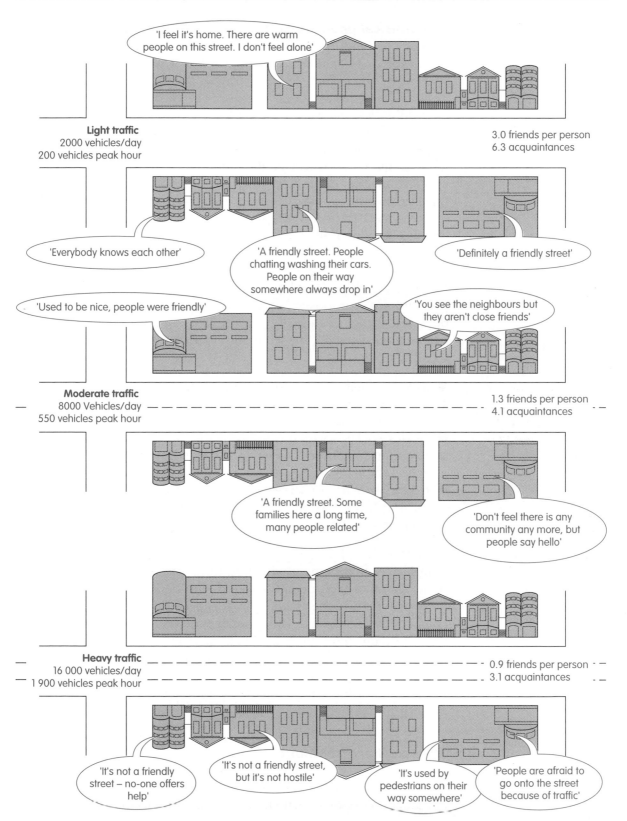

Figure 15.1 *The impact of traffic level on human interactions. From Appleyard & Lintell 1972.*

The physical environment

Changes in the environment, whilst they may seem minor in themselves, can have a major impact on local quality of life. Figure 15.1 shows the dramatic effect on neighbourhood life of changes in local transport networks.

Tackling issues such as dependency on private cars can seem a daunting proposition. UK car users, although a smaller percentage of the population than in other European countries, use their cars more frequently. However, the importance of weaning ourselves away from over-dependency on cars has been recognized in a number of policies and documents, ranging from the White Paper on Integrated Transport (Department of the Environment, Transport and the Regions 1998) to the 'Walking the Way to Health' campaign launched recently by the British Heart Foundation and the Countryside Commission. This campaign, which complements other initiatives, such as Healthy Living Centres and health improvement programmes, proposes setting up local schemes and locally designed walks. In addition to the undisputed benefits to health from regular walking, the campaign identifies the following benefits to communities:

- improves self-image and social relationships
- promotes neighbourliness and social interaction – helping to turn places into communities
- tackles social isolation
- discourages antisocial behaviour through more people being out and about
- is a reason to conserve wildlife and enhance the character of local places (British Heart Foundation and Countryside Commission 1998).

Graffiti, litter, boarded-up premises and dog mess are all signs of a neglected environment which, in turn, affects people's perception of the safety of their neighbourhood, and hence their willingness to be active participants within it. These issues often rank high on communities' agendas. The government has tackled these issues with funding through City Challenge and later through single regeneration budget monies which are available to revitalize degraded areas and build up community infrastructures. The Department of the Environment also produced a handbook of good practice in regeneration and health (DoE 1996).

The social environment

The quality of life in a community is a powerful determinant of health. By studying several healthy communities, Wilkinson (1996) has identified several factors which contribute to that quality of life:

> The small town of Roseto, Pennsylvania, USA (1600 people) is cited as an example of a community with markedly lower death rates from heart attacks than neighbouring areas. The population of Roseto is made up of Italian-Americans descended from migrants from the Italian town of Roseto in Southern Italy. It differed from other towns because it was 'remarkably close knit . . . with a sense of common purpose . . . [with] a camaraderie which precluded ostentation [and] . . . a concern for neighbours ensuring no one was ever abandoned . . . the family as the hub and bulwark of life provided a security and insurance against any catastrophe'. Roseto's considerable health advantage only seems explicable in relation to these social characteristics. As the younger people moved away, community and family ties broke down and people became more concerned with material values and conspicuous consumption.
>
> Source: Bruhn & Wolf 1979, cited in Wilkinson (1996, p. 116)

- social cohesion
- the existence of social networks
- active involvement in the community.

Social capital

Social capital refers to social cohesion and the cumulative experience of relationships, with both those known to us and those who are strangers, that are characterized by mutual trust, acceptance, approval and respect. People are social beings and the quality of social interaction is vital to both personal and communal well-being. Social capital provides the foundation for collective action in the public sphere for the public good.

> The story goes that if we basically trust each other, our relationships work better, whether with family, friends, neighbours, workmates . . . Any society which has too many distrustful members, who lack positive experiences and expectations, will have serious problems with compliance, crime, self-destruction, violence, poor health and other social indicators.
>
> (Cox 1997, p. 2)

Community networks may be built around activities associated with school, leisure or living in a particular locality. These networks may lead to the establishment of organizations. However, there is evidence that building social capital is only possible above a certain threshold of income. Work in Africa has shown that there may be levels of hardship experienced within homes below which it is impossible for family members to engage in social and civic activities (Moser 1996). If people are preoccupied with survival in its crudest meaning (i.e. ensuring they are fed, warm, sheltered and safe) they will be unable to focus beyond on broader communal issues. Social capital is also not always benign. Drug dealing and criminality on many housing estates rely on strong, closely integrated networks.

If social capital and trust are at the positive end of a neighbourhood quality of life spectrum, crime and fear of crime are at the opposite negative end.

Both crime and the fear of crime are health hazards and are associated with negative effects including depression and mental ill-health. It has been suggested that negative effects are both direct, e.g. stress and depression, and indirect, e.g. mental health linked to social isolation and feelings of vulnerability.

Crime and the fear of crime have a detrimental effect on people's health and are associated with poor mental health, decreased mobility and isolation and social exclusion. There is increasing evidence to suggest that social factors, in particular poverty, income inequality and lack of social cohesion, are important underlying causes of crime. Crime and the fear of crime are experienced disproportionately by certain disadvantaged groups (women, black and ethnic minority communities and gay people) and are often cited as the issues communities would most like to tackle. If you wished to promote community safety in a neighbourhood, what measures could you suggest?

Effective measures might include:

- Pre-school education, which has been shown to have a long-term effect on reducing criminal behaviour in adulthood
- Community policing which involves local communities and may itself promote social cohesion.
- Modifying the physical environment and increased surveillance, e.g. street lighting, concierge schemes.

Source: Acheson (1998), McCabe & Raine (1997)

Acts of thoughtlessness and disregard, such as excessive noise or petty disputes, whilst less severe than violence or the threat of violence, can have a large impact on quality of life. Loss of order and predictability is an important source of stress and worry.

The Jakarta Declaration (WHO 1997) emphasized the importance of community capacity building – in other words, increasing resources and developing personal skills to foster community activities.

Services

An adequate service infrastructure is essential to the health and life of a neighbourhood. If essential services, such as shops and post

Identify some examples of capacity building in a local community with which you are familiar.

Examples that you might have included are:

■ Managing services, e.g. tenants acting as housing managers
■ Creating jobs, e.g. business start-up schemes
■ Protecting the environment, e.g. local Agenda 21 schemes
■ Health and safety, e.g. community safety audits
■ Responding to poverty, e.g. credit unions.

In all these examples the neighbourhood has become the focus for the creation of networks and for linking health and regeneration.

offices, are not available locally, people are forced to travel outside the area, leading to a loss of social contacts as well as incurring additional costs (time and travel). This has been recognized by many communities fighting to retain local schools or shops and by the Social Exclusion Unit (1998) in its new deal for communities. However, many planning decisions appear not to recognize this fact. In particular, the increase in out-of-town supermarkets has had a severe impact on both small local shopping outlets and traffic rates.

There is great potential in building health into community activities, such as adult education, leisure activities and cultural activities. The following example shows how community arts can work together with health workers to promote neighbourhood health.

Community arts

The Bromley-by-Bow Centre, with funding from the King's Fund, has launched six 'Talking Art' projects:

■ Birthday cards, designed by community groups, to be sent to all children in the area including ideas such as invitations to 'vaccination parties' to improve immunization
■ Weekly groups run by a professional storyteller, interpreter and health promotion worker
■ Workshops for primary care workers to explore how art can be used to communicate health information
■ Singing courses offered to people with asthma to alleviate symptoms and reduce reliance on drugs
■ Dancing and movement courses offered to people with weight problems and people suffering from depression
■ A programme for people with eating disorders which looks at issues, such as low self-esteem, through presentation of self-images and discussion.

It could be argued that any neighbourhood development work has the potential to promote health by increasing social contacts and trust, or social capital. Additional spin-offs in terms of direct support for healthy lifestyles are common, as the following example shows.

 Community gardens

A scheme to tackle neglected gardens and increase neighbourliness works by linking volunteer gardeners with residents, often older people, who can no longer keep up their gardens to the standard they would wish. The linking is done via a community development worker based at the local community centre. Gardens may become sources of home-grown produce, which is shared between the volunteer and the resident. The scheme achieves several goals:

- Increased social contact
- Increased opportunities for exercise
- Increased availability of fresh fruit and vegetables
- Improved appearance of gardens.

Healthy Living Centres

A government White Paper 'The People's Lottery' (1997) announced a New Opportunities lottery fund which will provide £300 million to set up a network of Healthy Living Centres (HLC) nationwide. The intention is to fund new and additional services which will enable partnerships of communities and agencies to tackle inequalities in health. Funding will enable Healthy Living Centres to be accessible to the most disadvantaged 20% of the population. No central blueprint is being provided because the intention is to stimulate innovative and imaginative ways of responding to local needs.

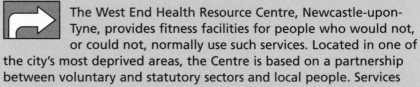 The West End Health Resource Centre, Newcastle-upon-Tyne, provides fitness facilities for people who would not, or could not, normally use such services. Located in one of the city's most deprived areas, the Centre is based on a partnership between voluntary and statutory sectors and local people. Services provided include:

- Structured health and fitness programmes for people with chronic health conditions including coronary rehabilitation courses
- Community health and preventive services, e.g. physiotherapy and speech therapy services
- Information on health and social services, health rights and welfare benefits
- Projects linking arts and health
- A meeting place and focus for links between people and statutory agencies.

Healthy Living Centres do not need to focus on a physical building, but may refer to a programme of activities. Organizations in the voluntary, private and public sectors are invited to bid for the fund money. The Healthy Living Centre projects are intended to:

- improve quality of life
- address the needs of the most disadvantaged
- encourage community participation
- complement relevant local and national strategies, e.g. health action zones.

Although there is no blueprint for a Healthy Living Centre, prototypes have been cited including the West End Health Resource Centre set up in Newcastle-upon-Tyne in 1996.

 Brockenhurst, a Healthy Village

Brockenhurst is a village (population 6500) in the New Forest, Hampshire. 25% of the population is aged over 65. Major health needs include loneliness, frailty, bereavement and transport problems. Among younger people, needs include a lack of jobs, isolation of lone parents, anxiety, depression and boredom and drug use. Derek Browne, a local GP, together with other residents, raised enough money to purchase the village hall in the 1980s, in an attempt to promote health through increased social networks. Partners for health include voluntary groups, charities, the local health promotion unit, the local health authority and regional health authority, parish, district and county councils, and the private sector. Dr Browne uses his contact with local people to 'prescribe' various activities including social clubs, joining the gym, badminton, yoga, dancing, music, cricket and golf. The gym at the local hotel takes referred patients who are prescribed exercise. Most of those involved in such activities are female, 70% are retired, 30% live alone and 62% are aged over 70.

In the project's first 2-year pilot scheme several hundred people were involved using community resources and facilities. Outcomes included:

- a local stroke club
- extension of the dial-a-ride scheme
- a new bathers' group
- new youth advisory services
- a local database on resources
- a new health and care forum and an identified resources coordinator.

Dr Browne comments that 'the strength of the project is that it was not imposed on the village but grew out of it'. There is a 70% success rate from the point of view of users, referrers and the providers involved. This project has been effective in building networks and establishing local cohesion as well as providing opportunities for more active lifestyles.

The concept of Healthy Living Centres is easier to translate to urban areas with transport and communication links. The Healthy Village approach has been seen as helpful to address the particular health needs of rural populations which have a high proportion of older people. Browne (1995) and Butler (1998) describe a process of networking in which a village coordinator uses existing community resources (e.g. churches, hotels, pubs, schools) to support the primary care team in promoting health.

Although the Healthy Village approach may help to provide support and services for certain groups, it is unlikely to tackle the economic aspects of deprivation that the Rural Development Commission (1998) has identified:

Is community-based healthy urban living a possibility in the 21st century?

- lack of services and transport
- low and seasonal income levels
- high cost of living, including housing costs
- limited job opportunities, especially for women.

Evaluating neighbourhood work

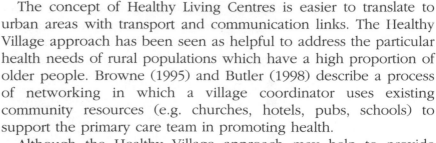

Possible indicators of social capital

Civic involvement, e.g.
- Awareness of local organizations
- Following current affairs
- Discussing current affairs with others

Participation, e.g.
- Involvement in local politics
- Fund-raising for organizations
- Committee work for organizations

Social trust, e.g.
- Gifts of time to community, e.g. volunteering work, involvement in local campaigns

Sharing space, e.g.
- Use of public space, e.g. parks
- Involvement in local cultural events
- Feel safe walking at night

Workplace related, e.g.
- Workplace perceived as fair
- Workplace perceived as secure and safe
- Workplace community

Personal, e.g.
- Social networks with family and friends
- Society perceived as fair
- Adoption of healthy behaviours

Source: Cox (1997)

Evaluation of neighbourhood work is difficult, involving long-term processes to promote social cohesion and participation. The funding of innovative projects should not be tied to inappropriate evaluation targets. Traditional evaluation of health interventions through the use of mortality and morbidity targets needs to be replaced with more appropriate short and medium measures of the impact of such interventions through, for example, the take-up and utilization of services and resources by the target population (SHEPS 1998). There is currently a lot of development work being carried out on how to measure social capital.

Conclusion

The neighbourhood provides a valuable setting for accessing many vulnerable groups including older people and people on low income. Neighbourhoods are real-life settings with the potential for priorities to be defined by residents rather than professionals. Addressing health on a neighbourhood basis is attractive because it means addressing core determinants of health, such as the social fabric and quality of people's lives. It is important that in the new focus on neighbourhood settings, the opportunity to address people's self-defined needs is taken. It would be easy to use neighbourhoods merely as a means of professional outreach work, but this would be to neglect one of the great strengths of this setting.

Many members of the primary care team (especially health visitors and GPs) regard themselves as working with neighbourhood communities. How might their role change if they were to focus on community capacity building and building social capital?

Whilst there are many advantages to working within a neighbourhood setting, it is not a universal panacea. Many factors which affect people's lives are determined at national level, e.g. level of benefit entitlement or availability of employment. However, the neighbourhood setting does offer opportunities for creative and imaginative ways of working which support the core principles of health promotion – participation, equity, empowerment and collaboration.

Questions for further discussion

- ■ What health promotion resources can neighbourhoods offer?
- ■ What are the advantages and limitations of using a neighbourhood setting for health promotion?

Summary

This chapter has identified neighbourhoods as a key setting for health promotion and discussed reasons for its popularity. Government initiatives focusing on neighbourhoods, such as Healthy Living Centres, have been considered. Examples of innovative practice centred on neighbourhood work have been given and the problems of evaluating such work discussed.

Further reading

Gowman N 1999 Healthy neighbourhoods. King's Fund, London.
Jones L, Sidell M 1997 The challenge of promoting health: exploration and action. Macmillan/Open University Press, Hampshire. *Part 1 on promoting health at the local level: the collective approach includes chapters looking at community action, working in partnerships, working with primary health care teams and evaluating local action.*
Wilkinson R G 1996 Unhealthy societies: the afflictions of inequality. Routledge, London. *This book looks at the evidence for social cohesion and the promotion of social equity as determinants of health.*

References

Acheson D 1988 Independent inquiry into inequalities in health: a report. Stationery Office, London

Appleyard D, Lintell M 1972 The environmental quality of city streets: the residents' viewpoint. Journal of the American Institute of Planners 38: 84–101

British Heart Foundation and Countryside Commission 1998 Walking the way to health. Newsletter, 1 December 1998

Browne D 1995 Healthy villages. In: Occasional Paper 71: Rural general practice in the United Kingdom. Royal College of General Practitioners, Exeter

Butler P 1998 The village people. Healthlines, October 1998. HEA, London

Cox E 1997 Building social capital. Health Promotion Matters 4: 1–4

Department of Culture, Media and Sport 1997 The people's lottery. Command Paper, Stationery Office, London

Department of Health (DoH) 1999 Saving lives: our healthier nation White Paper. Stationery Office, London

Department of the Environment 1996 Regeneration and health: good practice note. DoE, London

Department of the Environment, Transport and the Regions 1998 A new deal for transport: better for everyone. Stationery Office, London

McCabe A, Raine J 1997 Framing the debate: the impact of crime on public health. Public Health Alliance, Birmingham

Moser C 1996 Confronting crisis. Comparative study of household responses to poverty and vulnerability in four poor urban communities. Environmentally sustainable investment studies, monograms series 3. World Bank, Washington

Rural Development Commission 1998 Rural disadvantage – understanding the process. Rural Development Commission Rural Research Report No. 35. Rural Development Commission, Salisbury

Social Exclusion Unit 1998 Bringing Britain together: a national strategy for neighbourhood renewal. Stationery Office, London

Society of Health Education and Promotion Specialists (SHEPS) 1998 Healthy Living Centres: a response. SHEPS, Glasgow

Wilkinson R G 1996 Unhealthy societies: the afflictions of inequality. Routledge, London

World Health Organization 1997 New players for a new era: leading health promotion into the 21st century. 4th International Conference on Health Promotion, Jakarta, Indonesia 21–25 July 1997. Conference Report World Health Organization, Geneva/Ministry of Health, Indonesia

16 *Health promotion in primary health care and hospitals*

OVERVIEW

Primary health care and hospitals provide an important setting for health promotion and their role in promoting health is becoming more recognized. Whilst still focusing predominantly on treatment, health care settings provide an opportunity for building health gain into existing services. As a setting, health services provide unique advantages of access, trust and credibility.

The Government is committed to shifting the NHS towards a primary care-led service where primary care groups (PCGs) led by GPs commission services on behalf of their local populations (DoH 1997). Commissioning for health gain needs to be integrated into overall packages which include care and treatment services.

The potential of hospital settings to promote positive health has also been recognized, and in 1990 the World Health Organization Regional Office for Europe launched the Health Promoting Hospitals initiative. In this chapter, the potential of both the primary care and hospital setting to promote health is examined and examples of good practice are given to illustrate what can be achieved.

Introduction

The original goals of the NHS were to provide a comprehensive health service, to improve physical and mental health and to prevent, diagnose and treat illness. This has much in common with the goals of health promotion, although historically the cure and treatment of illness has taken precedence over the prevention of ill health, or the promotion of positive health. The health service is an important setting for health promotion because it offers a range of health professionals the opportunity to integrate health promotion into their practice, and thus to fulfil the early promise of a comprehensive and health-promoting health service.

309

In what ways does the health service provide:

- **Opportunity?**
- **Access?**
- **Credibility?**
- **Competence?**

There are other unique characteristics of the health service setting. Use of health services is universal, so that everyone at some point in their lives comes into contact with health service providers, and for many more vulnerable groups, such as people with long-standing limiting illness, contact is long term and frequent. Health practitioners enjoy high levels of trust and credibility amongst the general population and thus have the ability to affect people's knowledge, attitudes and beliefs. The NHS is the country's largest single employer and therefore workplace initiatives may affect a significant percentage of the workforce and their families. All these factors provide good reasons for prioritizing the health services as a setting for health promotion.

Why is primary health care a key setting for health promotion?

Primary health care (PHC) refers to the first tier of health provision, provided in local community settings by generalists. PHC 'is the first level of contact of individuals, the family and community with the national health system bringing health care as close as possible to where people live and work and constitutes the first element of a continuing health care process' (MacDonald 1993).

Primary health care is a key setting because:

Compare and contrast the primary health care and hospital settings for health promotion.

- most people have contact with primary health care practitioners
- 97% of the population is registered with a GP and over 70% consult their GP at least once a year
- primary service health promoters enjoy high status and credibility amongst the general public (Office of Health Economics 1994).

Primary health care has several advantages when compared to the more specialized services provided in the hospital sector. These are:

- Better access because services are provided in the community.
- Improved communications because service users and providers meet on more equal terms. Primary health care providers are generalists. They see people in their own homes as well as in health centres, clinics or surgeries. They see the same people over a number of years and have an understanding of how their health relates to the rest of their lives. These factors help to break

down the barriers between professional and client, and so improve communication.

■ Adequate provision of primary health care services will often mean that more specialized hospital-based services are unnecessary. For example, proper management and monitoring of chronic conditions such as diabetes and asthma should help prevent the development of crises which require hospitalization.

■ Primary health care and prevention is cheaper than hospital care.

■ As stays in hospital become shorter, the role of the primary health team becomes more important.

Primary health care has been highlighted as a key setting in both international and national health promotion policies. The WHO 'Health for All 2000' programme called for a reorientation of health care services away from the tertiary hospital sector and towards the primary sector: 'The focus of the health care system should be on *primary health care* – meeting the basic health needs of each community through services provided as close as possible to where people live and work, readily accessible and acceptable to all, and based on full community participation' (WHO 1985, p. 5, original emphasis).

The 1997 White Paper on the NHS (DoH 1997) introduced the concept of integrated care led by primary care groups (PCGs). PCGs are groups of GPs and community nurses who, working with local authorities, social services and lay representatives, take responsibility for commissioning, and possibly providing, services for their local population. There are four options or levels of PCG:

1. Minimum level, supports health authority (HA) in commissioning care, acts as an advisor
2. Takes devolved responsibility for managing the budget, acting as part of the HA
3. A freestanding body accountable to the HA for commissioning care
4. Includes (3) above, plus added responsibility for providing community services.

Recent policy changes emphasize the need for primary health care to be part of wider service provision. Local 3-year Health Improvement Programmes (HImPs) will be drawn up after consultation between PCGs, health authorities, NHS trusts and local authorities. HImPs offer the possibility of responding to specific local needs as well as collaborative working for health. The Care in the Community Act 1990 also impacts upon primary health services. This legislation requires social services departments and health authorities to liaise together to provide individualized care programmes for people in need.

Although PHC enjoys many advantages as a setting to promote health, there are barriers to a philosophy of health promotion permeating the service. The dominant medical model of health means that primary health care is still oriented to treatment rather than to prevention or health promotion. The policy and organizational context make sharing between members of the primary health care team difficult. Practical problems of time, space and large caseloads also make it difficult to prioritize health promotion. Figure 16.1 illustrates how the core health promotion principles of participation, collaboration and equity (WHO 1986) can be integrated into the primary care setting and some of the factors which might make this difficult.

Figure 16.1 *Health promotion in primary care. From Taylor et al 1998.*

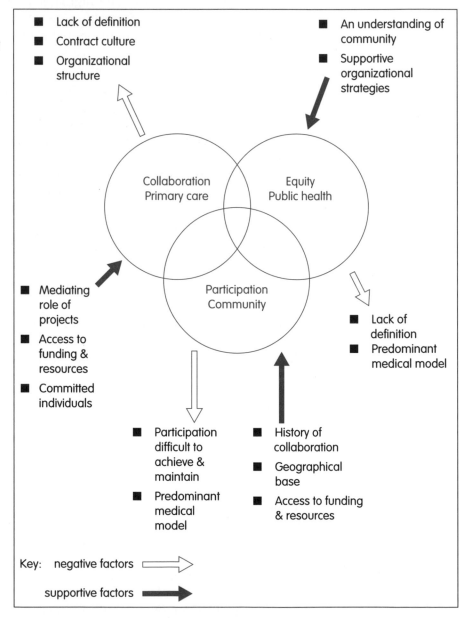

How can the primary health care setting become more health promoting?

Participation, collaboration and equity are core health promotion principles.

■ How can community participation be increased?
■ How can the contribution of each member of the primary health care team be enhanced and members encouraged to work together?
■ How can primary health care work towards addressing inequalities in the health status of the local community?

Responsibility for health promotion in primary health care

PHC professionals include independent contractors providing NHS care such as general practitioners (GPs) and dentists, as well as staff employed by them such as practice nurses. Other PHC staff, such as health visitors, district nurses and community psychiatric nurses, are employees of health trusts, and social workers are employed by local authorities. Other health practitioners such as physiotherapists and chiropodists may be employed by health trusts or on a sessional basis by GPs. Together, these professionals make up PHC teams who provide a range of health care services for everybody in the community (see Fig. 16.2). An outline of the main aspects of their health-promoting role is given in Chapter 8.

Primary health care provides a setting where health promotion at primary, secondary and tertiary levels takes place. An example of

Figure 16.2 *Primary health care services.*

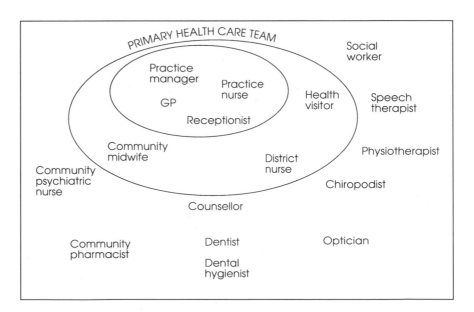

primary prevention, or preventing the occurrence of ill health, is the provision of child immunization services. Secondary prevention is preventing ill health becoming chronic and restoring people to their previous level of health. An example of secondary prevention is advising someone with bronchitis to give up smoking. Tertiary prevention, or helping people with chronic or irreversible ill health to cope with their condition and enjoy their maximum potential for health, is illustrated by the example of asthma clinics which teach people to monitor and manage their condition.

Much of the health promotion practised in PHC settings is carried out by nurses. Practice nurses, health visitors, midwives, district nurses and community psychiatric nurses have much scope for health promotion in their daily contact with the practice population. Much of this is opportunistic, and one survey found that three-fifths of practice nurses felt that they needed more training in how to plan and organize health promotion (Calnan & Williams 1992). Nurses are also responsible for collecting information on patients' health status and for health surveillance. Research has demonstrated the potential for community nurses to work in group and community settings to empower clients (Taylor et al 1998). However, the demands of their statutory duties and caseload size mean these types of health promotion activities tend to take a low priority.

A difficult but important goal of health promotion is empowerment. Many health workers use the term to describe patient education or any communication with a patient. Yet empowerment often necessitates organizational and environmental change (Kendall 1998). Figure 16.3 shows how empowerment and health gain can be built into nurse–client contacts.

- **What factors might make it difficult for primary care nurses to act in ways which empower their clients?**
- **How could primary care nurses enhance the empowering aspects of client contacts?**

Much of the health promotion that takes place in PHC settings is opportunistic. A client has a consultation or is referred to a member of the PHC team and is identified as 'at risk'. The practitioner may offer advice, information or a further referral. In some cases, the practitioner may start a series of brief interventions using motivational interviewing to identify the client's readiness to change (see Ch. 11).

Figure 16.3 *Health-promoting nurse–client contacts. Adapted from HEA 1998.*

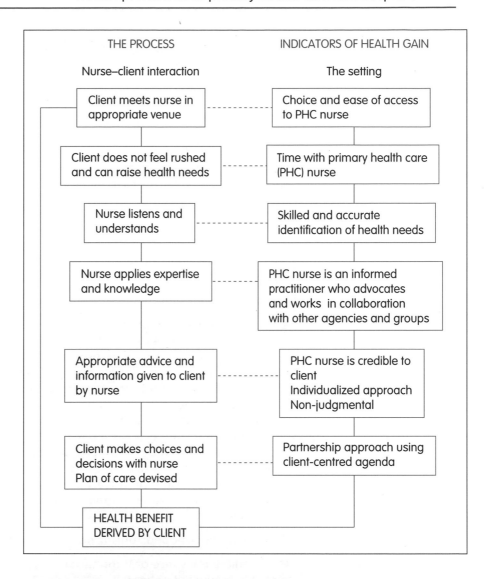

THE PROCESS

Nurse–client interaction

INDICATORS OF HEALTH GAIN

The setting

Client meets nurse in appropriate venue — Choice and ease of access to PHC nurse

Client does not feel rushed and can raise health needs — Time with primary health care (PHC) nurse

Nurse listens and understands — Skilled and accurate identification of health needs

Nurse applies expertise and knowledge — PHC nurse is an informed practitioner who advocates and works in collaboration with other agencies and groups

Appropriate advice and information given to client by nurse — PHC nurse is credible to client / Individualized approach / Non-judgmental

Client makes choices and decisions with nurse / Plan of care devised — Partnership approach using client-centred agenda

HEALTH BENEFIT DERIVED BY CLIENT

'Helping People Change' is a health promotion training and resources programme for primary health care professionals which was provided by the PHC Unit of the Health Education Authority. The aim of the project is to give PHC professionals the skills, knowledge and attitudes to:

■ Understand the concept of risk management
■ Understand the process of change and how to intervene effectively
■ Apply these principles to make brief health promotion interventions.

The following example illustrates the advantages of opportunistic health promotion, but there are also disadvantages.

A review of research investigating smoking cessation interventions concluded that:

'advice from GPs is more effective than no advice. On average, 5% of smokers will stop smoking, and stay abstinent for at least a year, following brief advice from a GP during one consultation ... The effectiveness can be increased by offering smokers literature on smoking, negotiating a date to stop smoking and making a contract with the smoker to stop on this date, and offering follow-up appointments to deal with problems in stopping smoking' (Sanders 1992, p. 11).

 How many advantages and disadvantages of opportunistic health promotion can you identify?

You may have included some of the following:

■ Opportunistic health promotion relies on the decisions of individual practitioners. This leads to patchy and uneven implementation, on a basis of chance rather than proven need.
■ Health promotion remains a marginalized luxury, to be tacked on at the end of a consultation if there is time. Research has shown that lack of time is an important factor limiting the amount of health promotion undertaken by both GPs and nurses (Littlewood & Parker 1992, Tapper-Jones et al 1990).
■ Doubts as to the value of opportunistic health promotion have been expressed. Almost half the community nurses in one study thought that raising the subject of smoking with patients consulting for unrelated problems made them annoyed (Littlewood & Parker 1992).

The advantages of opportunistic health promotion include:

■ Immediate relevance of information
■ Highly motivated patients
■ The ability to adapt and modify the input to suit individual needs.

The emphasis of recent policy has been on developing more planned and proactive health promotion activities. The introduction of HImPs stresses the need to address local priorities which have been defined after consultation with local agencies and communities as well as health professionals. There is evidence that planned health promotion interventions are effective, but there is disagreement as to whether or not this evidence justifies a move towards prioritizing such activities in primary health care settings (Family Heart Study Group 1994, OXCHECK 1995).

Primary health care is a social system with its own structure and culture which determines the way in which it tackles health and ill

Occupational health and primary care

The Camden Occupational Health Project (COHP) aims to raise the profile of occupational health issues in primary care by supporting patients and practice staff. The work of the COHP includes interviewing patients (referred by themselves, GPs or invited by the project) in GP surgeries to raise awareness and provide practical help, integrating information about occupational health issues into patients' records and advising and advocating on behalf of workers with occupational health problems. The COHP is funded by the local health authority.

Source: Jones & Sidell (1997)

health. Its partnerships tend to be client rather than population focused, and though based *in* communities, few practices work *with* communities. Primary health care is driven by a medical model of health rather than a social model, and evaluation is still often seen in terms of reduced morbidity and mortality, rather than in terms of health gain processes and outcomes. The priority in primary care is treatment, which means that often patient compliance is valued above patient autonomy and participation. Health promotion tends to be 'bolted on' to core tasks and is often delegated to practice nurses instead of being integral to everyone's work. Key health promotion activities, such as addressing health inequalities, are replaced by the need to respond to client demands, which may paradoxically have the effect of reinforcing inequalities by providing more services for more educated and articulate patients.

'There is a constant tension for practitioners between responding to demands for the treatment of symptoms and ill health on the one hand, and pressures to be proactive in preventing ill health or promoting health on the other' (Naidoo & Wills 1998, p. 143).

If general practice and primary health care are to be health promoting, *health* needs to be built in. Prevention in the form of immunization and screening has long been part of primary health care, but the social factors affecting health, such as housing, safety and transport, whilst perhaps acknowledged, are rarely addressed.

Why hospitals are a key setting for health promotion

In what ways could health be promoted in the hospital setting?

The hospital setting provides many opportunities for health promotion. There is a large workforce who have close contact with patients at a time of heightened awareness about health and illness, when they may be motivated to make major lifestyle changes. Research suggests that patient education is effective in the short term, through, for example, improving recovery rates and reducing anxiety (Latter 1996).

But a health-promoting hospital is not just a place where people are prompted to change the behaviour which may have brought them there. The health-promoting hospital is one in which health promotion is integral to the ethos of the institution and the way in which it is managed. Hospitals employ a large and varied workforce, whose health may be improved through the adoption of healthy workplace policies, whether this concerns healthy food in the canteen or holiday play schemes. Hospitals often have close links to their local communities and can use their role as exemplar to give the lead to other organizations. Outreach into the community is an essential part of patient care. Diabetic and coronary care involves partnerships with patients, their families, primary health care staff and voluntary groups.

The Health Promoting Hospitals (HPH) network, launched by the WHO European Regional Office in 1990, now operates in 47 countries on all continents. This initiative seeks to promote good practice by developing concepts and strategies, developing and disseminating model projects and networking via conferences and twice-yearly newsletters. The Health Promoting Hospital focuses on the health of staff, patients and its local community.

Hospitals accepted into the HPH network have to meet certain conditions:

- management agreement to the Ottawa Charter and the 1991 Budapest Declaration, which formally established the principles of the HPH Project (see Fig. 16.4)
- staff support for organizational change
- links with an independent academic or research institution for monitoring and evaluation purposes
- development of at least five sub-projects or 'intervention studies' to run for 5 years, which can be new initiatives or an extension of existing work
- links with other hospitals and similar institutions (networking) and with agencies outside the health service (health alliances).

To bring about change in a large and complex organization such as a hospital may require adapting management structures and facilitating greater participation by staff. Health-promoting hospitals may set up different projects but generally have the same overall aims:

- to make the hospital a healthier working and living environment for its large workforce and for patients
- to expand recuperation and rehabilitation programmes
- to provide information and advice on health issues

How might the need to reduce waiting lists and the consequent shortening of inpatient stays affect the ability of hospitals to be health promoting?

Beyond the assurance of good quality medical services and health care, a Health Promoting Hospital should:

1. Provide opportunities throughout the hospital to develop health-orientated perspectives, objectives and structures.

2. Develop a common corporate identity within the hospital which embraces the aims of the Health Promoting Hospital.

3. Raise awareness of the impact of the environment of the hospital on the health of patients, staff and community. The physical environment of hospital buildings should support, maintain and improve the healing process.

4. Encourage an active and participatory role for patients according to their specific health potentials.

5. Encourage participatory, health-gain orientated procedures throughout the hospital.

6. Create healthy working conditions for all hospital staff.

7. Strive to make the Health Promoting Hospital a model for healthy services and workplaces.

8. Maintain and promote collaboration between community based health promotion initiatives and local governments.

9. Improve communication and collaboration with existing social and health services in the community.

10. Improve the range of support given to patients and their relatives by the hospital through community based social and health services and/or volunteer groups and organisations.

11. Identify and acknowledge specific target groups (e.g. age, duration of illness etc.) within the hospital and their health needs.

12. Acknowledge differences in value sets, needs and cultural conditions for individuals and different population groups.

13. Create supportive, humane and stimulating living environments within the hospital especially for long-term and chronic patients.

14. Improve the health promoting quality and the variety of food services in hospitals for patients and personnel.

15. Enhance the provision and quality of information, communication and educational programmes and skill training for patients and relatives.

16. Enhance the provision and quality of educational programmes and skill training for staff.

17. Develop in the hospital an epidemiological database specially related to the prevention of illness and injury and communicate this information to public policy makers and to other institutions in the community.

Figure 16.4 *Health Promoting Hospital criteria (Budapest Declaration, WHO 1991).*

■ to shift the hospital from being solely a place of treatment to one where prevention and health gain are also valued and seen as part of its purpose.

Health Promoting Hospital Wards

The Aintree Hospital's Health Promoting Wards scheme arose from its participation in the HPH initiative. A steering group including directors, clinical staff, the HPH coordinator and health promotion specialists was set up to encourage grass roots health promotion activities at ward level. There is no dedicated budget, although funding has been provided by health trusts and the health authority. Achievements to date include an HRT (hormone replacement therapy) awareness day which led to the introduction of a weekly menopause clinic. There is an award scheme to encourage action with three stages – bronze, silver and gold.

The first stage, bronze, requires a link nurse/midwife to be identified. Staff and patients must have the opportunity to discuss healthy lifestyle needs and there has to be involvement in three specific health promotion events.

The second stage, silver, includes providing up-to-date health promotion displays, giving time to the link person to attend meetings and receive training, and proof of smoking cessation support given to staff and patients.

The third stage, gold, includes providing evidence of up-to-date health and safety staff training programmes, and patients' planned care programmes.

21 out of a possible 46 wards have signed up for the scheme.

Source: Prince (1998)

The health promotion principles identified above (equity, participation, collaboration and empowerment as well as sustainability) may also be applied to the hospital or ward setting (Coakley 1998).

Equity

Equity may refer to several different things at hospital level. Equity may mean ensuring adequate resourcing on the basis of need. Or it may mean egalitarian teamwork and non-hierarchical styles of communication between staff and between staff and patients. Equity may also mean taking special care to ensure that the needs of all groups are met. For example, many hospital routines are based on cultural norms which may not be shared by all patients. Diet and hygiene practices are often culturally specific, and being forced to adopt unfamiliar practices which may run counter to values and beliefs can be extremely distressing.

Participation

Participation refers to the ability to have a voice in how hospital

Patient Focus Project, Sheffield

The Northern General Hospital in Sheffield has adopted a Patient Focus approach to empower patients and staff. The project resulted from a patient satisfaction survey which produced some surprising results. For instance, a number of people said that they were lonely in hospital and had not been introduced to neighbouring patients or staff. A patient representative and patients' council was formed and care teams introduced to help staff build closer relationships with patients. Collaborative care protocols have been introduced, streamlining paperwork and allowing more time for individual assessment and care. Staff are involved through steering groups, open meetings and a regular newsletter. There is also more liaison with community and primary care colleagues resulting in shared-care protocols and outreach services.

services are organized. Patient panels and carer groups are examples of how community and lay representation may be encouraged. Relatives and carers can be encouraged to become involved in the care and recovery of patients. Hospital management and organization structures can seek to become more open and responsive to staff views.

Collaboration

Collaboration in a ward setting means making links within and beyond the hospital. Inside the hospital, interprofessional working which recognizes and validates the contribution of each member of the staff team is necessary. Voluntary groups whose members visit and support patients and carers, and hospital nurses' educational input into schools or voluntary organizations, are examples of collaboration with local communities.

For each of the following wards, identify other health and social care workers with whom a ward nurse might work:

- Medical geriatric
- Cardiac
- Paediatric
- Accident and emergency.

Empowerment

Empowerment means encouraging patients and relatives to share responsibility and decision-making. It also relates to staff and the removal of organizational structures which exclude some groups from decision-making at higher levels. If nurses are to empower patients, they themselves need authority and autonomy.

Identify some ways in which hospitals need to change in order to empower nurses. Some factors you may have included are:

■ Changes in timetabling and rotas which involve long hours, and shift work which impacts on family life
■ Pay scales which do not reflect the value of nurses' work
■ Hierarchical communication and administration structures which disempower student and staff nurses.

Think of a hospital with which you are familiar. Does it promote health in the ways outlined above? What do you think might be barriers to extending its health-promoting role?

Sustainability

Hospitals impact on the environment in numerous ways, through, for example, their high energy consumption, production of waste and use of transport systems. Hospitals can monitor the collection and disposal of clinical and domestic waste in order to eliminate extensive manual handling, and reduce the risk of spillage. Clinical waste can be incinerated and used to fuel extra boilers. Hospitals can negotiate with public transport companies to reduce employees' and patients' private car usage.

The health-promoting health service (HPHS)

The Health Education Board, Scotland, has launched a pilot HPHS project which seems to provide an overarching framework for health-promoting services in the acute and community sectors. Figure 16.5 shows how the framework builds on core health promotion principles and applies these to health service settings.

How could you use the framework to develop cardiac rehabilitation and aftercare?

■ Is there evidence to support a patient education programme?
■ What are the key elements of such a programme – diet, exercise, stress management, medication?
■ Are staff trained and motivated to deliver such a programme?
■ Does everyone know about the programme and understand their role in supporting it?
■ Is the ward and hospital environment supportive for both staff and patients, e.g. are there healthy food options on menus?
■ Do patients and their families participate in rehabilitation programmes and are their concerns acknowledged and addressed?
■ Are links made with local communities and services to support patients when they leave hospital?

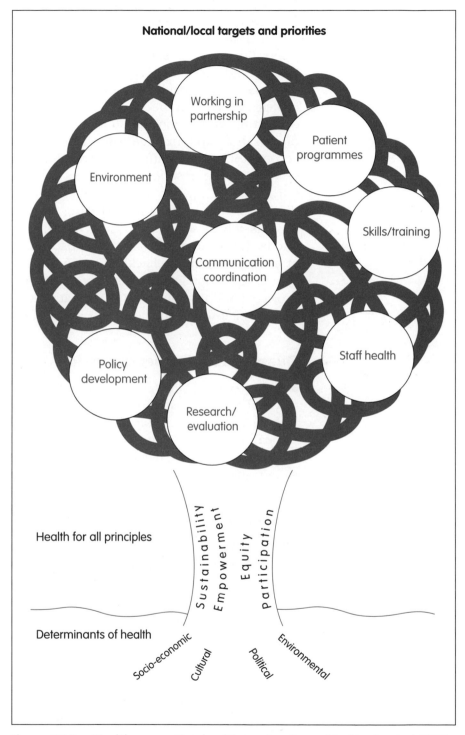

Figure 16.5 *Health-promoting health service. From MacHardy et al 1998.*

Conclusion

The health care services are an important resource for people's health. Primary care services are used by the vast majority of the population on a regular basis. The NHS is the largest employer in Britain and therefore has an enormous potential as a healthy workplace. The health services are undergoing rapid organizational change which can be experienced as stressful but also creates opportunities for innovation. Recent changes to health service organization and management have stressed the need for local accountability and partnership working. The necessity for health services to be responsive to users is now enshrined in policy (NHSME 1992). Whilst core activities remain medically focused on diagnosis, treatment, cure and care, there are many examples of projects which seek to integrate health promotion core principles into both primary health care and hospital settings. Initiatives can be at many levels, from checklists for individual practitioners to use to systematically integrate health promotion into client contacts, to pilot projects seeking to increase participation of users in various forums and hospital-wide schemes to promote health at ward level.

Questions for further discussion

■ Take one of the core health promotion principles (equity, collaboration, participation and empowerment) and consider how activities built on this principle could be integrated into a health service setting with which you are familiar.
■ What are the advantages and disadvantages of health promotion in primary health care and hospital settings?

Summary

This chapter has looked at the reasons for prioritizing primary health care and hospital settings for health promotion. Recent national and international policy developments which affect the delivery of health promotion in health service settings, and the range of professionals involved, have been identified. Ways in which health promotion principles may be applied in health service settings have been discussed and illustrated with examples.

Further reading

Jones L, Sidell M 1997 The challenge of promoting health: exploration and action. Macmillan/Open University, Hampshire. *Chapter 1 looks at the primary health care context, discusses dilemmas for health promotion in this setting and gives examples of good practice.*

Naidoo J, Wills J 1998 Practising health promotion: dilemmas and challenges. Baillière Tindall, London. *Chapter 7 looks at the policy context for health promotion in primary health care and evidence for its effectiveness. The dilemmas of practising health promotion in this setting are discussed and illustrative examples given of good practice.*

Scriven A, Orme J (eds) 1997 Health promotion: professional perspectives. Macmillan/Open University Press, Hampshire. *Section 2 on the health service looks at the potential for health promotion in different health service settings including primary health care and hospitals.*

Perkins E R, Simnett I, Wright L (eds) 1999 Evidence based health promotion. Wiley, Chichester. *Chapter 11 looks at the evidence for effective interventions in hospital and community settings.*

Health Promoting Hospitals Newsletter. WHO Regional Office for Europe, Copenhagen.

References

Calnan M, Williams S 1992 The role of general practitioners in coronary heart disease prevention in primary health care. A study commissioned by the Department of Health. HMSO, London

Coakley A L 1998 Health promotion in a hospital ward; reality or asking the impossible? Journal of the Royal Society of Health 118(4): 217–220

Department of Health (DoH) 1997 The new NHS: modern, dependable. Stationery Office, London

Family Heart Study Group 1994 Randomised control trial evaluating cardiovascular screening and intervention in general practice: principal results of British family heart study. British Medical Journal 308: 313–320

Health Education Authority 1998 Promoting health through primary health care nursing: a guide to quality indicators for purchasers. HEA, London

Jones L, Sidell M (eds) 1997 The challenge of promoting health: exploration and action. Macmillan/Open University Press, Hampshire

Kendall S (ed) 1998 Health and empowerment. Arnold, London

Latter S 1996 The potential for health promotion in hospital nursing practice. In: Scriven A, Orme J (eds) Health promotion: professional perspectives. Macmillan/Open University Press, Hampshire

Littlewood J, Parker I 1992 Community nurses' attitudes to health promotion in one regional health authority. Health Education Journal 51: 87–89

MacDonald 1993 Primary health care – medicine in its place. Earthscan, London

MacHardy L, Kerr A, Thomas D 1998 The health promoting health service: taking the concept into practice. International Conference Paper 'Working

together for better health'. Health Promotion Wales, Cardiff

Naidoo J, Wills J 1998 Practising health promotion: dilemmas and challenges. Baillière Tindall, London

National Health Service Management Executive 1992 Local voices: the views of local people in purchasing for health. Department of Health, London

Office of Health Economics 1994 Health information and the consumer. OHE Briefing No. 30. OHE, London

OXCHECK Study Group 1995 The effectiveness of health checks conducted by nurses in primary care: final results from the OXCHECK study. British Medical Journal 310: 1099–1104

Prince S 1998 Partnerships in health: health promotion on hospital wards. In: Healthlines, July/August. HEA, London

Sanders D 1992 Smoking cessation interventions: is patient education effective? Department of Public Health and Policy, London School of Hygiene and Tropical Medicine, London

Tapper-Jones L, Smail S, Pill R, Davis R 1990 Doctors' attitudes towards patient education in the primary care consultation. Health Education Journal 49: 47–50

Taylor P, Peckham S, Turton P 1998 A public health model of primary care – from concept to reality. Public Health Alliance, Birmingham

World Health Organization 1985 Targets for health for all. WHO Regional office for Europe, Copenhagen

World Health Organization 1986 Ottawa charter for health promotion. WHO, Geneva

World Health Organization 1991 The Budapest Declaration on Health Promoting Hospitals. WHO, Copenhagen

Working for Health Promotion

This section is concerned with the implementation of health promotion. How do we assess our clients' needs? Should health promotion interventions be targeted to particular groups? What strategies have been successful and what needs to be taken into account when planning a health promotion programme? Above all, how will we know if health promotion works?

17 *Assessing health needs*

OVERVIEW

The first phase in health promotion planning is an assessment of what a client or population group needs to enable them to become more healthy. This chapter explores the concept of need and how this may be perceived differently by different groups. The purpose of health needs assessment at national, regional or local level is twofold:

- to identify which improvements in health should have greatest priority
- to choose which particular groups or communities should have priority and so help in targeting interventions.

Recognition of the right to participate in defining health needs and health care was acknowledged in the 1978 WHO Alma Ata Declaration, and one of the underlying principles of 'Health For All' is community participation (WHO 1985).

The NHS reforms of the 1980s and 1990s also emphasized the participation of local people in setting priorities, signalling a philosophical shift from a paternalistic medical model to a participatory consumer-led model. This chapter considers the ways in which individual and local health needs are assessed and applied in planning for health promotion. It should be read in conjunction with Chapter 3 which outlines the principal sources of information about health status.

Key points

- Concepts of need
- Needs assessment strategies
- Relating needs to strategic planning
- Problems in assessing needs

Defining health needs

The concept of need is widely used but often not well understood. People may believe they 'need' a new coat because someone observed that their old one is worn out, or because it looks old compared to other people's coats, or simply because they would like one. A need may thus be something people want or something that is lacking in comparison to others.

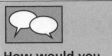

How would you distinguish between a need, a want, or a demand?

There are two different understandings of what constitutes a health need. It can be seen as:

■ a subjective, relative concept which is judged by an expert or professional and is influenced by whether the need can be met
■ an objective and universal concept which is a fundamental right.

Make a list of 10 important human needs:

■ Are some more fundamental than others?
■ Are these needs relative to a particular country or are they universal?

Economists tend to avoid the use of the term 'needs' altogether, arguing that it is overlaid with emotion and what is really meant by a health need is actually a matter of people's wants and demands, and these are limitless. Identifying health needs is therefore a question of identifying priorities. As Bradshaw notes, 'here questions are not what need is and who is in need, but who is to have first claim on limited resources and who is to judge that claim' (Bradshaw 1994, p. 48).

An alternative view is that there are universal needs. Maslow's famous hierarchy of needs (Maslow 1954) suggests that all human needs are in fact health needs (Fig. 17.1). For a person to be 'self-actualizing', physical, social and emotional needs must be met.

Figure 17.1 *Maslow's hierarchy of needs. From Oliver 1993.*

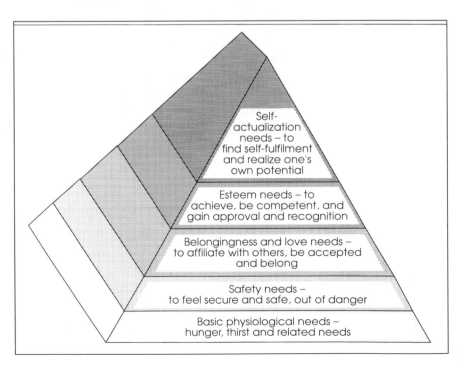

Doyal & Gough (1994) have similarly argued that the ultimate goal of human beings is to participate fully in society and to do this the basic needs for physical health and for autonomy must be met. These needs are not relative to a particular country or period of time but are fundamental rights. But they are not undisputed. How healthy do people have to be before we can say that their needs have been met? Similarly, how much autonomy do human beings need? Many older people and children are thought to be incapable of exercising autonomy (see Ch. 6 for more discussion of this).

Bradshaw (1972), in a widely used taxonomy, distinguished four types of health and social need:

■ normative needs as defined by experts or professional groups
■ felt needs as defined by clients, patients, relatives or service users
■ expressed needs when felt needs become a demand
■ comparative needs identified when people, groups or areas fall short of an established standard.

Normative needs

These are objective needs as defined by professionals. A normative need reflects a professional judgement that a person or persons deviates from a required standard. This may be against some external criteria such as occupational or legal requirements. Thus the manager of a restaurant is in need of training because he has not completed a course in food hygiene. Or it may be that a person deviates from what is defined as the range of 'clinically normal'.

 Normative need: child development

A health visitor decides that, according to a growth chart, an infant has failed to gain weight for some time and has fallen below the third centile. She deems the infant to be in need of supplementary feeding and suggests this is done by additional bottle feeding. Yet expectations of child development vary according to the place and time. This infant would not be regarded as failing to thrive in the USA or in the pre-war UK.

Normative needs are not absolute or objective 'facts' – they reflect the judgement of professionals which may be different from that of their clients. Health care workers will judge a need relative to what they are able to provide. For example, in an audit of the needs of carers, professionals identified more holidays and respite care, whereas carers saw their needs as extra money, advice and information (Percy-Smith & Sanderson 1992).

Felt needs

Felt needs are what people really **want**. They are needs identified by clients themselves which may relate to services, information, or support which can be termed service needs. Or it may be a need, experienced subjectively, of feeling unwell according to a person's personal standards of health which can be termed a health need. Armstrong (1982) describes felt needs as 'perceived needs' stemming from 'within' and not ascribed from 'without'. Moves towards bottom-up approaches in health and welfare have meant a greater acceptance of clients' views. However, needs may be limited by the perceptions of an individual. Individuals may not believe themselves to be in need simply because they do not know what is available in terms of treatment or services.

A GP practice is aware that a lot of patients are seeking consultations for their concerns about not getting pregnant. The practice decides to hold an evening talk on preconceptual care. The talk is advertised in the surgery. No one attends.

■ On what grounds did the practice decide that there was a need?
■ Why did the practice decide the need was for preconceptual care?
■ What other needs might patients have in this area?
■ What other response might the practice have to this patient need?

This is an example of a need identified by professionals. No consultation was involved.

The intervention was planned in the expectation that it would result in a saving of GP time, not as part of a programme to prioritize infertility. The intervention was poorly presented with no marketing, and no attempt to make it accessible for clients.

Expressed need

Expressed need arises from felt needs but is expressed in words or action – it has become a **demand**. Thus a client or group are expressing a need when they ask for help or information, or when they make use of a service. Sometimes people will use a service because it is all that is available, even if it does not adequately meet needs. The best example of expressed need (and unmet demand) is the waiting list. Some needs are not expressed, perhaps because of an inability or unwillingness to articulate the need. This could be due to language difficulties or a lack of knowledge. Expressed needs should not be taken as an indicator of demand because they exclude needs which are felt but not expressed. Tudor Hart's Inverse Care Law has been of vital importance in showing that just because a service or treatment is used less it does not mean that it is needed less (Tudor Hart 1971). Those who could most benefit from a service are often those least likely to use it. People may express different needs, and there is a tendency to listen to those with loud and powerful voices, such as views which come from an established group or views which appear to express a popular need.

Comparative needs

A person or group are said to be in need if their situation, when compared with that of a similar group or individual, is found 'wanting' or lacking with regard to services and resources. For example, if a person with schizophrenia in Area A was living in sheltered accommodation and receiving day care, but in Area B this was not available, we would say that schizophrenics in Area B were 'in need'. In the NHS, whilst people may be assessed to be in absolute need (normatively), in practice comparative needs assessment will often dictate whether their needs will be met. Areas may be compared on the basis of provision of services or length of waiting lists to see if the health needs of their populations are being met. In a sense, then, comparative need is about equity. It is about equal provision for equal need. This kind of analysis of need does, of course, assume that those in receipt of a service are receiving adequate provision and that their needs are being met.

Bradshaw's work is useful in showing that different groups in society hold different definitions of need. We can see that needs are not objective and observable entities to which we must just match our interventions The concept of need is a relative one and is influenced both by values and attitudes and by other agendas. Illich et al (1977) have argued that the essential nature of a profession is its possession of knowledge and authority to determine what people 'need'. Professionals may then offer a service to meet those needs, and in so doing maintain their own status and resources.

 Consider these interventions available to women in childbirth. Has medicine created these needs or are they needed improvements in technology?

- Prostaglandin to induce labour
- Epidural to reduce pain
- Electronic fetal monitoring
- Belt monitoring of contractions.

At first sight, these developments may be seen as the consequence of medical advances. However, medical interventions in childbirth can also be seen as an attempt to establish doctors' control over that of midwives. The range of interventions may, on the one hand, alienate women and make childbirth an uncomfortable and distressing experience and, on the other hand, the very availability of these services may create a need for them.

Background to health needs assessment

The process of assessing needs is nothing new. As we shall see in the next chapter, understanding needs is integral to a basic process approach to planning. Needs assessment including the collection of data is the first step, from which subsequent aims will be derived.

The NHS reforms of the 1990s required health authorities to assess the health and social needs of their local populations as a means of obtaining accurate and appropriate information on which to base priorities. This was in addition to epidemiological and demographic data on the amount and nature of mortality and morbidity and the demand for care in their area (see Ch. 3).

Need was defined as the population's ability to benefit from health services which range from prevention through care and treatment to rehabilitation. This basic principle has far-reaching implications. The NHS will assess health needs and then identify actions capable of being delivered by the NHS and which will achieve 'health gain'. The amount of need is thus not dependent on the size of the problem. The ability to benefit or to achieve health gain include interventions which:

- add years to life by reducing premature mortality
- add life to years by enhancing the quality of life and improving well-being.

 Which of the following NHS services contributes to 'adding years to life', and which to 'adding life to years'?

- Blood pressure screening
- Domiciliary nursing care
- Cervical cancer screening
- Community psychiatric nursing service
- Family planning services
- Day care centre for mentally ill people
- Accident and emergency departments
- Immunization
- Dental health services

Which other services contribute to 'Adding Years to Life' and 'Life to Years', and who is responsible for providing these services?

The concept of health gain is rooted in a medical model which sees health as the absence of disease. Consequently, health needs tend to be defined as problems which may be successfully met by services or treatment. Because need is seen as infinite and resources as limited, health authorities confine themselves to what is known to be effective care. Yet community surveys often show that the public define ill health far more broadly than simply problems requiring treatment by health services. Many priorities for health go beyond the narrow outcomes encompassed by adding 'years to life' and require health authorities to take account of the structural influences on health, such as housing, community safety and transport links (Carroll 1994).

A broader interpretation of the purpose of population needs assessment is provided by Pickin & St Leger (1993) who suggest that there are four possible reasons for assessing needs:

- to increase population health
- to maximize health potential
- to reduce variations and inequalities in health
- to establish equity in the use of resources.

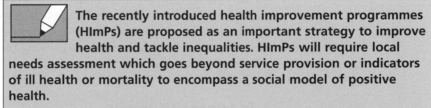

The recently introduced health improvement programmes (HImPs) are proposed as an important strategy to improve health and tackle inequalities. HImPs will require local needs assessment which goes beyond service provision or indicators of ill health or mortality to encompass a social model of positive health.

What sorts of information might be collected for a health improvement programme?

The purpose of assessing health needs

1. To help in directing interventions appropriately

A male patient who is young and fit has a heart attack. The nurse on the ward offers the patient advice on cardiac rehabilitation and information on healthy eating, exercise and safe drinking.

- Is the nurse meeting the patient's needs?
- Is health education information an appropriate intervention?

The medical and individualistic approach is adopted because it is a well-understood part of the nurse's professional role. The nurse understands coronary heart disease prevention as focusing on risk factors even though they are not relevant to this situation. The patient may have other health needs such as a concern about getting back to work or when he might be sexually active again. Assessing individual health needs means starting with the patient's own concerns.

2. To identify and respond to specific needs of minority groups, communities or sections of the population whose health needs have not been fully met

A district aims to reduce mortality from coronary heart disease and stroke in people under 65. Black and ethnic minorities comprise 35% of the population. It is well established in epidemiological data that the risk of CHD is high in Asians and that of stroke is high in African-Caribbeans (Balarajan & Raleigh 1993).

■ The District translates its literature into Asian languages.
■ GPs carry out opportunistic blood pressure checks on Black and minority ethnic patients.
■ A healthy eating booklet is produced which includes examples and photographs of Asian and Caribbean foods.

Is the District meeting the needs of ethnic minority groups? Or is it assuming that because epidemiology identifies Asians and African-Caribbeans as a high-risk group for CHD and stroke, all ethnic minorities are 'in need' of a CHD-prevention programme and their needs are the same?

3. To target risk groups

Targeting may be done in terms of diseases, life cycles, lifestyles, or social groups. The concept of risk groups has emerged as a means of directing health promotion activities to people who are most in need. Normative needs derived from epidemiological research, which identifies groups with poorer than average health, are often used to establish target groups. For example, lower socio-economic groups at most risk from ill health and premature death are a commonly identified risk group. Comparative need is used to identify at-risk groups who have low take-up rates of services. For example, travellers face specific difficulties accessing primary health care services and may, therefore, be a target group. A life cycle approach which identifies the health risks associated with different age groups has also been developed (Pickin & St Leger 1994).

However, a focus on high-risk groups can lead to 'victim-blaming'. Health problems are seen as specific to particular groups who may also be seen as responsible through their behaviour for their own ill health (Naidoo & Wills 1998). The example of HIV prevention illustrates this problem: gay men and injecting drug-users have been the subject of targeted health promotion campaigns. Yet it is not being gay which is a risk but certain sexual activities. Many health promoters also reject the notion of targeting because they prefer to work in partnership with groups and communities on the issues *they* define as important.

4. Resource allocation

The NHS was predicated on the notion that there was an untreated pool of sickness that, once treated by a national health service, would diminish. Experience shows that there can be unlimited demand for health care. As health care is provided, so expectations rise; as technology improves people with disabilities and chronic diseases live longer and demand more health care. General improvements in health and living conditions have led to people living longer and an increase in the percentage of older people in the population. It will not be possible to meet all these needs as resources are limited.

Most doctors and health care workers accept that some kind of priority setting or rationing of health care is inevitable. There have always been waiting lists but rationing is a more far-reaching concept. It entails decisions about how much money should be put into different forms of care or treatment. Not only does this raise issues about justice and equity, it also poses the huge dilemma about who decides the priorities for investment. Public views may be very different from those of doctors. For example, infertility treatment may have a high value to individuals but not to society as a whole. Osteoporosis screening (bone density measurement) may be rated highly by the public but not by doctors who have access to more information and are therefore able to question its effectiveness.

In Oregon in the USA a health commission of health care workers and the public devised a complex formula to prioritize health services and decided there were certain services that they would not provide. In the UK health care may no longer be free and available to all who need it. Health authorities are beginning to consider particular services which will not be provided as part of the NHS. Cosmetic surgery, for example, may no longer be provided except in exceptional circumstances such as when required as a result of burns or trauma (Smith 1994).

Bromley Health has undertaken a major exercise to elicit public views on health care priorities and changing provision to primary care, day-case surgery and the care of the mentally ill in the community. In-depth discussion groups were posed key commissioning dilemmas and asked their response (see p. 338).

The process of assessing need

Needs assessment can be carried out from the perspectives of professionals, the lay public and key informants (members of the community with a particular viewpoint, such as teachers or police officers). It can be carried out at different levels from that of the individual to specific groups (e.g. population groups, such as older

338 Working for health promotion

 Health authorities have limited resources. Consider the following typical costs of interventions. What factors would you take into account in deciding priorities?

Home visit by community psychiatric nurse 50.00
Tonsillectomy 1 250.00
Hip replacement 4 000.00
Place in group home for people with learning
  difficulties 30 000.00 per year
Pregnancy termination 200.00
Brief intervention of psychotherapy (10 weeks) 1 500.00
Day care for elderly mentally ill 200.00 per week

Some of the factors you may take into account are:

■ Costs – the relative costs of different services, and the 'opportunity costs' (i.e. if the money is spent on this, what is it not being spent on).
■ Numbers – how many people will benefit from the service and will it provide the greatest good for the greatest number?
■ Effectiveness – what are the likely outcomes of providing care or treatment?
  Will it promote health, prevent ill health, improve or cure ill health?
■ Quality – what areas of health-related quality of life (physical, mental, social, well-being, perception of pain, self-care) will be most affected by the service?

people or people with specific health problems) to local geographic communities to national populations.

In all cases assessing health needs should be guided by these common questions:

■ What do I want to know?
■ Why do I want to know this?
■ How can I find out this information?
■ What am I going to do with the information when I obtain it?
■ What scope is there to act on the information?

Individual needs

For those health promoters who work with individual clients, there is increasing recognition of the importance of client participation in the assessment of needs. Nursing practice, for example, has frequently been criticized for being too inflexible and routine – doing things *to* people rather than *with* them. Prescription has now given way to negotiation alongside the move from sick nursing to health nursing. Understanding the thoughts, feelings and experiences of individuals has become an important part of the therapeutic and nursing process.

For what reasons might clients find it difficult to express their needs in a clinical situation?

For each of these elements, list the main sources of information which would need to be accessed to complete a community profile. What are their strengths and limitations in providing a picture of the community?

Increasingly, health care workers seek to identify clients' views and perceptions about their health as part of their assessment. What they often find is that their perception differs from that of the client. Clients' need for information is often underestimated and in health care settings this may mean that information is confined to ward or clinic routines.

Despite the greater emphasis on being client-centred in all health, welfare and education work, health promoters tend to assess needs in relation to the service they provide. Very often client needs are seen as information because it is possible to provide this, whereas the satisfaction of physical needs (as in Maslow's hierarchy) may seem beyond their scope.

Community profiling

Community nurses have always worked with groups and communities to identify needs. The compilation of community profiles helps to provide a systematic assessment of needs rather than the subjective view of the health worker.

A community profile has been described as:

A comprehensive description of the needs of a population that is defined, or defines itself, as a community, and the resources that exist within a community, carried out with the active involvement of the community itself, for the purpose of developing an action plan or other means of improving the quality of life in the community.

(Hawton et al 1994)

Community profiles do not follow a standard format. Figure 17.2 shows a schematic representation of the main elements:

- the composition of the community, e.g. its age profile, the way the community is organized and its capacity to control its own health
- socio-ecological environment, e.g. extent of economic activity and unemployment, private car ownership, housing, transport links, green areas, air pollution
- availability, effectiveness and impact of health and social service provision
- local strategies for health, e.g. health improvement programmes, regeneration projects.

Public views

The NHS reforms of the 1990s emphasized the need to involve local people in all stages of the commissioning process. The Local Voices initiative aimed 'to give people an effective voice in the shaping of health services . . . Health Authorities have a dual responsibility to ensure that the voice of local people is heard. Firstly, they need to encourage local people to be involved in the purchasing process.

Figure 17.2
*Community
information profile.
From Annett & Rifkin
1990.*

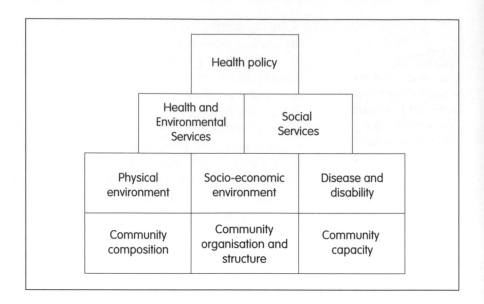

Secondly, they need to ensure that the providers take account of local needs in their activities' (NHS Management Executive 1992). For many health authorities this is part of a formal exercise conducted in a top-down way. Frequently the consultation is confined to issues relating to patient satisfaction with services and particularly the hotel aspects of care.

Ong & Humphris regard this as inadequate: 'It is not sufficient to see users as consumers who are satisfied or dissatisfied with services. The place of users is in the joint definition of need, priority setting and evaluation. This approach means a paradigm shift whereby the community perspective will be used as the guiding principle for setting priorities in health care' (Ong & Humphris 1994, p. 80).

The process of consultation is not always successful. It often views people as the passive providers of information and not as active participants in the process. The results of consultations may seemingly be ignored. The timing, location and publicity for public meetings may lead to a poor turnout. Those consulted may not be representative of the community or may be token representatives of particular groups.

Many health and local authorities are using a range of initiatives to achieve a wider picture of community needs than one-off consultations (see, for example, Barker et al 1997). These approaches represent a move away from traditional epidemiological data gathering towards techniques which reflect the importance of social and environmental factors and the involvement of the community in data collection. These include:

■ public meetings and focus groups
■ interviews with users and key informants

- using local media such as radio phone-ins
- community health panels and citizens' juries
- research techniques such as rapid appraisal, ethnographic studies and community development.

Rapid appraisal is a research technique applied to both urban and rural settings. It is geared to quickly identifying the health needs and priorities of a target population without great expense. Researchers interview people with knowledge of the area to identify problems and solutions. Key informants are:

- people who work in the community and have a professional understanding of the local issues (e.g. teachers, health visitors, police)
- people who are recognized community leaders and represent a section of the community (e.g. religious leaders, councillors, leaders of self-help groups)
- people who are important in informal networks and play a role in local communication (e.g. shopkeepers, bookmakers, lollipop persons).

List some of the advantages and disadvantages of rapid appraisal as a method of community needs assessment.

Rapid appraisal is useful if virtually nothing is known about the needs and priorities of the target population. It can give a deep understanding of the problems and issues in a community and provide a sense of local ownership. But it does not provide the quantitative analysis of the size of the problem which many public health departments require. It may also be difficult to get beyond personal agendas to find out the community's views.

Other sources of information might be existing written records, observations made in the neighbourhood or in the homes and workplaces of informants.

A locality management group held a focus group discussion on women's knowledge of the contraceptive pill as part of a series designed to improve client involvement in the assessment of health needs. The issues raised by the focus group have formed the basis for a questionnaire which is being given to women who present to their GP or family planning clinic for a repeat prescription of the contraceptive pill.

- **What reasons can you think of to explain why certain groups are hard to reach?**
- **Can you think of groups that might be hard to reach?**

Whose needs count?

Moves to participation either in community affairs or health care cannot involve everyone. There will be individuals and groups who are not able to take advantage of opportunities for expression. These are the potential and future users of a service; those who are not part of an established group; those who are not deemed sufficiently 'rational' to have a view such as children, people with learning difficulties and sometimes older people. Participation obviously favours those with the most influence and loudest voices.

It is very difficult to get a cross-section of a community and there are some groups of people who are hard to reach. These include homeless people, unemployed people, and people from Black and minority ethnic groups.

Some groups comprise individuals who may have a similar experience of health services because of a defining characteristic of being unemployed or homeless, but who do not have a collective voice or means of expressing their views. Other groups may be informal with no recognized meeting place. Many groups may be wary of formal and statutory bodies.

Williams & Popay (1994) describe examples of popular epidemiology where a community gets a health issue acknowledged by compiling evidence to substantiate their views. They term this a 'competing rationality'. For example, people in Camelford in Cornwall documented the symptoms they experienced when 20 tonnes of aluminium sulphate was accidentally tipped into the water tank supplying their homes.

Setting priorities

Since the publication of a national health strategy in *The Health of the Nation* and subsequently *Our Healthier Nation*, many health promoters will find that they are working to the key areas identified. The criteria used for setting these priorities are:

1. The area should be a major cause of premature death or avoidable ill health in the population as a whole or amongst specific groups of people.
2. There are marked inequalities in those who suffer ill health or premature death.
3. Effective interventions should be possible offering scope for improvements in health.

In addition, there may be locally determined priorities of specific health issues, such as diabetes, or particular population groups, such as older people.

We have seen in this chapter that people's identified needs may also be taken as the first step in the planning process. However, the

NHS tempers this subjective interpretation with economic priorities. People may express a need for interventions or treatment, the effectiveness of which is in doubt. The British Medical Association, for example, recently issued advice to all general practitioners on 'unnecessary prescribing' of antibiotics for simple colds or ear infections. For health promoters, therefore, a simple needs assessment may not be an adequate basis for setting priorities. There is a range of other influences which may determine what is included in a local health promotion plan:

- national targets of reducing disease
- a national theme, e.g. World Aids Day
- a major determinant of health in the area, i.e. age or poverty
- pragmatism on the basis of available skills and interests
- cost and staffing
- longer-term strategy
- existing activity
- cost-effectiveness and what is amenable to change and evaluation
- client choice
- professionals' views.

Conclusion

The process of encouraging consumerism and participation in public services by identifying and understanding individual and community needs has led to attempts to make such services more flexible. So we find as part of the nursing process, clients being encouraged to identify aspects of their situation that they deem harmful to their health. We find health authorities using a variety of methods to ascertain the views, beliefs and health behaviours of their population in addition to the objective measures yielded by epidemiology. We find voluntary and community groups being required as part of their funding to monitor not only their clients' use of the service but also their health needs.

The public sector, including the NHS, is seeking to integrate public views into the planning process. However, most of the information used to assess needs is gathered from a professional perspective which assumes a direct relationship between certain indicators and needs and which is embedded in a medical model of health. For example, if health statistics show an above average incidence of coronary heart disease, local health planners may well assume a need for greater provision of cardiac treatment and rehabilitation services and a health promotion programme to address risk factors for CHD. Health promoters have an important role to play in ensuring that needs assessment which feeds into planning takes account of public views and self-defined needs, and uses indicators to measure a social model of positive health.

Questions for further discussion

■ How useful is the concept of need as a basis for planning health promotion interventions?
■ How would you go about assessing the needs of:
  ❏ women who inject drugs?
  ❏ young asthmatics?
  ❏ carers of older people?

Summary

This chapter has discussed the ways in which need is defined. We have seen that perceptions of need vary according to whether these are client or professional views, and how the assessment is made – clients' expressed views; levels of service use; epidemiological and social data. The chapter concludes that need is relative, and influenced by values and attitudes as well as the historical context. It also considers the role of health promotion in identifying and meeting certain needs.

Further reading

Curtis S, Taket A 1996 Health and societies: changing perspectives. Arnold, London. *A comprehensive review of the ways in which health services throughout the world are responding to calls for more community involvement and participation.*

Doyal L, Gough I 1992 A theory of human need. Macmillan, London. *An important study exploring the concept of need and how this can be incorporated into health service planning.*

Popay J, Williams G (eds) 1994 Researching the people's health. Routledge, London. *Part Two looks at the theory of needs assessment including a review by Bradshaw of his taxonomy of need after 20 years.*

Robinson J, Elkan R 1996 Health needs assessment: theory and practice. Churchill Livingstone, Edinburgh. *A clear and readable account of the issues in health needs assessment. It looks at epidemiological approaches and locality commissioning.*

References

Annett H, Rifkin S 1990 Improving urban health. WHO, Geneva

Armstrong P 1982 The myth of meeting needs in adult education and community development. Critical Social Policy 2(2): 24–37

Balarajan R, Raleigh V S 1993 Ethnicity and health. Department of Health, London

Barker J, Bullen M, de Ville J 1997 A reference manual for public involvement. Bromley Health, Bromley

Bradshaw J 1972 The concept of social need. New Society 19: 640–643

Bradshaw J 1994 The conceptualisation and measurement of need: a social policy perspective. In: Popay J, Williams G (eds) 1994 Researching the people's health. Routledge, London

Carroll G 1994 Priority setting in purchasing health care. In: Smith R (ed) Rationing in action. BMJ Publishing, London

Doyal L, Gough I 1992 A theory of human need. Macmillan, London

Hawton M, Percy-Smith J, Hughes G 1994 Community profiling: auditing social needs. Open University, Buckingham

Illich I, Zola I K, McKnight J, Caplan J, Shaiken H 1977 Disabling professions. Boyars, London

Maslow A H 1954 Motivation and personality. Harper & Row, New York

Naidoo J, Wills J 1998 Practising health promotion: dilemmas and challenges. Baillière Tindall, London

NHS Management Executive 1992 Local voices: involving the local community in purchasing decisions. NHS Management Executive, Leeds

Oliver 1993 Psychology and health care. Baillière Tindall, London

Ong B N, Humphris G 1994 Prioritising needs with communities: rapid appraisal methodologies in health. In: Popay J, Williams G (eds) Researching the people's health. Routledge, London

Percy-Smith J, Sanderson J 1992 Understanding local needs. Institute for Public Policy Research, London

Pickin C, St Leger S 1993 Assessing health need using the life cycle framework. Open University Press, Milton Keynes

Smith R (ed) 1994 Rationing in action. BMJ Publishing, London

Tudor Hart 1971 The inverse care law. Lancet 1: 405

Williams G, Popay J 1994 Lay knowledge and the privilege of experience. In: Grabe J, Kelleher D, Williams G (eds) Challenging medicine. Routledge, London

World Health Organization 1978 Report on the Primary Health Care Conference: Alma Ata. World Health Organization, Geneva

World Health Organization 1985 Targets for health for all. WHO Regional Office for Europe, Copenhagen

18 *Planning health promotion interventions*

OVERVIEW

We have seen in Chapter 17 how needs assessment and targeting may be carried out, and the importance of carrying out this process and being clear about the context in which this is done. This chapter extends this discussion, and follows on from Chapter 17. First, definitions of planning are given and the reasons for planning discussed. Planning at different levels, from broad strategic planning through project planning to small-scale health education planning, is considered. Two planning models, the Ewles & Simnett (1999) and PRECEDE (Green et al 1980) are discussed in detail. A discussion of quality and audit and how this relates to planning follows.

Definitions

Planning is one of those terms which is used in many different ways. Other related terms are used in equally imprecise ways, so that often the same activity is labelled in different ways by different people. There are no hard and fast rules about the way terms are used, but the following definitions are presented as a means of clarifying the differences between related activities. These are the definitions we shall be using in this chapter.

- **Plan** – how to get from your starting point to your end point and what you want to achieve.
- **Strategy** – broad framework for action which indicates goals, methods and underlying principles.
- **Policy** – guidelines for practice which set broad goals and the framework for action.
- **Programme** – overall outline of action. The collection of activities in a planned sequence leading to a defined goal or goals.
- **Priority** – the first claim for consideration.
- **Aim** or **goal** – broad statement of what is to be achieved.
- **Objective** or **target** – specific goal to be achieved.

Judy has been given a remit to develop a health promotion *programme* with the aim of reducing the suicide rate. Her health authority's *policy* includes a commitment to equal opportunities. She decides her *priority* will be unemployed people, who are known to be at increased risk of suicide. Judy's *objectives* are (1) to set up a support group for unemployed people; and (2) to provide specialist counselling services. Her *strategy* is to network with existing community groups, and to recruit and train volunteer counsellors.

Reasons for planning

Health promoters usually have no problem in finding things to do which seem reasonable. Work areas are inherited from others, delegated from more senior members of the workplace or demanded by clients. It is possible to be kept very busy reacting to all these pressures, and planning health promotion interventions may seem a luxury or a waste of time. However, there are sound reasons for planning health promotion or being proactive in your work practice. Planning is important because it helps direct resources to where they will have most impact. Planning ensures that health promotion is not overlooked but is prioritized as a work activity.

Planning takes different forms and is used at different levels. It may be used to provide the best services or care for an individual client, as in the nursing process, or planning may be for group activities, such as antenatal classes. Planning may also refer to large-scale health promotion interventions targeted at whole populations.

The degree of formality of the planning process also varies. When planning a one-to-one intervention, the process is informal and may involve no-one else. Planning for a group intervention may involve liaising with other professionals as well as the target group, to find out what their aims and objectives are and what sorts of methods and resources are available and acceptable. A written plan may be produced to act as a guide and a statement of agreed outcomes and methods. Planning a large-scale intervention will usually involve more long-term collaborative planning. Often a working group (or task force or local forum) will be established early on to identify interested groups and gain their support and expertise. A written plan will usually be produced, outlining not only objectives and methods but also a timescale of what is to be achieved when, funding details and a budget, who is responsible for which tasks, and how the intervention will be evaluated and the findings reported back.

Rational planning

Rational planning models provide a means to guide choices so that decisions are made which represent the best way to achieve desired results.

'The "rational" approach suggests that the whole range of options should be identified and considered before a comprehensive programme is drawn up' (McCarthy 1982, p. 10).

Planning involves several key stages or logical stepping stones which enable the health promoter to achieve a desired result. The benefit is being clear about what it is you want to achieve, i.e. the purpose of any intervention. Planning entails:

1. An assessment of need.
2. Setting aims – what it is you intend to achieve.
3. Setting objectives – precise outcomes. Objectives should be SMART: specific, measurable, achievable, realistic, time-limited.
4. Deciding which methods or strategies will achieve your objectives.
5. Evaluating outcomes in order to make improvements in the future.

Some planning models are presented in a linear fashion. Others show a circular process to indicate that any evaluation feeds back into the process (see Fig. 18.1). The rational approach describes how decisions should be made. It does not take into account that there may not be agreement on objectives or the best way to proceed.

Figure 18.1
McCarthy's model for rational health planning. Reproduced with permission from the King's Fund Centre from McCarthy (1982).

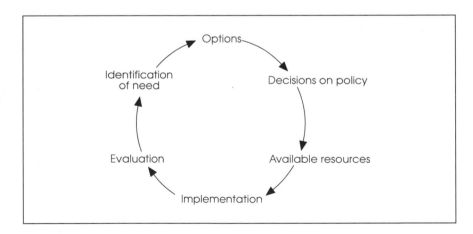

However, in real life, planning is often piecemeal or incremental. There is no grand design, but circumstances dictate many small reactive decisions:

What do you think would be the best starting point for planning an intervention or programme? Why?

Think of any planned activities you have been involved with. What was the starting point? Why?

The 'incremental' approach suggests that planning is necessarily based on limited information, and that the uncertainty of the future makes small decisions preferable to grand plans.

(McCarthy 1982, p. 10)

■ **Which do you think is preferable, rational or incremental planning?**
■ **Which are the most important factors to consider?**

Tannahill (1990) argues that what is needed is an integrated planning framework. Planning for health education is part of the broader task of health promotion and should seek to enhance good communication. Health-oriented health education is to be preferred to the narrower programmes which focus on diseases or risk factors. Tannahill states that disease-oriented or risk-factor-oriented health education tends to be prescriptive in tone and is apt to be duplicated by different professional groups. The public response may be to withdraw from the resulting proliferation of messages which are often inconsistent. He argues that integrated health-oriented health education which focuses on key settings and key groups is the preferred option (Fig. 18.2). This needs to be complemented by preventive and protective health promotion measures.

McCarthy (1982) and Tannahill (1990) argue that planning should be a rational, organized and integrated activity. French & Milner (1993) state that current health promotion practice is incapable of having a major impact on the health status of populations, and that planning to achieve these goals is illusory. In real life, planning is often carried out on a smaller scale and is subject to practical constraints. Planning health promotion interventions in practice is not always a neat unilinear process, but may be triggered by events at any stage in the planning process. For example, planning in real life often follows the allocation of resources instead of dictating resources.

The Managing Health Improvement Project (1993) also identifies a 'mixed-scanning approach' which involves listing options, reviewing the resource implications of each option, scanning

A university successfully bids for research funding to investigate the relative mobility and well-being of older people living at home and in residential care. They link up with a health promotion service whose work therefore becomes focused on older people.

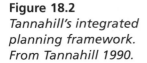

Figure 18.2
Tannahill's integrated planning framework. From Tannahill 1990.

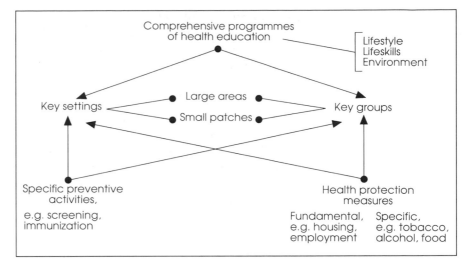

implementation according to costs, and review on a regular basis. In Chapter 17 we saw moves to incorporate health needs assessment into planning reflect the view that planning should be done *with* rather than *for* people and that the information which feeds into the planning process should take account of people's stated needs and priorities.

In reality, planning takes place within a larger context which includes many factors, such as the wider policy framework, as well as more pragmatic factors, such as expertise, experience and values. Any planning you as a health practitioner undertake will be affected by many different factors which may not always be consistent with each other.

Planning is used to cover activities which range from large-scale, such as strategic planning, to middle-scale project planning, and small-scale interventions, such as planning a health education session.

Strategic planning

Strategies describe desirable outcomes and broad ways of achieving these outcomes but do not necessarily go into details about methods or measuring outcomes. Strategic planning refers to planning a large-scale activity involving different partners and staged interventions. The English White Paper on public health (DoH 1999) refers to the need for integrated and inclusive policies. This is strategic thinking and planning for health which recognizes the contribution of other agencies and the need to have complementary strategies and activities which build on each other to achieve maximum outcomes. The Departments of the Environment, Transport and the Regions, Trade and Industry and

Education are all cited as having a major contribution to health through, for example, the creation of sustainable environments, integrated transport systems, full employment and educational achievement.

> The 'Health of the Nation' strategy for England (DoH 1992) set quantifiable targets with a timeframe for the reduction of diseases and risk factors. The 'Saving Lives: Our Healthier Nation' strategy for England (DoH 1999) sets fewer and broader targets. What are the advantages and disadvantages of setting measurable targets in a strategy?

Simnett (1995) described the following stages in developing a strategy:

1. **Identifying** likely partners.
2. **Diagnosis** – identifying where we are now and how we would like things to be different. What factors are likely to affect where we go?
3. **Vision** – where do we want to go? What outcomes do we want? What do other people want?
4. **Development** – what needs to change in order to get there? What programmes currently exist?
5. **Action plan** – planning what to do next.

These stages correspond to those of a rational model: assess – plan – do – evaluate.

Strategies may be local as well as national. For example, health improvement programmes (HImPs) require consultation between statutory and voluntary agencies and local populations to draw up an agreed 3-year plan to promote health in a defined locality. HImPs will include:

- detailed specification of services, projects and activities
- identification of costs, inputs and quality standards.

They may include targets (how achievement will be measured).

Project planning

Project planning is a smaller-scale activity and refers to planning a specific project which is time-limited and aims to bring about a defined change. Examples of small-scale health promotion projects include a project to raise the awareness of university students about meningitis, a project to train school nurses in presentation skills and a project to map safe routes to school for young children.

You are involved in a working group drawing up a local strategy to reduce alcohol use. Who would you want to be involved in the working group? What broad goals would be appropriate?

Broad goals might be framed in terms of:

■ Reducing availability of alcohol, e.g. alcohol-free policies in leisure places and workplaces, refusing licences for additional pubs or bars, clamping down on alcohol sales to young people.
■ Reducing the promotion of alcohol, e.g. banning advertisements for alcohol on local authority premises.
■ Teaching vulnerable groups about the effects of alcohol, e.g. sessions in youth clubs and community centres.
■ Training people to identify problematic alcohol use, e.g. sessions for GPs and practice nurses on early identification.
■ Increased health promotion coverage in local mass media linking alcohol to increased risk of accidents and violence.

The working group would need to involve a variety of partners in order to maximize its effectiveness. You might have identified representatives from the local authority, mass media, occupational health services covering workplaces, primary health care practitioners, mental health practitioners, teachers and youth workers, licensed victuallers, magistrates, the police service and voluntary agencies dealing with alcohol-related problems. The success of this strategy will depend on the different partners working together to achieve aims.

Ewles & Simnett (1999) define project stages as:

1. Start
2. Specification
3. Design and implementation
4. Implementation
5. Evaluation, review and final completion.

The start of the project is agreement that the project should take place, its overall aims and the allocation of a budget to support the project. Often the start is signalled by the formal adoption of a project proposal, indicating that an organization has given support for the development and implementation of a project.

Specification means setting objectives and quality criteria for how the project is to be delivered. Setting objectives is considered in more detail below. Quality and audit are discussed later in this chapter.

Design is the detailed planning of the training intervention. A Gantt chart (see Fig. 18.3) is a useful tool to use at this stage. A Gantt chart plots tasks and the people responsible for these tasks against a timescale in which these activities need to be undertaken. It portrays in a graphical form the interdependence of project tasks and how each single task contributes to the whole.

Implementation is the project activity, e.g. training sessions. Evaluation, review and final completion refers to the report on project outcomes and evaluation. It is useful to have a time-lag between completing the project and the final review in order to assess long-term as well as immediate outcomes.

The strategy outlined on page 353 includes a project centred on training GPs and practice nurses to identify problematic use of alcohol at an early stage. This project, which is part of the overall alcohol reduction strategy, would require careful and detailed planning, including:

■ Setting appropriate objectives. For example, would it be appropriate to set an objective of reducing problem drinking in the practice population? Why not?
■ How might objectives best be achieved? For example, should training be unidisciplinary or multidisciplinary? Should the training be accredited? Who would be the best person to run the sessions? What venue, day and time would be most acceptable? How would the sessions be funded? How long will the project last?
■ How would you evaluate the project? What criteria would you use to demonstrate success?

The kind of planning most health practitioners will be involved in will be on a much smaller scale. For example, you may want to plan a health education session with an individual client, or a series of sessions with a small group around a specific issue. Using the example above, you might want to plan a single session in detail. This would require you to:

■ set detailed objectives for participants to achieve by the end of the session, e.g. being aware of symptoms and behaviours (for example, poor attendance and time-keeping at work, especially in the mornings) which might be due to problematic alcohol use
■ investigate the range of resources available and select resources to use in the session
■ plan the session showing different activities and time allocated for each
■ plan a means of evaluating the session.

Planning models

Planning, whatever the scale of the activity, requires systematic working through a number of stages. The Ewles & Simnett (1999)

	March	April	May	June	July	August	September	October
Marketing and publicity	H&A							
Recruit participants		A						
Plan sessions				H	H			
Accreditation			H&A					
Pre-course needs assessment questionnaire				H&R				
Prepare materials, collect resources					H&A			
Check venue, timing, refreshments						A		
Action: training sessions							H	
Post-course evaluation								H&R
Evaluation report								H&R

Figure 18.3 *Gantt chart: planning training project. Three workers are involved: H (health promotion specialist); A (administrative officer); and R (researcher).*

Figure 18.4
Flowchart for planning and evaluating health promotion. From Ewles & Simnett 1999.

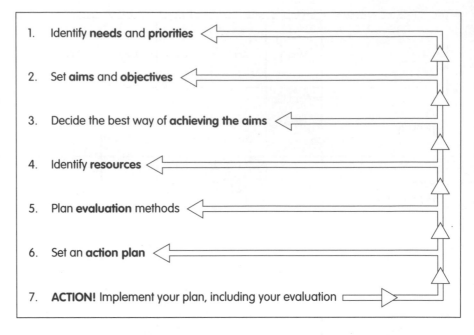

1. Identify **needs** and **priorities**

2. Set **aims** and **objectives**

3. Decide the best way of **achieving the aims**

4. Identify **resources**

5. Plan **evaluation** methods

6. Set an **action plan**

7. **ACTION!** Implement your plan, including your evaluation

planning framework presented below (see also Fig. 18.4) is a useful generic framework which can be adapted to a number of situations.

Ewles & Simnett (1999) planning model

Stage 1: Identifying needs and priorities

This may need local research and investigation, or may be the selection of particular clients from a caseload. Researching needs may require additional investigation. For example, local community profiles and local agencies might provide information on pressing local needs. Needs may already be defined for you, often on the basis of national or local epidemiological data reporting trends in illness and deaths. The previous chapter (Ch. 17) discusses this stage in more detail.

How could you find out what needs your clients have?

You might start a systematic enquiry, asking clients what issues they would like information and advice about. Or you might systematically go through caseload notes to identify what issues seem to be most common. For example, a health visitor might be aware that many parents are concerned about sleeping problems, leading her to set up a sleep clinic.

Other planning models start at different points. For example, Tones' planning model (Tones 1974, revised in Steel 1986) begins with a stated health promotion goal which is then analyzed to determine an appropriate educational intervention. This intervention is modified by referring to the characteristics of the target group, and a detailed educational programme planned. For example, an accident reduction programme identifies education about hazards in the home as a priority. The target group is older people. Based on evidence of other interventions with older people, it is decided that interpersonal communication would be most effective. Specific objectives are formulated concerning education about lighting and mobility aids. Whilst Tones' model focuses on educational interventions, the existence of national strategies for health promotion provides health promotion goals and aims which many practitioners may find themselves working to fulfil.

Berry's (1986) planning model starts with the setting up of a working group to review the problem and then identify a suitable health promotion project. This reflects an organizational context where procedures need to be established and agreed before any intervention can be planned. Health practitioners working in large organizations may find this starting point more realistic. The PRECEDE model discussed below starts with community-defined needs and goals.

Stage 2: Setting aims and objectives

Aims are broad goals concerned with improving health in a particular area, e.g. reducing the amount of alcohol-related ill health. Objectives need to be specific and should be statements that define what participants will have achieved by the end of the intervention. Objectives therefore need to be measurable in some way. There is a balance to be struck between setting objectives which are realistic but also challenging. Objectives can refer to educational, behavioural, policy, process or environmental outcomes.

Educational objectives may be divided into three categories:

- knowledge objectives concerning increased levels of knowledge
- affective objectives concerning changes in attitudes and beliefs
- behavioural or skills objectives concerning the acquisition of new competencies and skills.

Health promotion objectives may in addition include:

1. Behaviour change including changes in lifestyles and increased take-up of services, e.g. reducing the amount of binge-drinking or the prevalence of drink-driving,
2. Policy objectives concerning changes in policy, e.g. implementing alcohol-free policies in workplaces.
3. Process objectives concerning increases in participation and working together, e.g. increasing community participation and intersectoral working together.
4. Environmental objectives concerning changing the environment

Setting objectives for a training programme

Objectives for the training session on early identification of problematic alcohol use for GPs and practice nurses might include the following educational objectives:

1. Increasing participants' knowledge of the range of harmful effects and symptoms associated with problematic alcohol use.
2. Increasing participants' knowledge of the extent of problematic alcohol use and its association with social and demographic factors, e.g. gender, age, employment status, occupation.
3. Investigating participants' attitudes towards alcohol and public perceptions of alcohol use. Identifying the range between social drinker and alcoholic, with the many stages in between. Recognizing social and peer pressures to drink which contribute to many people's problematic usage of alcohol.
4. Enabling participants to use an assessment tool effectively to identify problematic alcohol use.
5. Enabling participants to use the Stages of Change Model to identify problem drinkers and appropriate interventions.

to make it more healthy, e.g. restriction on the advertising and sale of alcohol.

Objectives also reflect perspectives about the determinants of health and values about what are the most important things to achieve. These perspectives and values may be your own or may be derived from your organization.

Consider the different aims which may be included in a drug prevention strategy:

■ **To reduce the risks associated with drug-use and enable clients who do choose to use drugs to do so safely.**
■ **To reduce levels of harmful drug-use.**

What values and views about the determinants of drug-use are reflected in these different aims?

Stage 3: Identifying appropriate methods for achieving the objectives

This choice will be decided in part by external considerations, such as the amount of funding, or the particular expertise of the health promoter. However, the type of methods chosen should also reflect the objectives set. Certain methods go with certain objectives but would be quite inappropriate for other objectives. For example, participative small group work is effective at changing attitudes but a more formal teaching session would be more effective if specific

Consider the aims and objectives of the following two examples:

1. *Aim:* To hold an event to bring together people from Asian communities with experience of mental ill health, including people with mental health problems and carers, to share experiences, identify concerns and gauge interest in a self-help/support group.

   Objectives:

   1. To create a comfortable and positive atmosphere for participants.
   2. To ensure participation from representative groups of Asian communities.
   3. To ensure that diverse language and cultural needs are met appropriately and sensitively.
   4. To explore setting up a self-help/support group.
   5. To raise awareness about mental health issues amongst Asian communities.

2. *Aim:* To reduce suicides.

   Objectives:

   1. To establish a help-line and safe house for women in the next year.
   2. To ensure that within the next 2 years patients with schizophrenia managed in the community are reviewed at least monthly and more frequently when their state requires it.
   3. To set up a help-line and drop-in counselling service for young people.

- Are the aims and objectives specific and clear?
- What further information or details would be useful?

knowledge is to be imparted. Community development is effective at increasing community involvement and participation but would not be appropriate if local government policy change is the objective. The mass media are effective in raising people's awareness of health issues but ineffective in persuading people to change their behaviour. So the next stage in planning is deciding which methods would be the logical choice given your objectives. You may then find you have to compromise owing to constraints of time, resources or skills, but this compromise should concern the amount of input, or the use of complementary methods. It should not mean that you end up using inappropriate methods which are unlikely to achieve your objectives.

Stage 4: Identifying resources

When objectives and methods have been decided, the next stage is to consider whether any specific resources are needed to implement the strategy. Resources include funding, people's skills and

What would you need to include in a budget plan for the training sessions for GPs and practice nurses on early identification of problematic alcohol use discussed on page 358?

expertise, materials such as leaflets and learning packs and existing policies, plans, facilities and services.

You may find existing resources through libraries, organizations or your local health promotion service. You might also need to research the use and effectiveness of these resources. Or you may decide to adapt existing resources or even make your own, such as designing your own leaflet. Creating resources is a major task and should not be undertaken unless you are sure there is no available resource which is suitable.

Funding is an important issue for larger-scale interventions which require additional inputs over and above existing services and staff. For larger-scale interventions you may need to prepare a budget which is a statement of expected costs. This includes direct costs, which relate to the project, and fixed costs, which happen anyway.

Direct costs include:

- staff costs – salaries, superannuation, employer's National Insurance payments, annual increments
- capital costs, e.g. computer
- costs of specific activities, e.g. rental of community centre for training, buying resources to use in the training
- telephone, postage, photocopying
- travel and subsistence
- training and conferences to support staff development.

Fixed costs include overheads to cover accommodation, heating, lighting, telephone rental, etc.

A budget control system regularly monitors what is spent and what remains. This is usually done by monitoring the amount of money allocated, the amount of money spent, and the variance between the two (underspend or overspend) under each budget heading every month.

Stage 5: Plan evaluation methods

Evaluation must relate to the objectives you have set but can be undertaken more or less formally. You might just decide to ask participants their views at the end of the session, or spend some time noting your own perceptions of what went well and what could be improved next time. Or you might design a more formal means of evaluation, e.g. a questionnaire for participants to fill in anonymously, which is timetabled into the session. Evaluation is discussed in more detail in the next chapter.

Stage 6: Setting an action plan

This is a detailed written plan which identifies tasks, the person responsible for each task, resources which will be used, a timescale and means of evaluation. You might also include interim indicators of progress to show if you are proceeding as planned.

Stage 7: Action, or implementation of the plan

It is often useful to keep a log or diary to note unexpected problems and how you dealt with them, as well as unintended benefits. This information can then be fed into the evaluation process.

This framework may be used for planning a variety of interventions. Ewles & Simnett (1999) point out that in practice the planning process may begin at different stages, and that the whole process is cyclical, with experience and findings feeding into the different stages at different times.

PRECEDE

PRECEDE stands for predisposing reinforcing and enabling causes in educational diagnosis and evaluation. This model was developed by Green et al (1980) and has been used extensively in health education interventions. Figure 18.5 gives a diagrammatic representation of PRECEDE.

Phase 1 is the identification of a population's concerns and problems relating to their quality of life. The starting point is a

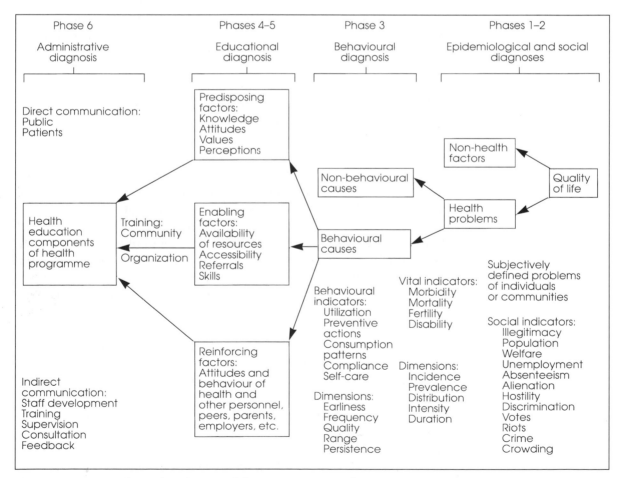

Figure 18.5   *PRECEDE planning model. From Green et al 1980.*

community's subjective perceptions, which may be determined in several ways. Chapter 17 considers a range of methods to identify community health needs.

Phase 2 is the identification and isolation of health problems from other social problems. A community's major concerns may relate to employment prospects or the effects of poverty, or law and order, rather than health. PRECEDE states that such issues are not within the remit of health promotion and excludes them from further consideration. Health problems are defined not only by reference to the community's perceptions, but also by reference to available epidemiological or medical data. Health as defined by the medical model is the focus for intervention.

Phase 3 is the behavioural diagnosis. Non-behavioural causes of health problems, such as unhealthy environments or policies, are excluded at this stage. Behavioural causes need to be carefully identified and ranked in order to progress to Phase 4, which is the identification of three categories of factors which affect behaviour. Predisposing factors are a person's beliefs, values and attitudes which will affect motivation to change. Enabling factors refer to the skills and resources which are necessary to allow the enactment of motivated behaviour. Social factors, such as income or accessibility of services, are also enabling factors. Enabling factors, if absent, will be 'barriers' which need to be overcome in order to enable behaviour change to occur. Reinforcing factors refer to the feedback received from significant others, which may help or hinder the process of behaviour change.

Phase 4 is the analysis of these three categories of factors and the selection of the most important factors.

Phase 5 follows automatically and is the decision of which factors are to be the focus of the intervention. The type and extent of resources available will help inform this decision. Phase 6 again follows logically from the previous phases, and is the development and implementation of an appropriate educational intervention. The management and administration of the intervention is also considered at this stage. Administrative diagnosis includes assessment of resources and organizational relationships, and the production of a timetable. Phase 7 is the evaluation of the intervention, although Green et al (1980) stress that this should be an integrated activity addressed throughout the planning process.

The intention is that using PRECEDE will guide the health educator to the most effective type of intervention. Using knowledge drawn from epidemiology, social psychology, education and management studies, the health educator can arrive at an optimum intervention. The model is said to be based on a complementary mix of expertise drawn from these different disciplines. Green et al (1980, p. 11) claim that PRECEDE 'has served as a successful model in a number of rigorously evaluated "real world" clinical trials'.

In practice, the model is often modified and is rarely used as illustrated. For example, it is unusual to begin the process of planning with as open an agenda as 'quality of life'. Priority topics, target groups or settings have more often been identified at the outset. For example, the 'Saving Lives: Our Healthier Nation' targets (DoH 1999) focus on specific diseases. So in practice PRECEDE often begins at the behavioural diagnosis rather than the needs assessment phase.

PRECEDE as a health education planning model mirrors the medical world. The planning process is dominated by experts. The general public may be involved in identifying problems, but the ways and means of tackling these problems are to be determined by experts. The focus is on achieving behavioural change at the level of individuals or groups. The social, political and environmental context of health is systematically screened out by the model in phases two and three. To some extent this may be explained by PRECEDE being a health education rather than a health promotion planning model. A model developed specifically for health education cannot be expected to apply to other forms of health promotion but, for most people, education, even if it does not include changing the environment, does include clarifying values, beliefs and attitudes, facilitating self-empowerment and supporting autonomy. In PRECEDE these activities tend to be subordinated to the primary aim of behaviour change. It could be argued that PRECEDE is a model dominated by social psychology and behavioural perspectives rather than educational perspectives, and that the label is therefore misleading. PRECEDE is, however, a highly structured planning model which ensures that certain issues are considered. If the objective is behaviour change, then PRECEDE is a useful model to follow.

Quality and audit

Why is it important to have a system of quality assurance in health promotion? Assessing the quality of practice through quality assurance, quality management or audit is an important aspect of professional practice. It helps to improve standards, identify cost-effective activities, demonstrate worth to outside agencies and ensure that activities meet stakeholders' requirements. It does this by focusing on three key dimensions: management quality, professional quality and participation by local people.

The core principles of quality have been defined as (Evans et al 1994):

■ equity – that users have equal access and/or equal benefit from services

Quality has been defined as: 'the totality of the features and characteristics of a product of service that bear on its ability to satisfy stated or implied need' (British Standards Institute 1992).

- effectiveness – that services achieve their intended objectives
- efficiency – that services achieve maximum benefit for minimum cost
- accessibility – that a service is easily available to users in terms of time, distance and ethos
- appropriateness – that a service is that which the users require
- acceptability – that services satisfy the reasonable expectations of users.
- responsiveness – that services adapt to the expressed needs of users.

Quality expresses a notion of 'fit for the purpose' but also conveys a notion of excellence. Applying the notion of quality to work practice is difficult. One means of trying to do this is through quality assurance or audit which has been defined as: 'a systematic process through which achievable and desirable levels of quality are described, the extent to which these levels are achieved is assessed, and action taken following assessment to enable them to be realised' (Wright & Whittington 1992).

Quality assurance is an ongoing process of continual assessment and improvement of practice. A quality system may include elements of quality assurance and quality management. Quality assurance involves setting standards which specify quality and ensure consistency. Quality management applies the emphasis on quality to everyone through increasing their control over their performance. Figure 18.6 gives a diagrammatic representation of the quality assurance or audit cycle.

Audit is a systematic process of scrutinizing a service or programme in order to improve performance. Audit may focus on a particular aspect, e.g. organization and management or training. Part of the purpose of an audit is to build a picture, providing evidence of gaps and areas for improvement by comparing what is done with agreed best practice. A key part of an audit is to see if a service meets the needs of its users, so it may involve gathering and acting on local people's views. Audit may involve an internal review or scrutiny by an independent, external auditor (e.g. the Audit Commission, OFSTED inspectors of schools).

Most service specifications now specify quantity, costs and quality. There has also been an increased emphasis on audit of public sector activities and clinical audit is well established. The

Identify one aspect of your health promotion work that would benefit from an audit.

Using the above criteria and any others you think are important, draw up a list of standards that might be relevant.

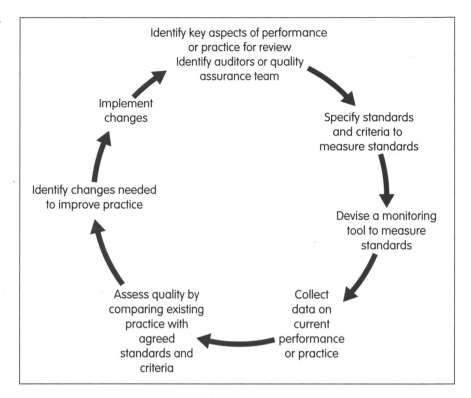

Figure 18.6 *A quality assurance or audit cycle. From Ewles & Simnett 1999.*

Identify key aspects of performance or practice for review
Identify auditors or quality assurance team

Specify standards and criteria to measure standards

Devise a monitoring tool to measure standards

Collect data on current performance or practice

Assess quality by comparing existing practice with agreed standards and criteria

Identify changes needed to improve practice

Implement changes

NHS White Paper 'The new NHS: modern, dependable' (DoH 1997) introduced a new National Institute for Clinical Excellence as well as national service frameworks and a Commission for Health Improvement in order to ensure high quality health services.

There are a number of audit schemes which are relevant to health promotion, e.g. the Society of Health Education and Health Promotion Specialists (SHEPS) external audit scheme for health promotion services. However, health promotion quality assessment or audit is particularly difficult because there is a wide range of activities and policies subsumed under the umbrella of health promotion which are carried out by many different agencies. Simnett (1995) stresses the importance of a wider audit of health promotion to ensure that it avoids duplication, moves forward to long-term goals and targets, and builds in accountability to local people.

Conclusion

There are sound reasons for adopting a planning model to structure health promotion interventions. Recognizing that health is a complex socially determined concept means that activities to promote health require careful planning, and often collaboration and working together with different agencies. Activities at different

What quality standards would be appropriate for general practice?

Quality standards for general practice might include:

- Patients' right to confidentiality.
- Patients' right to be seen within 24 hours.
- Patients should be greeted in a friendly, welcoming manner.
- Patients should be seen within 20 minutes of their appointment time.
- Patients' right to information about their own health, especially diagnosis, treatment options and side-effects, likelihood of recovery and how to prevent recurrence.
- Patients' right to ask questions and have these answered.
- Patients' right to a second opinion.
- Patients' right to see their records.
- Patients' right to be consulted about practice developments.

levels all benefit from planning, although the factors which need to be considered will vary according to the level of planned intervention. There are a variety of planning models for health promotion, two of which have been considered in more detail.

In reality, planning health promotion is a more complex process than the planning models suggest. This is because rational decision-making is only one factor in determining what happens. Many other factors are also important, including historical precedent, enthusiasms of key people and the political context. So it is unlikely that any health promotion intervention proceeds exactly along the lines indicated by a planning model, but this does not mean models are not useful. Models help structure activities and can act as a checklist to ensure that important stages are not missed out. They are there to be modified in the light of experience, not to act as strait-jackets.

Chapter 19 goes on to discuss the evaluation stage. Evaluating interventions, and being able to determine to what extent health promotion is successful in achieving its objectives, is the key to establishing health promotion as a central plank of health work.

Questions for further discussion

- What factors would you take into account when planning a health promotion intervention?
- How could you assess the quality of your health promotion work?

Summary

This chapter has clarified the terminology used in the planning process and has discussed the reasons for planning health promotion interventions. Planning happens at different levels, and an account of this has been given. Two planning models which have been developed specifically for health promotion have been discussed in greater detail. The assessment and evaluation of planning has been discussed through reference to quality assurance and audit cycles.

Further reading

Evans D, Head M, Speller V 1994 Assuring quality in health promotion. Wessex Institute of Public Health Medicine/Health Education Authority, Southampton. *A comprehensive and practical manual to help health promoters develop their quality assurance strategies and programmes.*

Ewles L, Simnett I 1999 Promoting health: a practical guide, 4th edn. Baillière Tindall, Edinburgh. *Chapter 7 gives further details and a practical guide to Ewles & Simnett's model. Chapter 8 discusses project planning in more detail.*

Simnett I 1995 Managing health promotion: developing healthy organisations and communities. Wiley, London. *A practical guide to developing health promotion strategies and improving practice.*

References

Berry J 1986 Project health: a step-by-step planning guide for health promotion and preventive medicine programmes. Health Education Journal 45: 109–111

British Standards Institute 1992 BSI handbook 22 quality assurance. British Standards Institute, Milton Keynes

Department of Health (DoH) 1992 The health of the nation. HMSO, London

Department of Health (DoH) 1997 White Paper: The new NHS: modern, dependable. Stationery Office, London

Department of Health (DoH) 1999 Saving Lives: Our healthier nation. White Paper. Stationery Office, London

Evans D, Head M, Speller V 1994 Assuring quality in health promotion. Wessex Institute of Public Health Medicine/Health Education Authority, Southampton

Ewles L, Simnett I 1999 Promoting health: a practical guide, 4th edn. Baillière Tindall, Edinburgh

French J, Milner S 1993 Should we accept the status quo? Health Education Journal 52: 98–101

Green L W, Kreuter M W, Deeds S F G, Partridge K B 1980 Health education planning: a diagnostic approach. Mayfield Publishing, Mountain View, California

McCarthy M 1982 Epidemiology and policies for health planning. King Edward's Hospital Fund for London, London

Managing Health Improvement Project 1993 Health Education Authority, London

Simnett I 1995 Managing health promotion: developing healthy organisations and communities. Wiley, London

Steel S 1986 Working in health education: a practical manual for the initial training of health education officers. HEC/Leeds Polytechnic, Leeds

Tannahill A 1990 Health education and health promotion: planning for the 1990s. Health Education Journal 49: 194–198

Tones K 1974 A systems approach to health education. Community Health 6: 34–39

Wright C, Whittington D 1992 Quality assurance: an introduction for health care professionals. Churchill-Livingstone, London

Evaluation in health promotion

OVERVIEW

There is great pressure on health promotion as a relatively new discipline to prove its worth through evaluation of its activities. In addition, the drive in the NHS to ensure that all practice is evidence-based affects health promotion as well as more clinical activities. In a situation where resources will always be limited, resource allocation depends on demonstrable effectiveness. There are thus many factors leading to a demand for evaluation of health promotion practice.

Evaluating health promotion is not a straightforward task. Health promotion interventions often involve different kinds of activities, a long timescale, and several partners who may each have their own objectives. Health promotion is still seen as belonging within the health services, where the dominant evaluation model is quantitative research centred on experimental trials. As a result, health promotion has been obliged to use unrealistic criteria to evaluate outcomes. As a new discipline, it has therefore suffered and its effects are seen as equivocal and its claim for resources unjustified. This chapter argues that health promotion is not only concerned with health or behavioural outcomes, but is broadly based with an emphasis on goals such as empowerment, equity, participation and collaboration, and a breadth of activities and settings.

This chapter considers what is meant by evaluation, looks at the evidence base for health promotion and discusses how to become a critical user of research. Different kinds of evaluation, focusing on outcomes, impact and processes are examined as well as the concept of cost-effectiveness. Pluralistic evaluation which addresses the multiple objectives of different partners is discussed. Several dilemmas inherent in evaluating health promotion practice are identified and considered.

Defining evaluation

As we have seen in the previous chapter, a planned approach to health promotion is based on a systematic assessment of the best available evidence regarding health needs and effective interventions. In practice, health promotion is often reactive, prompted by a need for an urgent or high-profile response.

Evaluation is a complicated process and uses resources which might otherwise be used for programme planning and implementation. Health promotion is an uncertain business and there are no guarantees that certain effects will follow certain inputs.

So why is it important to evaluate health promotion interventions? Evaluation is needed to assess results, determine whether objectives have been met and find out if the methods used were appropriate and efficient. These findings can then be fed back into the planning process in order to progress practice. However, given the fact that health promotion is a complex activity where there may be disagreement about values and priorities, evaluation is also about identifying the values or criteria which will be used to determine success.

> A young people's project results in more assertive and articulate young people who are prepared to question local and health authority decisions and demand appropriate services including additional leisure facilities and contraceptive and sexual health clinics.
>
> ■ What criteria of effectiveness might health promoters use?
> ■ What criteria might local and health authorities use?
>
> The health promoter might value and prioritize empowerment and autonomy; the statutory authorities might value and prioritize a visible change in behaviour from 'hanging around on streets' to being occupied and supervized within a youth centre. They might also see use and uptake of services as a positive outcome. This leads to the need for pluralistic evaluation strategies which take account of different people's agendas, which is discussed later in this chapter.

In all evaluation there are two fundamental elements: identifying and ranking the criteria (values and aims) and gathering the kind of information that will make it possible to assess the extent to which they are being met.

(Peberdy 1997, p. 269)

There are different criteria which can be used to judge the worth of a health promotion intervention:

■ effectiveness – the extent to which aims and objectives are met
■ appropriateness – the relevance of the intervention to needs
■ acceptability – whether it is carried out in a sensitive way

- efficiency – whether time, money and resources are well spent, given the benefits
- equity – equal provision for equal need.

> A well-man clinic is introduced in a primary health care practice. The aim is to monitor the health of middle-aged men in this age and to provide information and advice enabling them to adopt healthier lifestyles, so that in the longer term health risks such as high blood pressure or smoking are reduced. Over a period of time, the practice nurse invites all men aged 40–65 into the practice for a half-hour session where she checks vital statistics (weight, blood pressure), asks about lifestyle (e.g. diet, smoking, alcohol and drug use, sexual activity, exercise) and gives individually tailored information and advice about adopting a healthier lifestyle. This is followed up 1 year later by a questionnaire to find out if participants have made any lifestyle changes.
>
> Evaluation of the well-man clinic shows a 60% take-up rate of which 5% have introduced lifestyle changes 1 year later; 5% of the respondents were referred for further investigation or treatment; 80% of the participants found the session helpful, informative and useful. The practice nurse spent a large proportion of her time on this clinic and there were associated administrative costs.
>
> How could you use the evaluation criteria above to assess the worth of this programme?

Evaluation covers many different activities undertaken with varying degrees of rigour or reflectiveness. At its simplest level, evaluation describes what any competent practitioner does as a matter of course, that is, the process of appraising and assessing work activities. This includes the process of informal feedback or more systematic review of health promotion interventions. For example, noting how educational sessions have been received by the audience, or soliciting their comments, or those of peers and colleagues, is part of the evaluation process. Evaluation tends to mean a more formal or systematic activity, where assessment is linked to original intentions and is fed back into the planning process.

> Evaluation implies judgement based on careful assessment and critical appraisal of given situations, which should lead to drawing sensible conclusions and making useful proposals for future action.
>
> (WHO 1981, p. 9)

The professional development of health promotion practice depends on evaluation. Evaluating activities helps inform future plans and contributes to the building up of a knowledge base for health promotion. It also helps prevent the reinvention of the wheel, by informing other health promoters of the effectiveness of different methods and strategies. Health promotion has its own adherents and publicists. It is only through evaluation of different strategies and approaches that the health promoter is able to make informed choices about what methods to use and when. Evaluation is a necessary component of the reflective practitioner and enhances job satisfaction.

 A health promotion service uses two different methods to encourage dietary change – intensive group work and a mass-media campaign. The primary objective is to reduce fat consumption. The group work participants reduce their fat intake by 7% whereas the mass media audience reduce their fat intake by 3%.

On the basis of this evaluation, which form of intervention is the most efficient?

Although the group work participants have achieved a greater reduction of fat consumption, the mass-media campaign is most efficient because it reaches a much greater number of people.

Health promotion is not a technical strategy but a complex means of intervening in people's lives at different levels. The ultimate question of whether or not such activity is justified does not belong

A dental health project has been launched, and needs to be evaluated. There are two choices, either an 'in-house' evaluation conducted by the people involved in running the project, or an external evaluation conducted by outside researchers. These are some of the pros and cons of each option. Can you identify any others?

Insider evaluation
Pros   Knows background to project
           Cheaper
           Acceptable to everyone
Cons   Too involved in project
           No research expertise
           Biased to prove success

Outside evaluation
Pros   Unbiased attitude
           Research expertise
           Fresh perspectve
Cons   Expensive
           May appear threatening
           Unfamiliar with project

to practitioners alone, or managers, or funders, but must involve the whole community. Evaluation is one way of opening up the debate and of ensuring that everyone's voice is heard.

Evaluation may be carried out by practitioners or by outside researchers. The latter tend to be larger scale and more ambitious in their remit. There are advantages and drawbacks to each of these options.

Evidence-based practice

Evaluation helps build a basis of research and investigation to demonstrate which health promotion interventions succeed in meeting objectives. Evaluation therefore identifies effective health promotion practice which others can adopt. Evidence-based practice is firmly established in medicine and nursing, where randomized controlled trials of alternative treatment protocols are used to establish which form of treatment is most effective for most people. Evidence-based medicine is thus defined as 'the conscientious, explicit and judicious use of current best evidence in making decisions about the care of individual patients' (Sackett et al 1996). In health promotion, creating evidence-based practice is more problematic.

The randomized controlled trial is often not appropriate for health promotion interventions, where it is impossible to isolate the effect of the intervention, and where success is measured in part by its spread to other groups and populations beyond the immediate target group. However, this does not mean that there is no evidence on which to base health promotion work. Meta-analyses or systematic reviews of research studies pool together findings from different studies in effectiveness reviews.

Why might it be difficult to establish evidence-based health promotion practice?

The evidence base for health promotion

The following are two examples which demonstrate how the evidence basis for health promotion practice is developing:

1. Evidence reviews of research studies investigating suicide prevention strategies indicates that environmental modification of local suicide 'hotspots' is effective and worth implementing, but that maintenance of antidepressant and lithium therapy is more questionable.
2. Evidence reviews of skin cancer prevention strategies shows that primary health education about reducing skin exposure to the sun and sunbeds is effective, but that whole population skin cancer screening is more questionable.

Source: Gunnell (1994), Harvey (1995)

Meta-analysis takes quantitative research methodology as its model of evidence, with randomized controlled studies as the 'gold standard'. This bias towards quantitative research has been identified as a problem for health promotion, where change is often subjective, long term and related to many factors. Many commentators argue that health promotion needs to move towards a social science model of evaluation which acknowledges different 'stakeholders' who have different interests and viewpoints, and uses broader methodologies including more qualitative research (Naidoo & Wills 1998, Peberdy 1997). Effectiveness reviews are helpful but as Speller et al (1997) point out, the criteria for inclusion should refer to the quality of the health promotion intervention as well as the quality of the research.

A care worker observes that residents who are mobile suffer fewer infections and seem happier than those who are bed- or chair-bound. Many residents quickly lose mobility on entering the home. The care worker wants to set up a 'walking for health' scheme with a dedicated activity organizer. She wants to justify this proposal by having evidence of effective similar interventions.

What does she need to find out?

She needs to find the answer to the question of whether an intervention (promotion of regular walking) has a specific effect (reduction in infection and self-reported or observed well-being). Asking the right question is the most important step in evidence-based practice. She then needs to track down the best evidence and critically appraise it to apply her findings.

Evaluating research

Investigating what others have done and using their experience to feed into your own practice is one way of improving effectiveness. So it is important to be aware of how others' activities have been evaluated and to make your own assessment of whether or not the evidence they provide is persuasive. This involves developing your own critical reading of research. There are many sources of health promotion research; these are outlined below.

Critical reading of research studies involves examining the assumptions and biases of the authors, considering whether the methods they used are appropriate and rigorous, and deciding whether the conclusions they come to are justified by the evidence they provide. Below is a checklist of questions to ask when reading research critically (abridged from Naidoo & Wills 1998, p. 43).

Sources of health promotion research

- Professional journals, e.g. *Health Promotion International, Nursing Times, Health Education Journal, British Medical Journal.*
- Computerized databases on journals held in professional and educational libraries, e.g. CINAHL (Cumulative Index to Nursing and Allied Health Literature) and MEDLINE (reviews medical journals).
- Effectiveness bulletins and reviews, e.g. Effective Health Care Bulletins produced by the Nuffield Institute for Health, University of Leeds, and the NHS Centre for Reviews and Dissemination, University of York.
- Reviews of research produced by a variety of bodies e.g. Health Education Authority; Health Promotion Research Programme, University of Bristol; Social Science Research Unit, Institute of Education, London University.

Reading research critically: a checklist of questions to ask

1. When was the research carried out? In general, recent research is more useful.
2. Who carried out the research? Do they have particular interests, e.g. funding from particular bodies, involvement in the activity described.
3. Are aims and objectives clearly stated? Are objectives specific, relevant, measurable?
4. How was the research carried out? Was the methodology qualitative or quantitative or a combination of both? Was the methodology appropriate given the aims and objectives?
   - Was there before and after collection of data?
   - Were any research instruments used piloted?
   - How was the sample defined?
   - What was the extent of non-response? Were particular groups not represented owing to non-response?
5. Was the data analysis appropriate for the methodology? Was it systematic? If statistical analysis was used, was this appropriate and clearly explained?
6. Were appropriate conclusions drawn from the material presented?
7. Should this research be used to affect practice? In what ways?

Reasons for evaluation: the three Es

- To assess what has been achieved – did an intervention have its intended effects? (*Efficiency*)
- To measure its impact and whether it was worthwhile (*Effectiveness*)
- To judge its cost-effectiveness and whether the time, money and labour were well-spent (*Economy*)
- To inform future plans
- To justify decisions to others.

Process, impact and outcome evaluation

Evaluation is always incomplete. It is not possible to assess every element of an intervention. Instead, decisions are taken about which evaluation criteria to prioritize and also sometimes which objectives are to be assessed. A distinction is often made between process, impact and outcome evaluation. Process evaluation (also called formative or illuminative evaluation) is concerned with assessing the process of programme implementation. It addresses participants' perceptions and reactions to health promotion interventions, and identifies the factors which support or impede these activities. Process evaluation is therefore a useful means to assess acceptability and may also assess the appropriateness and equity of a health promotion intervention.

Evaluating outcome or process

Asian women have low uptake of some preventive services such as antenatal clinics and screening. A project has the aim of raising Asian women's awareness of their own health needs and the services available.

A bilingual link-worker based in a voluntary organization plans and runs a series of six health sessions for Asian women. A crèche is arranged and the sessions are held at the local community centre. The sessions are advertised by word of mouth and using local outlets, e.g. the mosque, corner shops. The linkworker spends the first session finding out what issues are of most interest to the women and modifies the planned course accordingly. Attendance varies from 10 to 19 women with a core group of 8 women who attend every session.

This project would rate highly on the criteria of acceptability, appropriateness and equity. It reaches a disadvantaged group, is accessible to that group, and is relevant to their stated needs.

Process evaluation employs a wide range of qualitative or 'soft' methods. Examples of such methods are interviews, diaries, observations and content analysis of documents. These methods tell us a great deal about that particular programme and the factors responsible for its success or failure, but they are unable to predict what would happen if the programme were to be replicated in other areas. Because process evaluation does not use 'hard' scientific methods, its findings tend to be more easily dismissed as unrepresentative. However, process evaluation is crucial to health promotion. We need to understand how health promotion interventions are interpreted and responded to by different groups of people and whether the intervention itself is health-promoting, and for this we need process evaluation.

Evaluation of health promotion programmes is usually concerned to identify their effects. The effects of an intervention may be evaluated according to its:

- *impact* – the immediate effects such as increased knowledge or shifts in attitude
- *outcome* – the longer-term effects such as changes in lifestyle.

Impact evaluation tends to be the most popular choice, as it is the easier to do. Impact evaluation can be built into a programme as the end stage. For example, a health promotion programme for secondary schools may include as the last session a review of the programme. Students may be invited to identify how they have changed since the programme began and how they think the programme will affect their future behaviour. Outcome evaluation is more difficult, because it involves an assessment of longer-term effects. Using the same example given above, outcome evaluation may be used to determine whether the programme did affect students' behaviour 1 year later. One way of ascertaining this would be to compare participants' health-related behaviour (e.g. smoking, alcohol and exercise) before and after the programme, but there are bound to be changes in students' behaviour over 1 year, irrespective of any health promotion programme. So it would be better to compare the students to another group of similar students who did not receive the programme. The second or control group of students is necessary to avoid the danger of attributing all behaviour change to the health promotion programme and therefore of overestimating its influence.

Outcome evaluation is therefore more complex and costly than impact evaluation. Going back a year later to the same students and getting new information from them will take up time and resources, as will obtaining a matched group of students to use as the control group. However, despite these problems, outcome evaluation is often the preferred evaluation method because it measures sustained changes which have stood the test of time. Results using data on impact or outcome are often expressed numerically, and this again increases credibility. Quantitative or 'hard' data are seen as more concrete or factual than the 'soft' data used in process evaluation.

Another way of categorizing different types of evaluation is by the type of objective set. Health promotion objectives may be about individual changes, service use or changes in the environment. The box below shows the range of possible objectives associated with smoking reduction interventions, each of which would need evaluation.

 Health promotion objectives for smoking reduction

- Increased knowledge, e.g. harmful effects of passive smoking
- Changes in attitudes, e.g. less willingness to breathe in others' smoke
- Changes in behaviour, e.g. stopping smoking
- Acquiring new skills, e.g. learning relaxation methods to reduce stress
- Introduction of healthy policies, e.g. funding to enable GPs to prescribe nicotine replacement aids for people on low income
- Modifying the environment, e.g. banning tobacco advertising and promotion, workplace no-smoking policies
- Reduction in risk factors, e.g. reduction in number of smokers and amount of tobacco smoked per person
- Increased use of services, e.g. take-up rates for smoking cessation clinics, number of calls made to quit smoking telephone helplines
- Reduced morbidity, e.g. reduced rates of respiratory illness and coronary heart disease
- Reduced mortality, e.g. reduced mortality from lung cancer

Although all these factors relate to health, they are quite separate, and there is no necessary connection between, say, increased knowledge and behaviour change. It is therefore inappropriate to evaluate a given objective (e.g. increased exercise rate) by measuring other aspects of an intervention (e.g. number of leaflets taken at a health fair or reported attitude change favouring exercise).

Cost-effectiveness

Part of the reason for evaluation is to determine whether desired results were achieved in the most economical way and whether allocating resources to health promotion can be justified. This involves different calculations. Cost analysis compares the costs of a health promotion intervention to the costs of competing activities. Cost-effectiveness is a comparison in monetary terms of different methods used to achieve the same outcomes. 'Cost effectiveness analysis can be used either to identify the intervention which achieves a specific target at lowest cost or that which achieves the greatest outcome for a given cost' (Tolley 1994, p. vii). For example, it might be necessary to look at the value of using resources for health promotion rather than for alternative uses; this is termed 'opportunity costs'.

Cost–benefit analysis is more complicated, and relies on pricing both the inputs and the benefits of a health promotion programme. An attempt is then made to calculate the cost of each benefit. This is known as a cost–benefit ratio. Putting a price on health outcomes or benefits is a very difficult exercise. One approach to this problem is to compare the cost–benefit ratio for a health promotion intervention with the cost–benefit ratio for some other health intervention. It is often assumed that prevention is cheaper than cure and that health promotion saves money, but this is not necessarily the case.

 An effective smoking prevention campaign is associated with the following costs.

Money is saved by:
■ Not having to treat people with smoking-related diseases on the NHS.
■ Not having to pay sickness benefit and disability pensions to people with smoking-related diseases.
■ Increased production in industry because fewer employees are off sick.

Money is lost by:
■ Retirement pensions paid to people who live longer.
■ Unemployment benefits to people in tobacco production and retail industry made unemployed due to fall in demand.
■ Loss of government revenue from tobacco taxation.

Overall, do you think this campaign is cost-effective?

Pluralistic evaluation

Evaluation is sometimes thought to be an unproblematic part of the health promoter's professional expertise. The assumption is that, faced with a certain set of findings, everyone would agree on their significance or meaning, but this is not necessarily the case. There may also be dispute about which findings are relevant or significant. The following example illustrates these points.

A road accident prevention programme is launched by a health authority and a local authority. The following groups are involved in the programme:

- Health authority
- Local authority
- Road traffic police
- The community
- The local cycling group
- Staff in the Accident and Emergency Department of the local hospital
- Teachers taking part in the schools programme.

Activities include road traffic calming measures, a primary school health education programme, and a free training course for young motorcyclists, as well as additional inputs into the national drink-driving campaign. A 6-month interim evaluation found good take-up (80%) of the motorcycle training course amongst 16- to 25-year-olds buying motorcycles. Teachers reported good results from the school programme. There was a 10% reduction in the number of drink-drive offences and road traffic accidents. However, out of this reduced number of accidents, the proportion of serious injuries to pedestrians and cyclists increased from 2% to 5%.

- What data would each group be most concerned with?
- Is this a success?
- What do you think the response of each group would be?

Success means different things to different groups of people, or stakeholders, who each have their own agendas and interests (Smith & Cantley 1985). Different stakeholders have unequal power to impose their evaluation agendas on others. Different groups of people engaged in health promotion interventions will each have invested something but may well be looking for different results. For example, funders of a project may be looking for efficiency or results which can be interpreted as cost-effective. Practitioners may be looking for evidence that their way of working is acceptable to clients and achieves the objectives set. Managers may be looking for evidence of increased productivity, measured by performance indicators. Clients may be looking for opportunities to take control over some health-related aspects of their lives.

It is therefore important to be clear at the outset about whose perspectives are being addressed in any evaluation. A starting point is simply to acknowledge that different vested interests are involved and try to identify them. The ideal is to then go on to represent the views of the different stakeholders by collecting data from each group. This process is called pluralistic evaluation (Smith & Cantley 1985). Using the process of methodological triangulation, which employs a wide range of data sources, an overall picture may be built up. Pluralistic evaluation which takes into account different stakeholders' views is more complete, although the findings may be complex and lack clarity. As Means & Smith (1988, p. 27) state:

> support for pluralistic evaluation requires bravery on the part of the funder. It not only lacks the same level of scientific respectability as the quasi-experimental design but more importantly it is likely to highlight conflicts of interest and perception between all the various groups that have to engage with any programme.

Dilemmas of evaluating health promotion

There are a number of difficulties surrounding attempts to evaluate health promotion. These are both theoretical and practical. In theoretical terms, the many meanings and definitions of the concept 'health' results in a lack of consensus about how best to evaluate it. For those who subscribe to the medical model of health, data concerning morbidity, disability and mortality are appropriate measures to use for evaluation purposes. For those who adopt a more social model of health, a much broader range of measures (including, for example, measures of socio-economic status or the quality of the environment) will be appropriate. For people who prioritize the educational model, measures of knowledge and attitude change will be paramount.

Practical difficulties arise when trying to obtain data and trying to combine different forms of data to provide an overall picture. Some relevant data are already available and accessible, for example morbidity and mortality data. Other data already exist and may be obtained, for example policy documents or health surveillance data. However, some data will need to be specially collected and, particularly in areas such as attitude change or empowerment, there are no easy or accepted means of doing this.

The following dilemmas flag up issues which are important to think through in relation to any evaluation you are planning of projects with which you are involved. They may also be used when looking at reports of other projects. Understanding these dilemmas helps health promoters to become more critical users of published research as well as being more confident that their own work is soundly based.

Dilemma 1: deciding what to measure
Deciding what to measure to assess the effects of health promotion is not easy. The golden rule must be to measure the objectives set during the planning process. (For more details on programme objectives, see Ch. 18 on programme planning.) Although this sounds straightforward, in practice it can be difficult, and a

surprising number of evaluation studies violate this principle. The objectives set may concern areas where there is a lack of consensus over appropriate measurement. For example, process objectives such as increased multiagency collaboration or increased community involvement are difficult to measure. To collect relevant data would require a special effort because they are not measured routinely. Change in people's attitudes or beliefs is particularly problematic to measure.

The success of a health promotion intervention is not solely about achieving behavioural changes or reductions in disease rates. For example, a needle exchange scheme should not be judged solely by a reduction in the rate of HIV infection among drug users. Other markers of success, such as the take-up rate, are also important. In many cases, expecting a clear change in morbidity from a behaviour change would be unrealistic. Although there is a link between needle-sharing and HIV infection, there are other risk factors, and expecting a preventive outcome from this initiative might be unwise.

A programme may have several different objectives, some of which are easier to measure than others. It then becomes tempting to measure the easiest objectives and extrapolate from these findings. But if the measurements are of different classes of events (e.g. combining behavioural, environmental and attitudinal objectives), it is not legitimate to do this.

A programme has been launched with the objective of reducing child accidents. The following have been suggested as suitable means of evaluating the programme. Are they all appropriate? Are they all feasible?

If the programme objectives included behaviour change, such as the adoption of safer routines in the home, how would this affect your response?

- Take-up of campaign literature
- Campaign awareness
- Sales of child safety equipment
- Establishment of local child accident prevention working groups
- Reduction in the number of accidents to children
- Reduction in the number of severe accidents to children that require hospitalization

---

Dilemma 2: how to be confident that results are due to the health promotion input

Because health promotion is a long-term process and because any situation is constantly changing, it can be difficult to be sure that any changes detected are due to the health promotion input, and not to any other factor. Health-related knowledge, attitudes and behaviour are constantly changing, regardless of health promotion programmes. Societies and environments are also changing in response to many different factors. How can the changes due to health promotion be isolated from everything else? There are two responses to this problem.

The classic scientific method of proof, the experiment, relies on controlling all factors apart from the one being studied. This can best be achieved under laboratory conditions. However, this is clearly impossible and unethical to achieve where people's health is concerned. Instead, the quasi-experimental design is usually the closest that can be achieved. This involves the use of a control group of people who are similar to the group receiving the health promotion input. Factors such as age, gender and social class are all known to affect health, so the control group needs to be matched as closely as possible to the input or experimental group with regard to these factors. Any changes detected in the input group are then compared to those found amongst the control group. Those changes which occur in the input but not the control group can then be attributed to the health promotion programme. Even this degree of scientific rigour is hard to achieve. Most health promotion programmes have spin-off effects and indeed are designed to do so. It is impossible to isolate different groups of people or to ensure that

A hospital nurse has set up a project to help cardiac patients to stop smoking. The intervention involved the identification of a key worker who was allocated time to interview patients to assess their smoking behaviour and draw up individual plans. After discharge, patients were followed up by a weekly telephone call for 6 weeks.

How could this project be evaluated so that any success in terms of smoking cessation in the target group could be shown to be due to the project?

What would be the strengths and limitations of the methods you identify?

1. Experimental evaluation would involve each smoking patient on arrival in the ward to be randomly allocated either to the experimental group (who receive the interview) or the control group (who do not receive the interview but get a care plan and general leaflet).
2. Single group time study evaluation would compare the number of smokers on the ward at a particular point in time with the number still smoking after 3 months.
3. Case study evaluation would interview patients about their involvement in the project and examine their knowledge, attitudes and reported behaviour.

programmes do not 'leak' beyond their set boundaries. However, the quasi-experimental design does mean that changes detected in the input group may be ascribed to the health promotion programme with a greater degree of confidence.

Macdonald et al (1996) argue that if we are to gain real insight into why initiatives succeed or fail we must have some 'illumination'. In other words, we need details on what is happening in initiatives and which features have been effective. This means using qualitative methods of evaluation. The health promotion initiative is treated as a case study and is intensively studied, using a variety of methods if possible. This enables the evaluator to get a detailed picture of how the programme has affected the people involved. These studies are typically small scale and findings are expressed in descriptive rather than numerical terms. Each case study is unique and findings cannot be generalized to other situations. Its strength as a method is that there is a high degree of confidence that identified effects are real and result from the programme. Both the quasi-experimental design and the case study are valid methods which can be used to isolate the effects of health promotion interventions. However, the quasi-experimental design has the higher status and is generally regarded as more respectable and credible than the case study.

Parlett & Hamilton (1987) describe evaluation which focuses on outcomes only as 'rather like the critic who reviews a production on the basis of script and applause meter readings, having missed the performance'.

Why is it important to use a broad range of methods to evaluate health promotion interventions?

Dilemma 3: when to evaluate

Health promotion programmes often have many different effects which will become apparent in different time periods following the intervention. For example, a CHD prevention programme may have the following six effects:

1. Improves people's knowledge of the risk factors for CHD.
2. Persuades more people to attend screening clinics.
3. Increases media coverage of CHD.
4. Prompts various organizations to adopt health policies including CHD prevention.
5. Persuades restaurants and cafes to provide healthier meal options.
6. Reduces premature mortality rate from CHD.

An immediate post-programme evaluation may identify only the first of these effects. An interim (e.g. after 3 months) evaluation may identify the second and third effects. The fourth and fifth effects may only be apparent at a later evaluation, e.g. after 6 months. 6 months after the programme, the increased attendance at screening clinics may no longer be discernible and attendance figures may have reverted to pre-programme levels. A reduction in the mortality rate may not be discernible for 5 years or more, by which time it will be difficult to attribute it to the health promotion programme. The assessment of the overall success or failure of a programme is therefore influenced by the timing of the evaluation.

Green (1977) has highlighted some of the ways in which the evaluation of outcomes of health promotion programmes may be influenced by timing:

1. The sleeper effect: the effects of a programme only become apparent a long time later and would be missed by immediate evaluation.
2. The backsliding effect: early changes which may be positive gradually disappear and after some time the situation may revert to how it was before the intervention.
3. The trigger effect: the programme sparks off a change which would have occurred spontaneously at a later date.
4. The historical effect: some or all of the changes could be due to causes other than the programme.
5. The contrast effect: a programme produces an effect opposite to that which was intended.

There is no solution to these problems, but the health promoter should be aware of the issues and try to time their evaluation so as to address those issues most relevant to their particular programme. If possible, evaluation should be carried out at different time periods following a programme, but this is often impossible to do.

Dilemma 4: knowing what constitutes success

A smoking cessation programme is launched which includes clinics for those wishing to give up smoking. A clinic run by a health promoter attracts 20 clients who attend all six sessions. At a 6-month evaluation, 25% of the participants have stopped smoking.

Is this a success?

The health promoter may be pleased with these results. People attend clinics often as a last resort, and 6 months is a reasonable time period to assess long-term behaviour change. However, the health promoter's manager may point out that 20% is an average success rate for people trying to quit, regardless of what methods are used. Clinics are time-consuming and 20 people is not a large group. 25% quitters is five people, four of whom might have quit using other less intensive or expensive methods. So one additional ex-smoker might be the result of the smoking cessation clinic.

In this case there is sufficient knowledge available for an informed assessment of success to take place, but in many other areas of health promotion, this is not the case. We do not know the degree of behaviour change which is likely to occur irrespective of any health promotion programmes, and in general we do not have information comparing different methods or strategies. So if specific objectives are set, they are often a 'shot in the dark', and may be either too ambitious or too modest.

Effectiveness reviews are a means of building up a knowledge base which can tell us what are reasonable expectations of success in health promotion. Success in health promotion is complicated because the aim is not just to change knowledge or behaviour, but to change the social determinants of health, and this requires qualitative as well as quantitative evaluation. This does not mean that it is impossible to find examples of successful health promotion interventions.

 Successful health promotion

The following strategies have been shown to be successful in reducing childhood road accidents.

■ Concerted campaigns to increase the use of child cycle helmets
■ Reducing vehicle speed, e.g. by introducing speed ramps and through legislation
■ Environmental modification through area-wide engineering schemes
■ Infant and child car restraints.

Source: Towner et al (1993), cited in Katz & Peberdy (1997)

The argument that 'health promotion doesn't work' because it is often inappropriate and impossible to find experimental evidence of its success is spurious. Health promotion is concerned with simultaneous change at many levels which requires a multi-pronged approach to evaluation which looks at processes as well as outcomes.

Dilemma 5: is evaluation worth the effort?

In the light of all the problems identified above, and given the fact that evaluation consumes limited resources, is evaluation worth the effort? Assessing the value of one's work is an important aspect of being a reflective practitioner. Deciding when a more formal or complete evaluation should be undertaken is not easy.

Ongoing routine work which is based on previously demonstrated effectiveness or efficiency is probably not worthwhile evaluating in depth. However, new or pilot interventions do warrant a more thoroughgoing evaluation because, without evidence of their effectiveness or efficiency, it is difficult to argue that they should

Why is it important to evaluate any projects or new interventions you undertake?

become established work practices. Other criteria that can be used to determine if evaluation is worth the effort relate to how well it can be done. If it will be impossible to obtain cooperation from the different groups involved in the activity, it is probably not worthwhile trying to evaluate. If evaluation has not been considered at the outset but is tacked on as an 'afterthought', the chances are that it will be so partial and biased as to be not worth the effort.

Evaluation is only worthwhile if it will make a difference. This means that the results of the evaluation need to be interpreted and fed back to the relevant audiences in an accessible form. All too often, evaluations are buried in inappropriate formats. Work reports may go no further than the manager, or academic studies full of jargon may be published in little-known journals.

Results of evaluation studies will be relevant to many different groups and it may be necessary to reproduce findings in different ways in order to reach all these groups.

> A district nurse has evaluated her health promotion activities. These include opportunistic one-to-one counselling and education, setting up a carers' support group, producing information leaflets on coping with dementia, and health surveys of people aged 75 and over.
>
> How could she make her findings known to her clients, her manager, her nursing colleagues, and other health and welfare workers?

Conclusion

Evaluation contributes to the accountability and development of evidence-based health promotion practice, and so is an important aspect of the health promoter's work. This involves becoming a critical user of published research as well as evaluating health promotion activity with which you are involved. There are often pressures to adopt unrealistic measures of success, such as reduced mortality rates or demonstrable cost benefits. Most health promoters are engaged in more modest activities which seek to achieve changes in knowledge, behaviour, attitudes, service take-up or the policy process. These are more appropriate outcomes to use for evaluation purposes.

Evaluation is a practical activity which feeds into the theoretical debate about the nature and purpose of health promotion. This debate cannot be confined to professionals, or those who hold managerial or financial power. It must include the public, those who are the targets of health promotion activity. This is why pluralistic evaluation, which enables participants to have a voice in determining effectiveness, is so important. Evaluation can be thought of as a bridge linking health promoters to others, including clients, funders, managers and colleagues.

Evaluation is not a simple activity and it consumes resources which might otherwise be spent on doing health promotion. The decision about whether, when and how to evaluate is therefore important. The question of evaluation should be considered at the outset of any planned health promotion intervention. If it is to be done, it should be done in the best possible way. If this is not feasible, then it is better to admit the impossible, and not attempt to evaluate. Ongoing monitoring may be the best one can do. This is acceptable, but there is a distinction between routine monitoring of activities through the use of performance indicators and a more thoroughgoing evaluation. It is important not to confuse the two and to be clear about which it is you are doing.

 The following have been suggested as guidelines for good practice in evaluation.

Which do you think should be included in a checklist 'Criteria to be met if undertaking evaluation'? Are there any other guidelines you would wish to add?

■ Evaluate early on before vested interests have had time to solidify.
■ Evaluate only if it will make a difference.
■ Evaluate only when it is appropriate.
■ Evaluate only when you can include the perceptions of different groups, e.g. only when you can do a pluralistic evaluation.
■ Publicize the results of evaluation widely in relevant formats.
■ Evaluate only when there is a chance of scientific accuracy.
■ If you cannot meet these criteria, do not evaluate.

Questions for further discussion

■ What factors would influence your decision about whether to evaluate a particular health promotion activity?
■ What factors would you wish to consider when evaluating a health promotion intervention?

Summary

This chapter has looked at how evaluation is defined and why health promotion needs to be evaluated. The concept of evidence-based practice has been discussed in relation to health promotion. Different kinds of evaluation have been identified, including process, impact and outcome evaluation. The concept of stakeholders, leading to the necessity for pluralistic evaluation, has been discussed. Finally, five central dilemmas in the practice of evaluation have been examined.

Further reading

Davies J K, Macdonald G (eds) 1998 Quality, evidence and effectiveness in health promotion: striving for certainties. Routledge, London. *Part 1 looks at assessing evidence and effectiveness for health promotion and examines experience from the USA, key settings and community-based work.*

Ewles L, Simnett I 1999 Promoting health: a practical guide, 4th edn. Baillière Tindall, Edinburgh. *Chapter 7 is a useful guide to using research in practice and carrying out small-scale research of your own.*

Katz J, Peberdy A 1997 Promoting health: knowledge and practice. Macmillan/Open University Press, Basingstoke. *Part 4 on evaluating health promotion is a detailed discussion on the reasons for evaluation and how to evaluate, which recognizes the different agendas of the different people who are involved.*

Muir Gray J A 1996 Evidence-based health care. Churchill Livingstone, London. *An accessible discussion of how to evaluate and use research to further practice.*

Naidoo J, Wills J 1998 Practising health promotion: dilemmas and challenges. Baillière Tindall, London. *Chapters 2 and 3 examine research, effectiveness and evidence-based practice in greater detail.*

Perkins E R, Simnett I, Wright L 1999 Evidence-based health promotion. John Wiley, London. *An interesting collection of contributions from different authors examining how the evidence for health promotion is assessed and used in different practice settings.*

References

Green L 1977 Education and measurement: some dilemmas for health education. American Journal of Public Health 67: 155–162

Gunnell D 1994 The potential for preventing suicide: a review of the literature on the effectiveness of interventions aimed at preventing suicide. University of Bristol Health Care Evaluation Unit, Bristol

Harvey I 1995 Prevention of skin cancer: a review of available strategies. University of Bristol Health Care Evaluation Unit, Bristol

Katz J, Peberdy A 1997 Promoting health: knowledge and practice. Macmillan/Open University Press, Basingstoke

Macdonald G, Veen C, Tones K 1996 Evidence for success in health promotion: suggestions for improvement. Health Education Research 11(3): 367–376

Means R, Smith R 1988 Implementing a pluralistic approach to evaluation in health education. Policy and Politics 16: 17–28

Naidoo J, Wills J 1998 Practising health promotion: dilemmas and challenges. Baillière Tindall, London

Parlett M, Hamilton D 1987 Evaluation as illumination: a new approach to the study of innovating programmes. In: Murphy R, Torrance H (eds) Evaluating education : issues and methods. PCP Education series, London

Peberdy A 1997 Evaluation design. In: Katz J, Peberdy A (eds) Promoting health: knowledge and practice. Macmillan/Open University Press, Basingstone, ch 17

Sackett D L, Rosenberg W C, Muir Gray J A, Haynes R B, Richardson W S 1996 Evidence based medicine: what it is and what it isn't. British Medical Journal 312: 71–72

Smith G, Cantley C 1985 Assessing health care: a study in organisational evaluation. Open University Press, Milton Keynes

Speller V, Learmonth A, Harrison D 1997 The search for evidence of effective health promotion. British Medical Journal 315: 361–363

Tolley K 1994 Health promotion: how to measure cost-effectiveness. Health Education Authority, London

World Health Organization 1981 Health programme evaluation: guiding principles. WHO, Geneva

Index

Page numbers in **bold** refer to tables; page numbers in *italic* refer to figures.

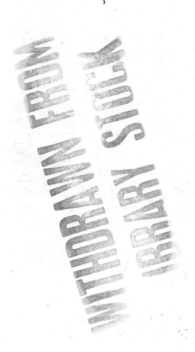